Investigative Techniques in Dermatology

Investigative Techniques in Dermatology

edited by

R. MARKS MB, BSc, FRCP
Reader and Consultant in Dermatology
Department of Medicine
Welsh National School of Medicine
Heath Park
Cardiff

BLACKWELL SCIENTIFIC PUBLICATIONS
OXFORD LONDON EDINBURGH MELBOURNE

First published 1979

British Library Cataloguing in Publication Data
Investigative techniques in dermatology.
  1. Skin—Diseases—Diagnosis
  I. Marks, Ronald
  616.5'07'5   RL105

ISBN 0-632-00365-0

Distributed in USA by
Blackwell Mosby Book Distributors
11830 Westline Industrial Drive
St Louis, Missouri 63141,
in Canada by
Blackwell Mosby Book Distributors
86 Northline Road, Toronto
Ontario, M4B 3E5,
and in Australia by
Blackwell Scientific Book Distributors
214 Berkeley Street, Carlton,
Victoria 3053

Set in Photon Times

Printed in Great Britain by The Whitefriars Press Ltd., London and Tonbridge

Bound by Kemp Hall Bindery, Oxford

Contents

Contributors

J. L. BURTON BSc, MD, MRCP
Consultant Senior Lecturer in Dermatology, University of Bristol, Bristol

C. D. CALNAN FRCP
Consultant Dermatologist, Institute of Dermatology, St John's Hospital for Diseases of the Skin, Lisle Street, Leicester Square, London WC2H 7BJ

J. J. CREAM BSc, MD, MRCP
Consultant Dermatologist, Charing Cross Hospital, London W6

W. J. CUNLIFFE MD, BSc, MRCP
Consultant Dermatologist, The General Infirmary at Leeds, Leeds LS1 3EX

G. H. ELDER MD MRCPATH
Professor of Medical Biochemistry, Welsh National School of Medicine, Heath Park, Cardiff CF4 4XN

R. FIFIELD BSc, MSc, PhD
Supra regional Protein Reference Unit, Cardiff Royal Infirmary, Cardiff

W. FRAIN-BELL MD, FRCP (Ed)
Consultant Dermatologist, The University of Dundee, Dundee

M. W. GREAVES MD, PhD, FRCP
Professor of Dermatology, Institute of Dermatology, Homerton Grove, London E9 6BX

P. S. HARPER MA, DM, MRCP
Reader and Consultant in Medical Genetics, Department of Medicine, Welsh National School of Medicine, Heath Park, Cardiff CF4 4XN

K. T. HOLLAND BSc, PhD
Lecturer in Microbiology, Medical School, University of Leeds, Leeds

J. A. A. HUNTER BA, MB, ChB, MRCP
Consultant Dermatologist, The Royal Infirmary, Edinburgh EH3 9YW

A. KOBZA BLACK MRCP
Clinical Lecturer in Dermatology, Institute of Dermatology, Homerton Grove, London E9 6BX

Ch. M. LAPIERE MD, PhD, MBAM (Belgium)
Professor in Dermatology, Hopital de Baviere, Boulevard de la Constitution 66, B–4020 Liege, Belgium

RONA M. MACKIE MD, MRCP
Professor of Dermatology, University of Glasgow, Western Infirmary, Glasgow G11 6NT

R. MARKS MB, BSc, FRCP
Reader and Consultant in Dermatology, Department of Medicine, Welsh National School of Medicine, Heath Park, Cardiff CF4 4XN

N. MOORE
Research Assistant, Department of Crystallography, Birkbeck College, Malet Street, London WC1E 7HX

W. C. NOBLE MSc, PhD, FIBiol, MRCPath
Reader in Bacteriology, Institute of Dermatology, London E9 6BX

F. S. WUSTEMAN BSc, DIC, PhD
Department of Biochemistry, University College, Cardiff

Preface

Many of the questions that repeatedly form in the minds of practising dermatologists and daily torment them, are capable of solution. This book is intended for those who hope to tackle one or several of these questions. It is also meant for those who for one reason or another cannot participate but wish to sit 'on the side lines' to learn something of the problems, pitfalls, facts and artefacts of the many new techniques in dermatological research. I sincerely hope that some of this latter group will be encouraged by reading this book to move off the side lines and on to the field of play.

The contents are loosely based on a series of lectures and demonstrations given during a course entitled *Investigative Techniques in Dermatology* held at the Welsh National School of Medicine in Cardiff in June 1975 and October 1977. No attempt at a comprehensive cover of all possible techniques was made on the course or in the present volume, but it is hoped to cover other subjects in other publications at later dates. The theoretical bases of the techniques are only briefly reviewed. The practical aspects of the various topics are covered in more detail although the 'Cookery book' approach has been avoided. Particular emphasis is given to the technical difficulties, the applicability of the methods described and the significance of the results obtained using the various tests.

It is a regrettable fact that many medical graduates still regard laboratories as places where 'scientists' and 'technicians' practise some dark art rather than as ideal places to obtain the answers to many clinically-based questions. This attitude is to be deprecated and throughout the book the 'team approach' is emphasized.

Dermatology is becoming an integral part of scientific medicine and I trust that the kind of information contained in the chapters that follow will in the near future be necessary for the best kind of dermatological practice.

R. Marks

1

Looking at skin lipids

J. L. BURTON

The major impetus to the study of skin lipids has been provided by the investigation of acne vulgaris. The severity of acne relates to the degree of seborrhoea (Pochi & Strauss 1964; Cunliffe & Shuster 1969b; Cotterill *et al* 1972) and free fatty acids have been thought to play a role in its pathogenesis, since they are both irritant and comedogenic (Kligman *et al* 1970; Ray & Kellum 1971; Strauss & Pochi 1965; Stillman *et al* 1975). Some doubt has been cast on the importance of free fatty acids in the pathogenesis of acne (Voss 1974; Fulton *et al* 1975) but the techniques which have been developed to study the skin lipids in acne are applicable to a variety of other problems.

SOURCES OF SKIN LIPIDS

The lipids which occur in the skin of humans differ markedly from those of animals (Nicolaides *et al* 1968) and the following account refers to human skin, except where otherwise stated.

Active lipid formation (lipogenesis) is undertaken by two types of cell in the skin, namely the sebocytes in the sebaceous glands and the keratinocytes in the keratinizing epidermis. The lipids formed by these two cell types differ chemically and probably fulfil separate physiological functions (Nicolaides 1965). Cutaneous lipogenesis is thus the net result of two separate processes under individual control.

In the human, skin surface lipids are derived from the following sources:
1 The sebaceous glands.
2 The keratinizing epidermis.
3 Exogenous lipid sources such as soaps, cosmetics, pomades and topical medicaments. There may also be contamination with small quantities of saturated petroleum hydrocarbons from the atmosphere (Downing & Strauss 1974; Gloor *et al* 1974).

THE SEBUM EXCRETION RATE

The sebaceous glands produce sebum by a holocrine process, in which the cells synthesize lipid as they move towards the centre of the gland and eventually

1

disintegrate. The lipid cell contents are then discharged via the sebaceous duct into the pilosebaceous follicle, whence they are excreted to the skin surface as sebum. Autoradiographic studies have shown that it takes 2 or 3 weeks for a tritium-labelled cell to travel from the basal layer of the sebaceous gland to the sebaceous duct, and a further week or so for the sebum to reach the skin surface (Epstein & Epstein 1966; Weinstein 1974; Plewig & Christophers 1974). There is in addition a large reservoir of sebum in the pilosebaceous orifice, so that the rate of delivery of sebum to the skin surface may not accurately reflect metabolic events in the glands themselves. Nevertheless, changes in sebaceous gland size or mitotic activity of the sebaceous basal layer will eventually affect the sebum excretion rate. Normally this remains reasonably constant in a given subject and therefore the rates in individual subjects can be compared, and changes, as a result of experimental procedures, can be measured.

A wide variety of ingenious and ingenuous methods have been used to study the sebum excretion rate (Burton 1971) including the nephelometric estimation of sebum washed from a glass cylinder applied to the skin by suction and the estimation of the carbon dioxide liberated after combustion of a sebum sample. The monomolecular layer technique (Jones *et al* 1951) is based on the assumption that water insoluble fatty acids on an aqueous surface form a film which is one molecule in thickness, the carboxyl groups extending into the water. The area occupied by each fatty acid molecule is constant, independent of the number of carbons in the molecule, and so the surface area of the film increases and decreases with the number of fatty acid molecules present. A lipid film of this kind will displace a hydrocarbon film on a watery surface. Thus, a standard film of mineral oil on the surface of water can be displaced by placing a drop of skin lipid solution in ether on the film. After the ether has evaporated the sample displaces an area of oil which, according to Jones *et al* (1951), should be proportional to the fatty acid concentration of the sample. Harber *et al* (1957) found that with this method there was no correlation between the absolute quantity of lipid and the extent of the spreading, but lipid specimens collected repeatedly from the same skin area in the same subject did show reproducible spreading values. It seems likely, therefore, that this method reflects differences in lipid composition rather than the absolute quantity of lipid. Other methods of assessing sebaceous activity have included planimetric measurements of gland size in biopsy specimens, and photodensitometry of the black spots produced by the osmic acid treatment of sebum absorbed on filter papers.

The most reliable method, however, is a simple gravimetric method in which sebum is collected on to absorbent papers held in contact with an area of cleaned forehead skin (Strauss & Pochi 1961). This area is delineated with adhesive tape and a rubber headband is used to hold the papers in place. After a timed collection period, the lipid is extracted with ether into a preweighed container which is again weighed after evaporation of the ether. This method, though technically simple, gives inaccurate results unless considerable care is taken to avoid the many sources of error. The method has been described in detail elsewhere (Cunliffe & Shuster 1969a; Cunliffe & Cotterill 1975) and the following remarks amplify some possible causes of inaccuracy:

1   Subjects should wash their hair on the evening prior to the test and apply no makeup or other topical application thereafter, but the face should be washed with soap in the normal way on the morning of the test. Earlier workers suggested that the accumulation of surface lipid can produce a 'feedback' inhibition of sebum excretion and there is good evidence that such inhibition does occur in the rat (Archibald & Shuster 1973). Until further evidence in man is available it seems reasonable to standardize conditions of skin cleansing for the 12 hours or so prior to the test.

2   The samples should, where possible, be collected at the same time of the day, since there may be circadian variation in both rate of sebum excretion and its composition (Burton *et al* 1970; Cotterill *et al* 1973).

3   The room should be ventilated and should not be too hot because sweat reduces the capacity of the papers to absorb lipids. For the same reason the subjects should not be allowed to take hot drinks during the test. Environmental temperature can have a marked effect on the apparent sebum excretion rate (Cunliffe *et al* 1970), probably by its effect on sebum viscosity (Burton 1970), but a room temperature of about 20–24°C is satisfactory.

4   The type of absorbent paper used is critical, because there is considerable variation in the amount of sebum absorbed by different papers, and even between different batches of paper from the same maker. The paper originally used by British workers is no longer available but a suitable alternative is the 'Special velin tissue, non-fluff', obtainable from the Koch-Light Laboratories, Colnbrook, Bucks., England (Cunliffe *et al* 1975).

5   The papers must be degreased prior to use by immersing them in Analar ether for about $2\frac{1}{2}$ hours. A small, but progressive decrease in absorbency is found if the papers are immersed for more than 6 hours (Cunliffe & Shuster 1969a). Thereafter, the paper must be handled with forceps, and it can be stored conveniently in ether-cleansed tinfoil. Some types of tinfoil treated with ether readily shed fragments of the shiny surface which stick to the papers, so it is best to use the dull surface.

6   The adhesive tape used to delineate the collection area on the forehead must be clean. Occasionally the adhesive sticks to the outer surface of the roll of tape and if this is not noticed it will be transferred to the collection papers.

7   The skin must be prepared, prior to the timed collection, by the serial application of preliminary absorbent papers until the accumulated surface lipid has been removed and only a 'follicular' pinpoint pattern of freshly excreted sebum is visible. Novice sebum-collectors usually underestimate the time required for this preliminary procedure and staining of their 'follicular patterns' with osmic acid vapour will often show that the papers are still heavily lipid-laden. The time for the skin preparation varies for each subject, but most will require four or five changes of paper at 5-minute intervals.

8   The investigator should check the position of the collection papers periodically throughout the test, as many subjects inadvertently move their rubber headbands.

9   The collection time should be standardized to about 3 hours. The hourly output of collected sebum decreases with time and it could be argued that the greater rate in the early hours is spurious and should be disregarded. The sebum collected during the first and subsequent 3-hour collection periods is linearly related however, and the first collection appears to produce a valid index of sebaceous activity (Cunliffe & Shuster 1969a). This observation emphasizes that the method does not directly measure the rate of secretion from the sebaceous glands to the follicular reservoir.

10   The ether used to extract the sebum from the papers should be evaporated in a rotary vacuum evaporator (eg Buchi Rotavapor). This reduces the fire risk and increases the accuracy of the subsequent weighing by reducing condensation of water vapour and contamination with dust.

11   Good weighing technique is vital. The balance must be accurate to 10 µg (eg Mettler M5) and it should preferably be kept in a draught-free balance room built with a concrete floor over a main structural crossbeam of the building. Room temperature should be constant, and humidity inside the balance should be controlled by the use of silica gel. The effects of static electricity can be reduced by the use of aluminium cups in place of glass.

Normal values for the sebum excretion rate by this method for subjects of different ages and sex have been given by Pochi and Strauss (1965) and Burton *et al* (1975), but obviously each worker must obtain his own normal range. It should be noted that the experimental error of the method is proportionally larger with low sebum excretion rates, and the variance of the method should therefore be determined at each end of the range.

Even if a technically satisfactory measurement of sebum excretion rate is obtained, the result can still be misleading, due, for example, to the subject taking a drug such as an oral contraceptive which affects sebaceous activity. Hormonal and other factors known to affect the rate of sebum production in man have been previously reviewed (Burton 1972; Pochi & Strauss 1974; Shuster & Thody 1974).

When comparing groups of subjects, difficulties can arise in the choice of suitable controls. Some degree of acne is almost universal during adolescence (Burton *et al* 1971) and the more severe grades of acne are associated with seborrhoea (Burton & Shuster 1971). The seborrhoea persists into middle age, long after the acne has become quiescent (Cunliffe & Shuster, 1969b) and since most middle-aged subjects have no reliable recollection of the severity of their adolescent acne the selection of control subjects with or without a previous history of acne is unreliable. Since the sebum excretion rate has such a wide range in the normal population, evidence of previous acne (eg scarring) should not necessarily preclude a subject from acting as a control. If a control group for the study of sebum production excludes subjects with acne or previous acne a falsely low sebum production figure will result (Pochi & Strauss 1974).

The sebum excretion rate is usually expressed in terms of the area of skin studied, but it could be related to the number of functioning glands by applying the 'replica' technique (Sarkany & Gaylarde 1968) in which a hardened plaster of Paris (dental grade) replica of the skin surface is stained with 0.25% osmium tetroxide. This allows the number of patent follicular orifices to be counted, and it also produces a permanent record of their position in relation to other microscopic features of the skin surface. Cunliffe and Cotterill (1975) have described an alternative technique in which a red dye (saturated Oil Red O) is used to stain the follicular orifices, followed by direct microphotography of the skin surface.

SKIN SURFACE LIPID COMPOSITION

The composition of skin surface lipids in the human varies in different parts of the body, but in sebaceous-rich areas such as the face, scalp and upper trunk, about 95% of the lipid consists of sebum (Greene *et al* 1970). The epidermal contribution consists mainly of triglycerides, cholesterol and cholesterol esters. The sebum as it is formed in the sebaceous glands consists predominantly of triglycerides, wax esters and squalene, with little or no free fatty acid proteolipids. There are large differences in skin surface lipid composition between individuals, but in each subject the lipid composition remains constant from day to day (Downing *et al* 1969).

Since the surface lipid is a mixture derived from sebaceous glands and keratinocytes, its composition varies with the anatomical site of origin, the areas with a lower density of sebaceous glands having a higher cholesterol content and a lower squalene content than the sebaceous-rich areas (Greene *et al* 1970). The composition also varies with the age of the subject, and before puberty, when sebaceous gland development is minimal, the epidermis contributes the major source of the surface lipid.

Our limited knowledge of the complex biosynthetic pathways of human surface lipids has been reviewed by Downing and Strauss (1974).

Sampling techniques

It will be obvious from the above that the apparent composition of the skin surface lipid will vary to some extent with the sampling technique used, according to the relative proportions of epidermal and sebaceous lipid obtained. The three methods most commonly used to sample surface lipid have been the use of absorbent papers (Cotterill *et al* 1971), wiping with a polyurethane sponge soaked in solvent (Ramasastry *et al* 1970) and the direct application of solvent in a glass cylinder pressed firmly to the skin surface (Greene *et al* 1970). The three techniques have been compared by Cunliffe *et al* (1971) who found that the samples obtained by the sponge method had a greater free fatty acid content than those obtained by the other methods, possibly due to increased bacterial contamination. The paper collection method appears to yield a sample with a lower epidermal contribution, and it has the advantage that the sample can be weighed before analysis to allow the sebum excretion rate to be measured in the same investigation. It may be unsatisfactory for the analysis of free fatty acids however, as the percentage recovery of standard solutions of fatty acids added to such papers is low, presumably because of binding to the papers (Strauss *et al* 1964; Kanaar 1971). For these reasons the cylinder method, using hexane or ether as the solvent, may be preferable. The cylinder used must have a smooth edge to avoid injury to the skin and, when used on the forehead, a pad should be placed over the eyes in case of leakage of solvent. Large cylinders are particularly susceptible to this complication as they overlap the forehead wrinkles, but this hazard can be avoided by taking multiple collections, using a small cylinder (eg 1 cm diameter) and a Pasteur pipette to transfer the solvent. The quantity of epidermal lipid extractable from the forehead skin by this technique is only 5–10 $\mu g/cm^2$, compared with 150–300 $\mu g/cm^2$ of sebum (Greene *et al* 1970). The influence of the epidermal lipid contribution, moreover, is diminished by virtue of the fact that its major constituent, triglyceride, is present in approximately the same proportion in sebum.

Large quantities of scalp lipid can be collected by pouring 500 ml ether over the scalp into a basin. Great care must be taken to exclude accidental ignition of the ethereal vapour during the collection procedure (e.g. by a spark from an electrical switch). The solution is filtered and the ether is then removed in a rotary evaporator.

Solvents differ in their extraction properties (Hodgson-Jones & Wheatley 1952; Nicolaides & Kellum 1965) and a non-polar solvent such as hexane might be expected to remove less epidermal cell lipid than more polar solvents such as chloroform:methanol mixture, which will penetrate to remove lipids deep in the epidermis. In practice, however, the choice of solvent makes little or no difference to the results (Downing & Strauss 1974).

Another factor which affects the composition is the interval between the preparatory skin cleansing and the collection and analysis of the sample (Wilkinson 1969). The increased free fatty acid content seen in the samples from a delayed collection or analysis is presumably related to triglyceride lipolysis by the bacterial contamination of the samples.

Storage of lipid samples

The samples should be analysed as soon as possible to avoid lipolysis subsequent to collection. If they have to be stored overnight it is probably best to keep them in a solvent in a sealed container at −20°C. Downing (1970) has demonstrated changes in the composition of stored lipid even when it is stored under nitrogen.

Analysis of lipid samples

The earliest analysis of lipid composition was performed by chemical estimation of the various lipid classes (Sobel 1949) but chromatographic techniques (t.l.c. and g.l.c.) have proved to be far more rapid, sensitive and accurate.

Types of chromatography

Chromatography is a separation technique which owes its name to the fact that many of the compounds first separated by this method were coloured. In a chromatographic separation it is necessary to have a *stationary* phase and a *mobile* phase. The stationary phase may be either a liquid or a solid whereas the mobile phase may be a liquid or a gas. Thus there are four main types of chromatography:

Mobile-stationary
1   Liquid-liquid.
2   Gas-liquid.
3   Liquid-solid.
4   Gas-solid.

In liquid-liquid or gas-liquid chromatography the components of the mixture to be separated partition themselves between the liquid stationary phase and the gas or liquid mobile phase, and this is, therefore, called *partition chromatography*. Separation will not, of course, be possible unless the solutes in the mixture have different partition coefficients.

In liquid-solid and gas-solid chromatography the solid stationary phase acts as a selective retardant to the components of the mixture to be separated, in other words, the components of the mixture are selectively adsorbed by the solid. This is called *adsorption chromatography*. In *thin layer chromatography* the stationary phase is in a solid which is held on the surface of a plate as a thin layer and the mobile phase (normally a liquid) is passed through it. In *column chromatography* the stationary phase is a solid which is held in a tube and the gas or liquid is passed through the tube.

Gel-filtration chromatography is in essence a form of liquid-liquid chromatography in which the liquid stationary phase is within the pores of the gel held in a tube. Small molecules have access to this liquid (usually water) while larger molecules have only limited access or are completely excluded. Many crosslinked polymers are available (eg Sephadex) in different grades and these are invaluable in separating molecules according to their size.

Thin layer chromatography (t.l.c.)

This versatile technique, which can be used for both preparation and analysis, is particularly useful in the separation of lipid mixtures. The solid phase must be of uniform thickness and should be sufficiently robust to stand up to the subsequent development (ie separation) and visualization procedures (q.v.). Materials which are widely used for the solid phase are silica gel, alumina, kieselguhr and cellulose. The stability of the thin layer can be increased by adding a binder such as starch or plaster of Paris. Alumina is a good adsorbant for non-polar basic mixtures and silica gel is good for non-polar acidic or neutral mixtures. Polar mixtures on the other hand are better separated on silica gel, kieselguhr or cellulose. The properties of these adsorbants can be modified by adding small amounts of other chemicals such as buffers, acids or bases. The addition of silver nitrate, for example, can be used to bind double-bonds to separate saturated and unsaturated fatty acids.

Preparation of plates

Silica gel provides a satisfactory stationary phase for lipid separation and suitable plates can be obtained commercially (eg from E. Merck & Co.). A cheaper alternative is to coat 20 × 20 cm glass plates with a 0.25 mm layer of silica gel using a plate-spreader (eg Shandon 'Unoplan').

Silica Gel G, which contains calcium sulphate as a binding agent, produces a fairly durable stable phase, but if quantitative radio-labelling experiments are to be performed it is better to use silica gel H which has no binding agent. This can more easily be scraped off the glass plate following separation of the lipid classes for subsequent analysis by scintillation counting. It is essential that the plates are thoroughly cleaned before preparation (eg by chromic acid followed by distilled water) otherwise the silica will not adhere to the glass satisfactorily. A suitable slurry is made by mixing 30 g in 50 ml of distilled water and this is sufficient for five plates. A 'feeler' gauge can be used to check the setting of the plate-spreader. After drying, the plates can be stored for a few days in a desiccated cabinet until required. The silica gel adsorbant must be activated for 30–60 minutes at 100°C just before use. Oxidizable impurities contained in the silica gel can be removed by 'washing' the blank plates by developing them with ether prior to use. In this way the impurities are eluted beyond the solvent

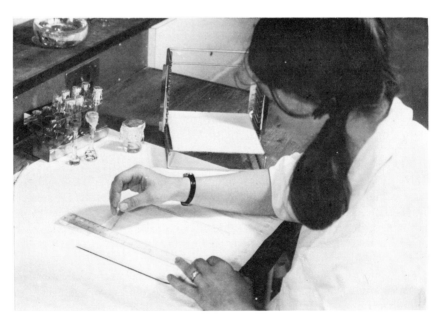

Fig. 1.1 Dividing the t.l.c. plate into lanes, using a needle to scratch the lines. Note that the ruler is supported by a block at each end to hold it just clear of the plate.

front of the subsequent analytical run. The silica plates are then divided into narrow lanes (eg 7 mm) by using a needle (see Fig. 1.1). The lanes must be narrow to maintain constancy of the densitometer response over the whole length of the eventual chromatogram (Downing 1968).

'Spotting' of samples

Prior to analysis the solvent used to obtain the SSL sample is evaporated by heating to 35°C while nitrogen is blown over the surface. The sample is then redissolved in an appropriate volume of chloroform:methanol to give a final concentration of 50 μg lipid in 5 μl of chloroform:methanol. Polar solvents should not be used for the sample application as they allow the lipid samples to spread too widely, thus resulting in poor resolution. The samples are 'spotted' onto the base of each lane using constricted microlitre pipettes (Marburg). Care is required to avoid disturbing the thin layer. A suitable volume for each lane is 3–20 μl. This low loading gives better separation of the closely running compounds, but if minor components are being sought, a higher total loading may be required. The samples should of course be 'spotted' a little way up the plate to ensure that they do not dip in the solvent mixture when the plates are being developed, and it is found that more reproducible results are obtained if the samples are applied as a horizontal linear 'streak' rather than a circular 'spot'. Semiautomatic applicators are available which apply the sample streak from a syringe.

Development

Thin layer chromatography plates are normally developed by ascending chromatography. The solvent is placed in the bottom of a closed tank that is allowed to become saturated with its vapour. The tank should have a lid, preferably sealed by suitable longitudinally split silicone rubber tubing, in order to reduce to the minimum any change in the composition of the developing solvent resulting from differential evaporation to the atmosphere. The tank is lined with thick filter paper dipping in the solvent as this helps to keep the tank saturated with vapour and the plate may be allowed to stand in the tank prior to the separation in order that the solid layer may become saturated with the vapour. To develop the plate, its bottom edge is placed in the solvent, which is allowed to flow 10–15 cm up the plate before the latter is removed, dried and visualized (q.v.). The tank should be kept away from sunlight, radiators and draughts as a slight temperature differential is enough to produce an irregular solvent front. Vibrating machinery should be switched off during the development.

The choice of a solvent system to separate a particular mixture is to a certain extent empirical, and indeed t.l.c. can be compared with cooking. Published recipes are by no means infallible, and the results they produce seem to vary from one laboratory to another, presumably due to differences of temperature, pressure and humidity in the environment. One method of finding a solvent with the right polarity to separate the mixture is to place spots of the mixture on the thin layer and add different solvents from a capillary to the centre of the spots. The position of the solvent front is then noted, the solvent dried off and the spots visualized. A solvent that moves most of the components of the mixture about halfway from the centre of the spot to the solvent front is satisfactory. The ratio of the distance travelled by a substance to the distance travelled by the solvent front is called the R_F value. More polar compounds have a low R_F value and tend to remain near the source, but they can be made to travel further up the plate by using a more polar solvent. Sometimes a mixture of solvents is required, but the mixture should be kept simple to avoid changes in its composition during use. Minor adjustments of the concentration of the most polar solvent will often have a marked effect on the R_F value. The addition of a small quantity of acid (eg acetic acid) may prevent compounds from tailing or smearing due to the presence of more than one ionic species. The following series lists some commonly used solvents in order of increasing polarity:

Petroleum ether.
Cyclohexane.
Benzene.
Chloroform.
Diethyl ether.
Acetone.
Ethanol.
Methanol.
Water.

For the separation of skin surface lipids, multiple development with a sequence of solvents is required. The solvents used must be Analar grade and should be redistilled before use. The less polar solvent systems should be used before the more polar solvents to avoid spot distortion. The most widely used solvent sequence is probably that described by Downing (1968) which is as follows:

1   Hexane.
2   Benzene.
3   Hexane:ether:acetic acid (70:30:1).

The excellent separation which this sequence produces is shown in Fig. 1.2. This sequence may not suit all climates, however and other suitable development sequences have been described (Kellum 1967; Nicolaides *et al* 1968; Cotterill *et al* 1971; Pye *et al* 1976). All these methods give good separation of tryglycerides and free fatty acids, but they do not always provide a clear demarcation between cholesterol esters and wax esters, nor between diglycerides and cholesterol.

Free fatty acids can be further separated according to their degree of unsaturation by a silver ion t.l.c. method (Wilkinson 1973). This process separates saturated fatty acids (no double-bonds) from monenes, dienes and a fourth band of 'polyenes' which contain polyunsaturated fatty acids (PUFA) with three to six double-bonds.

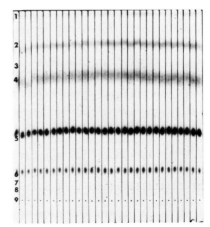

Fig. 1.2 Appearance of the thin layer chromatograms after charring; 1, paraffin hydrocarbons; 2, squalene; 3, cholesterol esters; 4, wax esters; 5, triglycerides; 6, free fatty acids; 7, cholesterol; 8, diglycerides; 9, origin. Reproduced from *Journal of Investigative Dermatology* (1969) **53**, 323.

Phospholipids and glycolipids form only a small proportion of the cutaneous lipids, but they are essential structural components of the cellular membrane system and they may be involved in the process of keratinization. Total lipids from the skin may be separated into (a) netural lipids (b) acidic phospholipids and glycolipids and (c) choline-containing phospholipids by column chromatography, using silica gel H (Gray 1967). The phospholipids and glycolipids can then be further separated by two-dimensional t.l.c. (Long 1976) (Fig. 1.3).

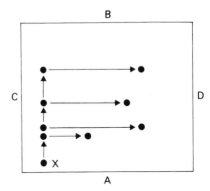

Fig. 1.3 Two dimensional t.l.c. A mixture is applied at spot X, and the plate is developed in the first dimension from A to B and then in the second dimension from C to D.

Visualization

If the components of the mixture to be analyzed are colourless, the developed plate must be treated with a visualizing agent to show up the position of the separated components as coloured spots. If necessary the layer can be treated first with a solution of dichloro-dimethyl-silane to increase its stability to subsequent spraying or washing with aqueous solutions. Most colourless compounds can be visualized by spraying with a specific reagent. Amino acids, for example, can be visualized by spraying with ninhydrin solution and heating at

110°C in an oven. Some reagents such as iodine will detect a wide range of compounds. The plate may either be sprayed with 1% methanolic iodine or stood in a jar containing iodine crystals. Spots stained by iodine will, however, quickly fade. Another general reagent used to locate spots is fluorescein-bromine. The developed plate is sprayed with 0.05% aqueous fluorescein and while still damp exposed to bromine vapour. This method, which depends on the ability of the organic compound to stop the thin layer becoming wet, will produce fluorescent spots on a dark red background.

Organic compounds such as lipids can be visualized by charring the separate components to elemental carbon. For the charring of lipids most workers recommend the use of sulphuric acid, either as a 50% spray, or by immersing the plates momentarily in 10% sulphuric acid and then drying before heating the plates at 180–220°C for 20–30 minutes in a ventilated oven. This method, which produces unpleasant fumes, is potentially dangerous, and it is better to incorporate a 5% ammonium sulphate solution into the plates when they are made (Walker 1971). By this method the use of sulphuric acid is unnecessary, since it is generated when the plates are heated in the oven.

Absolute cleanliness is of course essential at all stages for accurate t.l.c. work, but snags can arise in unexpected ways. I particularly like the story of the workers who found incredibly high squalene levels every Wednesday. Frenzied investigation eventually revealed that a neighbouring technician popped into their laboratory every Tuesday to heat his pork pie lunch in their oven.

Densitometry

The weight of each lipid fraction can be estimated by photodensitometry, since the size and optical density of each spot varies with the weight of carbon it contains. A suitable instrument for this purpose is the Chromoscan recording, integrating and reflectance photometer (Joyce Loebl). The area under each peak is proportional to the amount of carbon in each spot, and these areas can be measured either by planimetry, or by cutting out the peak from the recorder chart and weighing the paper. Occasionally the charring of the plate produces a background colour which varies slightly along the length of the plate. This produces a variation in the baseline reading, but this can be overcome by adjusting the baseline of the reading to zero for each lipid fraction.

The principles of densitometry relating to t.l.c. analysis of lipids have been discussed by Downing (1968). The proportion of carbon which a compound contains (the 'carbon density') will govern the maximum yield of elemental carbon it can produce on charring. Most lipid fractions give a carbon yield which is proportional to the weight of the lipid present, but cholesterol and free alcohols enhance the carbon yield and the cholesterol peak must be reduced by an arbitrary correction factor of 0.66 to allow for this.

An alternative to t.l.c. which has been used to measure sebum excretion rate and to analyse lipid mixtures is infra-red spectroscopy with internal reflectance (Fulton *et al* 1971). The principles underlying this method, which relies on the stretching and deformational vibrations associated with covalently bound atoms, have been discussed by Davenport (1971). From the patient's point of view the technique is simple, since it only involves a crystal being pressed on the skin, but the apparatus required is expensive and the reproducibility between instruments is not good. The method is less accurate than t.l.c. which can detect changes in concentration of 5% or more, whereas the range of variation with infra-red spectroscopy is 10–40% (Shalita *et al* 1975).

Gas-liquid chromatography (g.l.c.)

The basic apparatus (see Fig. 1.4) used for g.l.c. involves a liquid-stationary phase in a column mounted in a thermostatically controlled oven. At one end of the column is fitted the sample injection unit and at the other end is the sample detector. The carrier gas enters the column and carries the injected sample through to the flame-ionization detector. The components of the mixture are separated on the column and pass out one by one through the detector which produces an electrical signal that after amplification works a potentiometric recorder. The oven provides accurate temperature regulation to ensure reproducible retention times of the various components on the column. The use of temperature programming, in which the temperature is increased during the run, decreases the retention time and sharpens the peaks produced on the recorder.

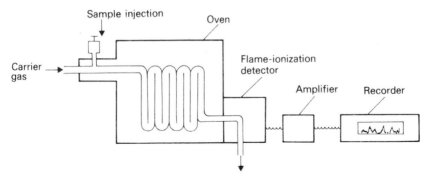

Fig. 1.4 Gas-liquid chromatography apparatus.

Lipids are usually chemically converted to their methyl esters before analysis, mainly because considerable experience has accumulated in the interpretation of the peaks which methyl esters produce. Several procedures for the conversion of lipids to their methyl esters are described in textbooks of organic chemistry, but the diazomethane method is to be avoided because it can produce artefactual peaks and the chemicals may explode when concentrated.

Methods of g.l.c. analysis of skin surface lipids have been described by various authors including Krakow *et al* (1973) and Cunliffe and Cotterill (1975). The method described by Cunliffe and Cotterill (1975) for the analysis of free fatty acids and triglycerides may be outlined as follows:

Skin surface lipid samples are separated into five main constituents by t.l.c. and the free fatty acid and triglyceride fractions are scraped off the plate and extracted from the silica gel by serial washing in diethyl ether. The samples are then evaporated to dryness under a stream of nitrogen prior to methylation.

The methylation of free fatty acids is accomplished by adding 0.5 ml of BF_3/Me OH solution to each tube and incubating at 80°C for 2 minutes. Distilled water (2 ml) is added, the free fatty acid methyl esters ('fames') are extracted by two washings with pentane, and the sample is evaporated to dryness.

Triglycerides are methylated by adding 1 ml of 0.25 M solution of sodium methoxide in methanol to each tube and incubating at 60°C for 1 hour. Water (1.5 ml) is added and the esters are extracted as before.

The esters are injected in 10 ml pentane, using nitrogen at 40 ml/min as the carrier gas. The temperature is progressively increased from 110°C to 215°C, increasing at the rate of 0.75°C per min. The area of each peak is recorded by a digital electronic integrator and the results are expressed as the percentage contribution of each peak to the total free fatty acid or trigylceride fraction.

Gas-liquid chromatography of cutaneous lipids has been used mainly for the detailed analysis of fatty acids and triglycerides, but other lipid fractions can also be analysed by g.l.c. Chromatography of intact wax esters is possible, and sterols can be chromatographed as esters or trimethylsilyl ethers. Direct g.l.c. of unfractioned lipids has been attempted but the chromatograms are too complex to be of value. It is inadvisable to identify specific fatty acids through g.l.c. procedures alone, although analysis on two or more stationary phases and under various operating conditions may allow a structure to be tentatively assigned to a particular peak.

Gas-liquid chromatography can also be used to determine the chain length of individual fatty acids and to determine whether or not the chain is branched. It is also possible to say whether a particular compound has an odd or an even number of carbon atoms. The degree of saturation can be measured by performing the g.l.c. analysis before and after the unsaturated compounds have been obliterated by bromination. The application of these sophisticated analytical techniques to cutaneous lipids is illustrated by the study of Krakow *et al* (1973). Previous workers had found a significant increase in the concentration of a minor fatty acid in the facial skin of acne patients (Kellum & Strangfeld 1972), and Krakow *et al* (1973), using complex g.l.c. techniques identified this as octadeca-5,8 dienoic acid. Further work is now required to determine whether this finding is more than an epiphenomenon.

The use of g.l.c. apparatus and the errors likely to arise in the quantitative analysis of lipids by g.l.c. have been reviewed by Lewis and Hayward (1971), and Johnson and Stock (1971). The effects of variation in instrument design and operating conditions on quantitative g.l.c. of fatty acids have been discussed by Horning *et al* (1964) and computerization of g.l.c. data with special reference to fatty acids has been described by Boyne *et al* (1970).

Highly radioactive compounds separated by g.l.c. can be estimated by continuously counting the effluent. However, if a compound is only weakly radioactive this is not possible and discrete fractions must be collected and subsequently counted. Alternatively the compounds issuing from the g.l.c. apparatus can be collected onto a moving paper strip, thus retaining the advantages of continuous operation as in a flow system (Yardley & Long 1972).

THE STUDY OF CUTANEOUS LIPOGENESIS
in vitro

The study of cutaneous lipogenesis *in vivo* is limited by technical problems of sampling etc, and in man there are further limitations imposed by ethical considerations relating to the use of drugs, hormones and radioactive isotopes. For these reasons, several groups have developed techniques applicable to the direct study of cutaneous lipogenesis *in vitro* (Griesemer & Thomas 1966; Hsia *et al* 1966, 1970; Wilkinson 1970; Summerley & Woodbury 1971; Summerley *et al* 1976; Cooper *et al* 1974, 1976). Much of our knowledge of the sites of lipid synthesis, the substrates used, and the pathways of lipogenesis has been derived from these *in vitro* techniques (Wheatley 1974).

In these methods one or more small skin biopsies are taken, the subcutaneous fat is carefully trimmed away and the intact skin is then incubated in a buffer at 37°C with a suitable radioactive substrate for a given time (usually several hours). The buffer contains antibiotics to prevent bacterial contamination and it is usually oxygenated by bubbling a constant stream of oxygen through it. A large variety of substrates have been tested (lactate, acetate, proprionate, butyrate, etc) and it has been found that, in animals at least, glucose is the major lipid precursor (Wheatley *et al* 1971) and so C^{14}-labelled glucose is a very suitable substrate to use. An additional advantage of using glucose is that is stimulates lipogenesis, and its incorporation parallels the absolute rate of lipogenesis (Wheatley *et al* 1971). Many workers have used C^{14}-acetate as the substrate, but this is an unphysiological precursor which can upset metabolic pathways at high concentrations. Even glucose may be unsuitable for studies of regulatory mechanisms if it is used in concentrations exceeding 2 mM. The addition of serum or insulin to the culture medium will increase the uptake of the substrate, (Wilkinson 1973; Long 1976) but according to Wheatley *et al* (1970), lipogenesis most closely follows the *in vivo* metabolic pathways with a phosphate buffer without additives. Other difficulties inherent in this type of incubation experiment have been discussed by Wheatley *et al* (1970).

Following incubation the sebaceous glands can be harvested intact to allow the incorporation of radioactivity into the appendage-freed epidermis, sebaceous glands and dermis to be measured separately. This can be achieved by soaking the skin samples in a concentrated salt solution (eg 2 M sodium iodide or calcium chloride) for 3 hours at room temperature, and then peeling off the epidermis and the attached sebaceous glands, which can then be further separated by microdissection (Kellum 1966). Chemical separation of the epidermis from the dermis is dependent on the swelling effect on collagen by the salt ions. Another way of separating the epidermis and the sebaceous glands is by producing suction blisters. The blister roof is then composed of epidermis and the sebaceous glands remain in the dermis (Hsia *et al* 1970). An alternative technique which leaves the sebaceous glands *in situ* in the dermis is to soak the skin for 3 hours in 0.5% acetic acid, after which the epidermis can be peeled off (Cooper *et al* 1976).

It is also possible to study *in vitro* lipogenesis in isolated epidermal cells in man (Wilkinson 1970) and in animals (Prottey *et al* 1972; Long 1976). Suspensions of epidermal cells can be prepared by treating the epidermis with a 0.1% solution of trypsin, filtering the suspension through a nylon gauze and resuspending the cells in a solution of phosphate-buffered saline. The sterility of the cell suspension can be checked by plating out, and cell viability can be assessed by checking that the cells exclude the dyes nigrosin and eosin. In the rat, the addition of serum to the medium altered the pattern of substrate incorporation into the various lipid classes, and changes in the density of the cell suspension also altered the pattern of incorporation (Long 1976). A similar method has been applied to pig epidermal slices in culture (Long 1977).

The total lipids present in the tissue (including the radioactive proportion) can be extracted by the method of Folch *et al* (1957), and separated into the main lipid classes by t.l.c. After charring the various fractions can be scraped from the plate and the radioactivity in each is measured by a scintillation-counter. The lipid fractions extracted in incubation experiments can also be measured gravimetrically (Summerley *et al* 1976). After chromatography and autoradiography the silica gel is scraped from the areas on the plates which correspond to the various lipid fractions. The lipids are then recovered from the silica by serial extraction with chloroform:methanol which is then evaporated under nitrogen. Each extract is then redissolved in a small volume of chloroform and absorbed on previously weighed paper which is dried and weighed again to give the weight of lipid.

These methods are likely to find increasing use in the study of the physiology and pathology of cutaneous lipogenesis but the results must be interpreted with caution. The composition of dermal lipid produced by the sebaceous glands varies with the rate of lipogenesis (Cooper *et al* 1976). The rate of lipogenesis is increased by the ingestion of 100 g of glucose (Hsia *et al* 1970) whereas it is decreased by 18 hours of fasting prior to the biopsy (Hsia *et al* 1966). The composition of the lipid produced by sebaceous glands is also related to the gland size. In the larger sebaceous glands proportionately more of the labelled substrate is incorporated into squalene at the expense of triglycerides (Summerley *et al* 1976). It is essential therefore that due attention should be given to the nutritional state of the skin donor and the size of the sebaceous glands being studied when the results of *in vitro* experiments are being interpreted.

The highly contrasting patterns of lipid synthesis in the sebaceous glands and the appendage-freed epidermis have enabled an *in vitro* technique to be used to confirm that epidermoid cysts originate from the epidermis and are not of sebaceous origin, whereas sebocysts (steatocytomata) produce two lipid patterns, one which resembles isolated sebaceous glands and one which resembles appendage-freed epidermis (Summerley & Woodbury 1971).

REFERENCES

ARCHIBALD A. & SHUSTER S. (1973) A non-endocrine control of sebum secretion. *Archiv fuer Dermatologische Forschung* **246**, 175.

BOYNE A. W. & DUNCAN W. R. H. (1970) Computer treatment of gas-liquid chromatographic data with special reference to fatty acid methyl esters. *Journal of Lipid Research* **11**, 293.

BURTON J. L., CUNLIFFE W. J. & SHUSTER S. (1970) Circadian rhythm in sebum excretion. *British Journal of Dermatology* **82**, 497.

BURTON J. L. (1972) Factors affecting the rate of sebum excretion in man. *Journal of the Society of Cosmetic Chemists* **23**, 241.

BURTON J. L., CUNLIFFE W. J., STAFFORD I. & SHUSTER S. (1971) The prevalence of acne vulgaris in adolescents. *British Journal of Dermatology* **85**, 119.

BURTON J. L. & SHUSTER S. (1971) The relationship between seborrhoea and acne vulgaris. *British Journal of Dermatology* **84**, 600.

BURTON J. L., PYE R. J., MEYRICK G. & SHUSTER S. (1975) The sebum excretion rate in rosacea. *British Journal of Dermatology* **92**, 541.

BURTON J. L. (1970) The physical properties of sebum in acne vulgaris. *Clinical Science* **39**, 757.

BURTON J. L. (1971) Sebaceous glands—some observations on their physiology and pathology in man. MD Thesis, University of Manchester.

COOPER M. F., MCGRATH H. & SHUSTER S. (1976) Sebaceous lipogenesis in human skin. Variability with age and with severity of acne. *British Journal of Dermatology* **94**, 165.

COOPER M. F., THODY A. J. & SHUSTER S. (1974) Hormonal regulation of cutaneous lipogenesis—effects of hypophysectomy, posterior hypophysectomy and melanocyte stimulating hormone treatment. *Biochimica et Biophysica Acta* **360**, 193.

COTTERILL J. A., CUNLIFFE W. J., WILLIAMSON B. & FORSTER R. A. (1971) A semiquantitative method for the biochemical analysis of sebum. *British Journal of Dermatology* **85**, 35.

COTTERILL J. A., CUNLIFFE W. J., WILLIAMSON B. & BULUSU L. (1972) Further observations on the pathogenesis of acne. *British Medical Journal* **3**, 444.

COTTERILL J. A., CUNLIFFE W. J. & WILLIAMSON B. (1973) Variations in skin surface lipid composition and sebum excretion rate with time. *Acta Dermato-venereologica* **53**, 271.

CUNLIFFE W. J., BURTON J. L. & SHUSTER S. (1970) The effect of local temperature variation on the sebum excretion rate. *British Journal of Dermatology* **83**, 650.

CUNLIFFE W. J. & COTTERILL J. A. (1975) In *The Acnes; Clinical features, pathogenesis and treatment*, p.293. W. B. Saunders Co Ltd, London.

CUNLIFFE W. J., COTTERILL J. A. & WILLIAMSON B.(1971) Variations in skin surface lipid composition with different sampling techniques. *British Journal of Dermatology* **85**, 40.

CUNLIFFE W. J. & SHUSTER S. (1969a) The rate of sebum excretion in man. *British Journal of Dermatology* **81**, 697.

CUNLIFFE W. J. & SHUSTER S. (1969b) Pathogenesis of acne. *Lancet* i, 685.

CUNLIFFE W. J., WILLIAMS S. M. & TAN S. G. (1975) Sebum excretion rate investigations—a new absorbant paper. *British Journal of Dermatology* **93**, 347.

DAVENPORT J. B. (1971) Infra-red spectroscopy of lipids. In *Biochemistry and Methodology of Lipids*, Eds. Johnson A. R. & Davenport J. B., p.231. Wiley, New York.

DOWNING D. T. (1968) Photodensitometry in the thin layer chromatographic analysis of neutral lipids. *Journal of Chromatography* **38**, 91.

DOWNING D. T. (1970) Lipolysis by human skin surface debris in organic solvents. *Journal of Investigative Dermatology* **54**, 395.

DOWNING D. T., STRAUSS J. S. & POCHI P. E. (1969) Variability in the chemical composition of human skin surface lipids. *Journal of Investigative Dermatology* **53**, 322.

DOWNING D. T. & STRAUSS J. S. (1974) Synthesis and composition of surface lipids of human skins. *Journal of Investigative Dermatology* **62**, 228.

EPSTEIN E. H. & EPSTEIN W. L. (1966) New cell formation in the human sebaceous gland. *Journal of Investigative Dermatology* **46**, 453.

FOLCH J., LEES M. & SLOANE-STANLEY G. H. (1957) A simple method for the determination and purification of total lipids from animal tissues. *Journal of Biological Chemistry* **226**, 497.

FULTON J. E., WEEKS J. G. & McCARTY L. (1975) *The inability of a bacterial lipase inhibitor to control acne vulgaris (Abstr).* Joint Meeting of S.I.D. and European Society of Dermatological Research, Amsterdam.

FULTON J. E., ANDERSON A. & RANDALL S. (1971) Sebum excretion: analysis by infra-red spectroscopy. *Journal of Investigative Dermatology* **56**, 413.

GLOOR M., JOSEPHS H. & FRIEDRICH H. C. (1974) Influence of air pollution on paraffin content of skin surface lipids (German). *Archiv fuer Dermatologische Forschung* **250**, 277.

GRAY G. M. (1967) Chromatography of lipids. I. An improved chromatographic procedure for the quantitative isolation of the neutral ceramide-containing glycolipids from mammalian tissues. *Biochimica et Biophysica Acta* **144**, 511.

GREENE R. S., DOWNING D. T., POCHI P. E. & STRAUSS J. S. (1970) Anatomical variation in the amount and composition of human skin surface lipid. *Journal of Investigative Dermatology* **54**, 240.

GREISEMER R. D. & THOMAS R. W. (1966) Lipogenesis in human skin. IV. *In vitro* rate studies. *Journal of Investigative Dermatology* **47**, 432.

HARBER L. C., HERMAN F., MANDAL L. & SULZBERGER M. (1957) Lipid studies on the human skin surface by means of the monomolecular layer method. *Journal of Investigative Dermatology* **29**, 55.

HODGSON-JONES I. S. & WHEATLEY V. R. (1952) Studies of sebum. 3. Methods for the collection and estimation of small amounts of sebum. *Biomedical Journal* **52**, 460.

HORNING E. C., AHRENS E. H., LIPSKY S. R., MATTSON F. H., MEAD J. F., TURNER D. A. & GOLDWATER W. H. (1964) Quantitative analysis of fatty acids by gas-liquid chromatography. *Journal of Lipid Research* **5**, 20.

HSIA S. L., DRIEZE M. A. & MARQUEZ M. C. (1966) Lipid metabolism in human skin. II. A study of lipogenesis in skin of diabetic patients. *Journal of Investigative Dermatology* **47**, 443.

HSIA S. L., FULTON J. E., FULGHUM D. & BUCH M. M. (1970) Lipid synthesis from acetate C[14] by suction blister epidermis and other skin components. *Proceedings of Society for Experimental Medicine and Biology* **135**, 285.

JOHNSON A. R. & STOCK R. B. (1971) Gas-liquid chromatography of lipids. In *Biochemistry and Methodology of Lipids,* Johnson A. R. & Davenport J. B. p.195. Wiley, New York.

JONES K. K., SPENCER M. C. & SANCHEZ S. A. (1951) The estimation of the rate of sebum secretion in man. *Journal of the Investigative Dermatology* **17**, 213.

KANAAR P. (1971) Variations in skin surface lipid composition. *British Journal of Dermatology* **85**, 600.

KELLUM R. E. (1967) Human sebaceous gland lipids. Analysis by thin layer chromatography. *Archives of Dermatology* **95**, 218.

KELLUM R. E. & STRANGFELD K. (1972) Acne vulgaris. Studies in pathogenesis: fatty acids of human surface triglycerides from patients with and without acne. *Journal of Investigative Dermatology* **58**, 315.

KELLUM R. E. (1966) Isolation of human sebaceous glands. *Archives of Dermatology* **93**, 610.

KLIGMAN A. M., WHEATLEY V. R. & MILLS O. H. (1970) Comedogenicity of human sebum. *Archives of Dermatology* **102**, 267.

KRAKOW R., DOWNING D. T., STRAUSS J. S. & POCHI P. E. (1973) Identification of a fatty acid in human skin surface lipids apparently associated with acne vulgaris. *Journal of Investigative Dermatology* **61**, 286.

LEWIS C. A. & HAYWARD, BARBARA J. (1971) Human skin surface lipids. In *Modern Trends in Dermatology,* vol. 4, ed. Borrie, P., p.89. Butterworths, London.

LONG V. J. W. (1976) Incorporation of 1–¹⁴C-acetate into the lipids of isolated epidermal cells. *British Journal of Dermatology* **94**, 243.

LONG V. J. W. (1977) Incorporation of 1–¹⁴C-acetate into epidermal lipids. A comparison between epidermal cells and epidermal slices. *British Journal of Dermatology* **97**, 139.

NICOLAIDES N. (1965) Skin lipids. II. Lipid class composition of samples from various species and anatomical sites. *Journal of American Oil Chemists' Society* **42**, 691.

NICOLAIDES N. & KELLUM R. S. (1965) Skin lipids. I. Sampling problems of the skin and its appendages. *Journal of American Oil Chemists' Society* **42**, 685.

NICOLAIDES N., HWEI C. F. & RICE G. R. (1968) The skin surface lipids of man compared with those of eighteen species of animals. *Journal of Investigative Dermatology* **51**, 83.

PLEWIG G. & CHRISTOPHERS E. (1974) Renewal rates of human sebaceous glands. *Acta Dermato-Venereologica* **54**, 177.

POCHI P. E. & STRAUSS J. S. (1964) Sebum production, casual sebum levels, titratable acidity of sebum and urinary fractional 17-ketosteroid excretion in males with acne. *Journal of Investigative Dermatology* **43**, 383.

POCHI P. E. & STRAUSS J. S. (1965) The effect of ageing on the activity of sebaceous glands in man. In *Advances in Biology of Skin*, vol. VI, ed. W. Montagna, p.121. Pergamon Press, New York.

POCHI P. E. & STRAUSS J. S. (1974) Endocrinologic control of development and activity of the human sebaceous gland. *Journal of Investigative Dermatology* **62**, 191.

PROTTEY C., HARTOP P. J. & FERGUSON T. F. M. (1972) Lipid synthesis in rat skin. *British Journal of Dermatology* **87**, 586.

PYE R. J., MEYRICK G. & BURTON J. L. (1976) Skin surface lipid composition in rosacea. *British Journal of Dermatology* **94**, 161.

RAY T. & KELLUM R. E. (1971) Acne vulgaris. Studies in pathogenesis: free fatty acid irritancy in patients with and without acne. *Journal of Investigative Dermatology* **57**, 6.

RAMASASTRY P., DOWNING D. T., POCHI P. E. & STRAUSS J. S. (1970) Chemical composition of human skin surface lipids from birth to puberty. *Journal of Investigative Dermatology* **54**, 139.

SARKANY I. & GAYLARDE P. (1968) A method for demonstration of the distribution of sebum on the skin surface. *British Journal of Dermatology* **80**, 744.

SHALITA A., LEWIS S. & LEE W. (1975) *Methods for analysis of sebum composition* (Abstr). Joint Meeting of S.I.D. and European Society of Dermatological Research, Amsterdam, June 1975.

SHUSTER S. & THODY A. J. (1974) The control and measurement of sebum secretion. *Journal of Investigative Dermatology* **62**, 172.

SOBEL H. (1949) Squalene in sebum and sebum-like materials. *Journal of Investigative Dermatology* **13**, 333.

STILLMAN M. A., MAIBACH H. I. & SHALITA A. R. (1975) Relative irritancy of free fatty acids of different chain length. *Contact Dermatitis* **1**, 65.

STRAUSS J. S. & POCHI P. E. (1961) The quantitative gravimetric determination of sebum production. *Journal of Investigative Dermatology* **36**, 293.

STRAUSS J. S. & POCHI P. E. (1965) Intracutaneous injection of sebum and comedones: histological observation. *Archives of Dermatology* **92**, 443.

STRAUSS J. S., POCHI P. E., MASUCCI F. J. & MAITHENY E. J. (1964) Titratable acidity of sebum as determined by a micropotentiometric technique. *Journal of Investigative Dermatology* **4**, 349.

SUMMERLEY R. & WOODBURY S. (1971) The *in vitro* incorporation of ¹⁴C-acetate into the isolated sebaceous glands and appendage-freed epidermis of human skin. *British Journal of Dermatology* **85**, 424.

SUMMERLEY R., YARDLEY H., RAYMOND M., TABIOWO A. & ILDERTON E. (1976) The lipid composition of sebaceous glands as a reflection of gland size. *British Journal of Dermatology* **94**, 45.

VOSS J. G. (1974) Acne vulgaris and free fatty acids. *Archives of Dermatology* **109**, 894.

WALKER B. (1971) A novel charring technique for the detection of lipids on thin layer chromatograms. *Journal of Chromatography* **56,** 320.

WEINSTEIN G. D. (1974) Cell kinetics of human sebaceous glands. *Journal of Investigative Dermatology* **62,** 144.

WHEATLEY V. R. (1974) Cutaneous lipogenesis. Major pathways of carbon flow and possible inter-relationships between epidermis and sebaceous glands. *Journal of Investigative Dermatology* **62,** 245.

WHEATLEY V. R., HODGKINS L. T., COON W. M., KUMARASIRI M., BERENZWEIG H. & FEINSTEIN J. M. (1971) Cutaneous lipogenesis precursors utilized by guinea-pig skin for lipid synthesis. *Journal of Lipid Research* **12,** 347.

WHEATLEY V. R., HODGKINS L. T. & COON W. M. (1970) Cutaneous lipogenesis—evaluation of model systems and the utilization of acetate, citrate and glucose as compared with other tissues. *Journal of Investigative Dermatology* **54,** 288.

WILKINSON D. I. (1970) Incorporation of acetate $-1-^{14}C$ into fatty acids of isolated epidermal cells. *Journal of Investigation Dermatology* **54,** 132.

WILKINSON D. I. (1973) Some factors affecting C^{14} –acetate incorporation into polyunsaturated fatty acids of skin. *Journal of Investigative Dermatology* **60,** 188.

WILKINSON D. I. (1969) Variability in composition of surface lipids. The problem of epidermal contribution. *Journal of Investigative Dermatology* **52,** 339.

YARDLEY H. J. & LONG V. J. W. (1972) Radio-gas chromatography by collection of radioactive compounds issuing from a gas chromatograph on a moving strip of paper. *Journal of Chromatography* **73,** 235.

FURTHER READING

JOHNSON A. R. & DAVENPORT J. B. (1971) *Biochemistry and Methodology of Lipids.* Wiley, New York.

SHELLARD E. J. (1968) *Quantitive Paper and Thin layer Chromatography.* Academic Press, New York.

Special Issue on Sebaceous Glands and Acne Vulgaris. In *Advances in Biology of Skin,* vol. XIV, eds. Montagna W., Bell M. & Strauss J. S. Pergamon Press, New York. Also published in *Journal of Investigative Dermatology* (1974) **62,** 118–339.

STAHL E. (1970) *Thin Layer Chromatography—Laboratory Handbook.* Allen & Unwin, London.

2

Methods for microbiological investigation of acne

K. T. HOLLAND & W. J. CUNLIFFE

This chapter details techniques which although of help in the investigation of acne may be applicable to certain other diseases. The main part of the chapter is related to microbiological techniques but a description of surface micro-scopy of the skin, the stratum corneum sampling technique of Marks and Dawber (1971) and isolation of sebaceous glands (Kellum 1966) are included. The final sections include the clinical grading of acne, and a scheme which is possibly of value if the investigator wishes to evaluate a drug for acne.

MICROBIOLOGY OF ACNE

Acne is a disorder of the pilosebaceous follicles and within these follicles as well as on the adjacent skin surface there are large numbers of microorganisms. Many dermatologists believe that these organisms play an important role in acne. However, as yet, there is no irrefutable evidence to confirm or deny this view. For those who support this thesis *Propioni-bacterium acnes* is considered to be the most important. This may be a dangerous assumption because *P. acnes* is just one type in the ecological system. Staphylococci, micrococci, sarcina and yeasts are present also, and shifts in their numbers or types might well affect the physiology of the pilosebaceous unit and so predispose to acne.

It is obvious that further investigations should proceed to identify the in-teraction of these organisms in this environment and to ascertain their impor-tance in acne.

The problems

Microbiological investigations are beset with various technical difficulties.

Controls and animal model

In any investigation the need for controls is essential and within the age range 13–22 years old the number of people with no acne whatsoever is low (Cunliffe, Ead & Gould, Unpublished observations, 1976). To circumvent this problem it is possible to compare data from subjects with different grades of acne. Comparison of data obtained from prepubertal subjects and those subjects whose acne has now regressed may also help. An animal model is very desirable but sad to say one does not exist.

Sampling

The microorganisms of interest are those situated in the pilosebaceous units, and probably to a lesser extent those on the surface of the skin which aggregate in microcolonies. Fig. 2.1 illustrates the position of the microorganisms in a normal pilosebaceous duct. The bacteria are also sometimes seen in the proximal part of the sebaceous gland. Clearly, there are technical difficulties associated with removing all the microorganisms from the entangled keratin of the pilosebaceous duct, and from the uneven skin surface. Therefore, short of taking a biopsy there is no method available that will remove all the microorganisms.

There are added difficulties concerned with reproducibility of the methods. Most methods sample many pilosebaceous units, some of which may be normal and some acne prone follicles. The number and size of units vary in any area (Cunliffe *et al* 1976) and consequently the number of microorganisms that could be supported will be different. However, the two ways of indicating reproducibility of methods are to compare samples obtained from the symmetrical parts of the body or to compare adjacent sites. At present there is no reliable way of testing whether all microorganisms are removed.

A perfect sampling system would remove all the microorganisms, leave the skin intact, be painless, disperse the clumps of organisms for accurate enumeration, be reproducible and be sensitive, ie estimate low numbers. No method available at present has all these advantages.

Sampling methods

The discussion of the sampling methods includes a general description of the technique, its advantages and disadvantages and its area of main use in investigations. The reader is advised to consult the references for precise details (see pp. 34–35). Methods 1–4 sample almost exclusively surface organisms only; 7–10 ductal organisms and methods 5 and 6 sample the surface and the upper parts of the duct.

1   *Nutrient medium contact (Ulrich 1964)*

A sterile solidified medium in a suitable holder is placed against the skin and then removed for incubation. The position of the colonies on the agar surface indicates the distribution of the skin surface microcolonies. It is of no use for enumeration but the general types of microorganisms can be identified.

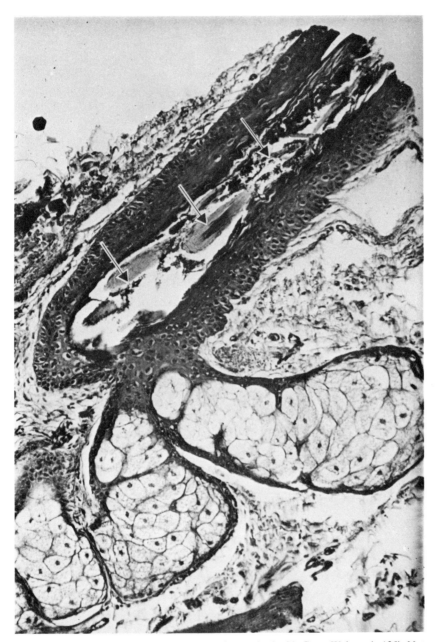

Fig. 2.1 Sebaceous gland and pilosebaceous duct stained with Gram-Weigart (×125). Note that the arrows indicate many microorganisms at all levels of the pilosebaceous duct.

2   *Velvet pad method*

This surface method is a copy of the replica plating method (Lederberg & Lederberg 1952) in which a sterile velvet pad is pressed on the skin surface and then on to suitable solid media (Verdon 1961); alternatively, the pad can be agitated in a fluid to disperse the microorganisms (Reibel *et al* 1967). The cloth acts as a set of multiple inoculation needles which transfer the microorganisms. This technique is useful for demonstrating the distribution of bacteria on the skin surface and allows identification of the major types. However, it is unsuitable for the enumeration of microorganisms even with agitation, because the sample obtained would represent only a small percentage of the total microorganisms on the skin. It will not sample microorganisms from the follicles.

3   *Sellotape stripping technique (Evans et al 1950)*

Sterile tape is placed on the area of skin to be sampled and then on to a suitable medium. This method has all the disadvantages of the velvet pad method and also only one type of medium or incubation environment can be used per stripping. This will limit the range of types of microorganisms isolated. However, it can be used to isolate types from just below the skin surface in the follicles by taking repeated samples from the same site.

4   *Surface swabbing*

A moistened sterile cotton wool swab on a stick is wiped over a known area of skin, replaced into sterile 5 ml nutrient broth in a test tube and agitated on a Rotamix. This will remove many microorganisms off the wool. The method is suitable for identifying the types of bacteria on the surface but not within the follicles. It gives a low count, 20% of the total and below (Roberts 1975). There are two reasons for this; firstly, it does not remove all the bacteria from the skin surface, and secondly, not all the bacteria can be removed from the cotton wool. However, it is the most suitable method for clinical use to identify the types of bacteria on the skin and then to determine their antibiotic sensitivity.

5   *Scrub technique (Williamson & Kligman 1965)*

In this method 1 ml buffered non-ionic detergent (Triton X 100) is pipetted into a glass or metal cup (see Fig. 2.2A) held in position on the skin. The skin is rubbed with a smooth Teflon abrader for 1 minute and the fluid removed. This procedure is repeated with a fresh 1 ml of Triton X 100, the two fractions are pooled and the viable bacterial count performed. This is a good method for enumerating and typing microorganisms from the skin surface but it will not remove all microorganisms from the deeper regions of the pilosebaceous

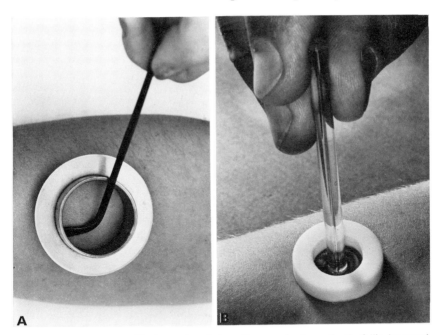

Fig. 2.2 A, apparatus used in the scrub technique; B, apparatus in use for the follicular sampling technique.

ducts. It is a superior method to the previous four because the clumps of microorganisms will be dispersed and a more realistic count obtained. However, reproducibility may be affected by the force and speed of rubbing with the rod which will differ from operator to operator and even by the same operator. Also, differentiation between surface and pilosebaceous duct organisms cannot be achieved. Despite this disadvantage it is a commonly used and recommended technique for investigations.

6   *Ultrasonic method (Stringer & Marples 1976)*

This method was introduced as a modification of the scrub technique to ensure standardized agitation on the skin. The method is similar to method 5 except that the Teflon abrader is replaced by an ultrasonic probe immersed in 2 ml of Triton X 100; the probe does not touch the skin. By experimentation it was found that a power of 90 W for 10–15 seconds was most satisfactory. However, above this power, pain was experienced. Overall, the method did not give an improvement on the scrub technique.

7   *Comedo extractor (Smith & Waterworth 1961;*
Izumi et al 1970)

A sterile comedo extractor is used to express the comedo which is then homogenized in a detergent to release the microorganisms for a viable count.

This method is limited to blackheads and whiteheads and cannot be used for normal skin and inflammatory lesions. However, it does have the advantage of sampling only one follicle.

8   Surgical sampling (Marples & Izumi 1970; Shalita & Rosenthal 1972)

Pustules can be sampled by expressing the pus with a sterile blade. Ths pus is processed but this method is limited to pustules and fluctuant nodules.

9   Follicular sampling (Holland et al 1974)

A Teflon disc is placed over the skin to be sampled and one drop of cyanoacrylate gel is placed within the discs. A glass sampler (see Fig. 2.2B) is held in the disc for 30 seconds and removed. The sampler removes the surface keratinocytes and part of the pilosebaceous duct keratin. The sampling process can be repeated with other samplers at the same site. The authors usually sample twice at one site and both samples are treated in the same way. In order to disperse the bacteria and remove them from the horn, the sampler is rotated on its longitudinal axis at 6000 rev/min for 1 minute in 12.5 ml Tween 80 broth with 2.5 ml No. 9 Ballotini beads. Viable counts are performed on the fluid. This method is easy to perform, can be used on normal skin and has the advantage that it samples specifically from the pilosebaceous duct. It has been shown that surface microorganisms are not sampled because they are locked between the cyanoacrylate gel and the surface keratinocytes. The disadvantage is that the method should not be used near the eye because of the adhesive properties of the cyanoacrylate. Further-more, any microorganisms lying a few micrometres beneath the cyanoacrylate gel and stratum corneum surface are not released into the fluid. *Pityrosporum ovale* may be located at this site and this method is perhaps not suitable for its isolation.

All the methods so far described have two common disadvantages. They all sample an area of skin which includes involved and non-involved pilo-sebaceous units. The follicular sampling method can be adapted to overcome this problem by dissecting and then homogenizing the individual pilosebaceous ducts. In this way not only can the number and types of microorganisms be related to the acne pilosebaceous units but also to the in-dividual units. Secondly, no method can effectively remove all the material from the pilosebaceous units and consequently the numbers of microorganisms isolated will be lower than the total.

10   Isolation of the pilosebaceous units (Puhvel et al 1975)

After a skin biopsy and calcium chloride treatment (Kellum 1966) the epidermis and the sebaceous glands can be separated from the dermis. The in-dividual glands can be micromanipulated and added to separate 1 ml quantities of 0.01% Triton X 100 in phosphate buffer. The complete individual unit can then be homogenized to release the microorganisms. This method is excellent for research purposes but would be of little use for routine needs because a biopsy is required and the method is difficult and time-consuming. It is doubtful as to whether the technique would be feasible with acne lesions.

Enumeration of microorganisms

Two types of count may be performed. A total count includes those alive and dead and a viable count estimates only those capable of division. In skin microbiology it is usual to perform viable counts but dead organisms may be important due to the release of intracellular products.

Total count

A useful method is to place a drop of the sample fluid in a Halber counting chamber with a coverslip and using phase contrast microscopy count the microorganisms. The results are expressed as cells per ml which can be related back both to the original sample volume and thereby to the skin surface area. The major types in the sample can be differentiated by their morphology as cocci and rods. *Pityrosporum ovale* and *P. obiculare* can be differentiated from the bacteria by their size and by staining the sample fluid with 1:1 Quink Blue Black ink : 30% KOH (Midgley G., Personal communication, 1976). This method works well because bacteria are not stained and the two *Pityrosporum* species can be differentiated (see pp. 29–30). The authors have modified this procedure for use with detergent and/or lipid present in the sample fluid. The fluid should be shaken with approximately equal volume of ether and after formation of two layers the top ether layer is pipetted off. The remaining ether is evaporated off by incubation at 37°C for 5 minutes. The proportion of stain to sample fluid can be varied to suit the user, but a ratio 5:1 is suitable.

Viable count

In all the methods which are designed for counting microorganisms the sample is dispersed in a fluid usually with a non-ionic detergent such as Triton X 100 or Tween 80. From this fluid serial tenfold dilutions can be prepared in sterile diluent, and from these dilutions volumes inoculated and spread on suitable solid media. Readers are referred to standard microbiology textbooks for various procedures for viable counting (eg Cruickshank *et al* 1975). After the appropriate incubation the separate colonies can be counted, and from the dilution factors the number of colony forming units isolated from the area of skin calculated. A colony forming unit may consist of a single cell or an aggregate.

Analysis of results

Analysis of numbers of microorganisms from a set of individuals usually shows a skewed distribution towards those carrying high numbers of organisms. Therefore, in order to compare numbers of microorganisms in groups of people, say controls and test groups, two types of statistical analysis are useful:

1   Wilcoxon Ranking Method (Wilcoxon 1945).

2   A statistical method such as the 't' test or analysis of variance can be used by logarithmically transforming the counts to give a normal distribution.

Differentiation of microorganisms

Three microorganisms have been implicated in acne. *Propionibacterium acnes, Staphylococci* and *Pityrosporum ovale,* the former probably being the most important. These will be considered in turn.

Propionibacteria

These bacteria are Gram-positive non-motile rods with typical diphtheroid appearance, ie club shaped and in some cases show evidence of rudimentary branching. They are described as anaerobic and have been given the name anaerobic diphtheroids and *Corynebacterium acnes* (Bergey 1975). They are now designated *Propionibacterium* and three species have relevance *P. acnes, P. granulosum* and *P. avidum* the latter being less important. A simple set of tests are given in Table 2.1 to differentiate these species. It should be noted that not all strains fall readily into the groups but this system is very useful (see Cummings & Johnson 1974; Marples & McGinley 1974; Bergey 1975, for more detailed descriptions and comments on classification). There is confusion in the literature over nomenclature and information in Table 2.2 may be useful. *P. avidum* is usually found only in the axilla, whilst *P. granulosum* is found more frequently on the face than the back. *P. acnes* is always found and failure to isolate this bacterium is indicative of a failure in the technique. Puhvel *et al* (1975) using individual normal follicles isolated up to 10^7 cells per follicle and within acne affected follicles the number could be higher. Using other methods 10^7 bacteria per cm^2 of skin for the face and 10 to 100 times lower for the back

Table 2.1 Simplified scheme for the identification of skin *Propionibacteria* species from Marples and McGinley (1974)

Group	Colony colour	Phage sensitivity	Indole production	Casein hydrolysis	Nitrate reduction
P. acnes	Cream	+	+	+	+
P. avidum	Pink	−	−	+	−
P. granulosum	Pink	−	−	−	−

Table 2.2 Nomenclature of the skin anaerobic diphtheroids. There are three main groups

1	*P. acnes*	= *C. acnes*	= *C. acnes* type 1
2	*P. avidum*	= *C. avidum*	= *C. acnes* type 11a
3	*P. granulosum*	= *C. granulosum*	= *C. acnes* type 11b

have been shown (Marples *et al* 1974; Holland *et al* 1976).

Isolation requires incubation at 37°C for 7 days (to differentiate colony type) under anaerobic conditions. An anaerobic jar is preferable. Many routine complex media may be used; Brain Heart Infusion and Reinforced Clostridial Medium have been found satisfactory by the authors. After primary isolation many of the strains may be grown under aerobic conditions provided the medium is heavily inoculated.

Culture of *P. acnes* may lose viability after subculture due to infection with bacterophage which is found in the nose and on the skin. Therefore, care should be used when subculturing these strains. The method for the isolation of the bacterophage used in the differentiation tests is given by Marples and McGinley (1974).

Micrococcaceae

Detailed classification is given in Bergey's Manual (1975) for the Gram-positive cocci. It is common to use the Baird Parker Classification (1974) or the Schleifer and Kloos (1975) and Kloos *et al* (1974) Classification. The former divides the bacteria into *S. aureus* biotypes A–F, *S. epidermidis* biotypes 1–4, *S. saprophyticus* biotypes 1–4 and micrococci. The latter uses 10 species of *Staphylococcus* and 7 species of *Micrococcus*. The International Sub-Committee for Staphylococcus Taxonomy (Hill 1976) recommend a simplified scheme based on the work of the above authors. It can be appreciated that the classification of the staphylococci has yet to be crystallized. The authors use the Scheifer and Kloos (1975) classification employing 9 biochemical tests. All groups of bacteria may be grown on nutrient agar but the authors have found it an advantage to use heated blood agar because this helps differentiation. Other recommended media include trypticase, soya, yeast extract and agar (Marples 1974). It is important to realize that after anaerobic culture for the propionibacteria on Brain Heart Infusion or Reinforced Clostridial Medium staphylococci will also grow. However, since they are in lower numbers and have flat white to yellow colonies compared to the more domed brown to pink colonies of the propionibacteria there should be no confusion.

The most common type of *Staphylococcus* isolated is *S. epidermidis* biotype 1 (Baird-Parker 1974) known as two different species, *S. epidermidis* and *S. hominis* in the Schleifer and Kloos (1975) system. Other staphylococci and micrococci may be isolated but at a much lower frequency.

These bacteria are isolated at 37°C aerobically for 2 days incubation. On the acne sites the numbers are 100 to 1000 less than propionibacteria but there is an indication that their numbers may be higher in the follicles of acne lesions compared to normal follicles (Puhvel *et al* 1975). Work by Roberts (1975) suggests that the numbers are higher on the skin surface of some acne lesions.

Pityrosporum ovale

Two principal species are *P. ovale* and *P. obiculare* and the former is probably considered to be more important in acne (Marples 1974). *P. obiculare* are more spherical in shape compared to *P. ovale,* and also usually have thicker cell walls which can be seen by the ink staining method (see p. 27). *P. ovale* has two main morphological types, one more rod shaped and the other more ovoid. They are Gram-positive and grow on similar media producing a distinct fruity smell resembling aldehyde C_{14} undecalactone (Van Abbe 1964).

Isolation of these organisms for quantitative work is very difficult because they adhere to the stratum corneum and thus low counts are produced. Secondly, no medium seems totally adequate. A synthetic medium (Shifrine & Marr 1963) with asparagine as the nitrogen source and glucose as the carbon source with myristic or palmitic acid will grow stock strains, but is not suitable for primary isolation. A more successful method used by the authors, but not used enough to be recommended yet, is incubation for 7 days at 36°C in 5% CO_2, 95% air on a medium of peptone, glucose and oxbile at pH 6.0 with penicillin present as a bacterial inhibitor. Other workers (Midgley G., Personal communication, 1976) use similar media but include chloramphenicol as a bacterial inhibitor and actidione as an inhibitor for the saprophytic fungi. At present the most satisfactory method is total counting by staining and microscopy (see p. 27).

Gram-negative organisms

Gram-negative rods, in particular *Enterobacter-Klebsiella* and *Proteus* species are occasionally found in patients as a complication of oral and topical antibiotic treatment. The *Enterobacter-Klebsiella* group may produce pustules whereas the *Proteus* species may cause a severe nodular cystic acne during the course of such treatment (Fulton *et al* 1968). These organisms grow well on reinforced clostridial medium and heated blood agar. In cases of acne not responding to treatment therefore, it is important that the clinician asks his laboratory colleagues to culture not just for the propionibacteria and staphylococci but also for these Gram-negative organisms.

In summary, for routine clinical needs, a swab soaked in the appropriate media is a suitable means of sampling but close liaison is required with the bacteriologist because of the difficulties in growing *P. acnes.* For clinical trials the scrub technique of Kligman and Williamson (1965) is adequate. For research needs several techniques are applicable, the sampling technique of Kligman and Williamson (1965) ideally modified, and for specifically sampling the sebaceous duct the techniques of Holland *et al* (1974) and the biopsy technique of Puhvel *et al* (1975) are helpful.

IN VIVO MICROSCOPY OF THE SKIN SURFACE

Dermatologists can still learn a great deal by detailed *in vivo* examination of the skin. The Leitz MZ Microscope is used for this purpose (see Fig. 2.3); it magnifies either 25 or 50 times, is light and compact and has two major advantages (Williams *et al* 1974). It is simple to keep the skin site in focus, the microscope being hand held on the skin and therefore, moving in time with the patient's movements. Secondly, it can be used at any skin site. With this microscope the choice of illumination is important; too bright a light results in excessive glare on the skin. Although a light attachment is available with this microscope this reduces the versatility and the authors recommend a cold fluorescent lamp.

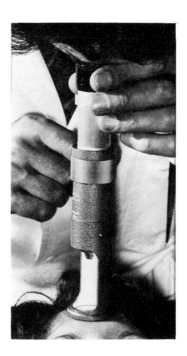

Fig. 2.3 Surface microscope in use.

Although the Leitz MZ Microscope is not ideal for normal skin it gives reasonable visualization in many common dermatoses such as psoriasis, eczema, icthyosis, warts, purpura and haemangiomas.

Normal skin, and in particular the normal looking skin of acne patients, was viewed by stripping the skin twice with 3M sellotape and staining with a lipophilic stain (saturated solution of Oil Red O in equal parts of 70% acetone and alcohol). This technique reduces the surface glare by removing the surface lipid which otherwise is a problem in the seborrhoeic areas.

A graticule can be placed in the eyepiece of the microscope, allowing measurements of the size of scales and pilosebaceous duct orifices. Acceptable photographic results have been obtained by adapting a Leica MDa Body and Leica view finder to the microscope, and by using high speed Ektachrome film ASA 160 with a multiblitz 50E flash gun at a distance of two feet.

SKIN SURFACE SAMPLING TECHNIQUE OF MARKS AND DAWBER (1971)

This method samples the stratum corneum which can then be investigated using the techniques of microbiology, histochemistry, electron microscopy and scanning electron microscopy. The materials required for sampling are:

a Cyanoacrylate gel (Permabond) obtainable from Staident Products Limited, 33 Clarence street, Staines, Middlesex, England.

b Microscope slides.

c Acetone.

The method is as follows:

a Place a drop of cyanoacrylate gel on to the skin.

b Press the slide on to adhesive for 20 seconds.

c Slowly 'peel' the slide off the skin; this is not a painful process.

d The sample can then be processed for the purpose of the study.

e Remove excess gel from the skin with acetone.

It is advisable not to use the adhesive on the face because of danger to the eyes. Whatever analysis is performed on the sample it is never certain as to how much has been left behind. Clearly the force used by the investigator in removing the sample will be a determining factor.

ISOLATION OF SEBACEOUS GLAND (KELLUM'S TECHNIQUE, 1966)

This technique is of value in:

a Assessing drug localization to the sebaceous gland.

b Assessing sebaceous gland lipogenesis (by the *in vitro* incorporation of radioactive tracers such as glucose or amino acids—Cooper *et al* 1976).

c To quantify the number of microorganisms in the pilosebaceous duct (Puhvel *et al* 1975).

The materials and methods are as follows:

a Perform a 0.5 × 1.0 cm biopsy and immerse the skin in 10 ml 2N calcium chloride.

b The time of exposure to 2N calcium chloride depends upon the age and site of the sample and is usually in the order of 2–3 hours at room temperature.

c With fine forceps peel off the stratum corneum and the attached pilosebaceous units.

d Examine the sample on a slide with a dissecting microscope.

e The sebaceous glands and pilosebaceous duct are easily seen and removed with operating scissors for further studies.

CLINICAL ASSESSMENT

The main value of grading is in the clinical evaluation of a new drug but this technique is also of some help in routine clinical assessment.

Overall grading

Several methods of overall grading exist (Pillsbury *et al* 1965; Burton *et al* 1971). A good light is essential, too bright a light blanches some of the smaller spots; a cold fluorescent lamp is recommended. The authors divide the patients into twelve grades of inflammation 0–11; this is a subjective assessment. The scale represents one of increasing severity; zero is a normal skin and grade 11 represents the most severe grade imaginable. Grade 1 is but a few blackheads, usually found around the nose and chin; the subjects with Grade 2 have in addition a few small inflamed lesions. Grades 1 and 2 represent the physiological type of acne seen in the majority of adolescents—the so-called acne minor (Kligman 1974).

Most patients with acne who present to the United Kingdom skin clinics have Grades 3–7. The difficulty of expressing the classification in words is almost selfevident. For example, a patient with fifty small papules may have a far less degree of acne than a patient with only six deep nodules and six succulent papules. The state of activity of the lesion is also important in assessing the overall grade. It is naive to assume that an inflamed lesion looks the same throughout its natural history. A resolving nodule looks less active than one which has reached its peak of inflammation. Even a perfect colour photograph, although of help, cannot accurately reflect the true situation since palpation of the skin is an important part of the overall grading. Despite the apparent difficulties the art of overall grading is one which is easily learned.

Spot counting

Spot counting has many disadvantages but if done correctly is of considerable value. It is better to avoid counting non-inflamed blackheads around the nose and on the chin because of the occurrence of small and insignificant comedones. The following lesions which represent the entire spectrum of acne lesions could be counted.

a Open comedones (blackheads).
b Closed comedones (whiteheads).
c Inflammatory papules.
d Superficial pustules.
e Deep pustules.
f Nodules.
g Cysts.
h Resolving papules, this may represent a papule, superficial pustules, deep pustule or nodule in the resolution phase.
i Macules (usually represent a resolving inflammatory lesion).

However, at times it may be easier and adequate to group the lesions into:
a The non-inflamed lesions, ie blackheads and whiteheads.
b Superficial inflamed lesions, ie papules and pustules.
c Deep inflamed lesions, ie deep pustules, nodules and cysts.

DRUG EVALUATION

In the evaluation of a drug in the treatment of acne, whether it be for research or for trial work, it is advisable to perform two baseline investigations either within a few days of each other or at one month apart; this is to avoid difficulties brought about by the premenstrual flare. Assessment at one, two and three months of treatment should be adequate. If the drug has not produced any effect after three months then it is of no value in acne.

The technique to be used along with clinical assessment would depend on the possible action of the drug. If the drug is aimed at reducing sebum excretion then the methods described on pp. 2–5 are required. Most drugs available at this time reduce the microbial population and so the reader is referred to pp. 22–28. Since a reduction in microorganisms is associated with a reduction in triglycerides and lipolysis, measurement of surface lipid composition as described on pp. 5–15 may also be indicated.

From an analysis of the information above, it can be seen that some of the existing techniques are less than adequate and therefore, more work needs to be instigated to refine these methods and to develop new ones. In this way more reliable data will be generated and hopefully the condition of acne better understood.

REFERENCES

BAIRD-PARKER A. C. (1974) The bases for the present classification of staphylococci and micrococci. *Annals of the New York Academy of Sciences* **236,** 7.

BERGEY'S (1975) *Manual of Determinative Bacteriology,* 8th edn., eds. Buchanan R. E. & Gibbons N. E. Williams & Wilkins Co., Baltimore.

BURTON J. L., CUNLIFFE W. J., STAFFORD I. & SHUSTER S. (1971) The prevalence of acne vulgaris in adolescence. *British Journal of Dermatology* **85,** 119.

COOPER M. F., HAY J. B., McGIBBON D. & SHUSTER S. (1976) *Androgen metabolism and sebaceous activity in clonal acne.* Data presented at the European Society of Dermatological Research, Amsterdam.

CRUICKSHANK R., DUGUID J. P., MARMION B. P. & SWAIN R. H. A. (1975) *Medical Microbiology, II.* Churchill Livingstone, Edinburgh.

CUMMINGS C. S. & JOHNSON J. L. (1974) *Corynebacterium parvum* synonym for *Propionibacterium acnes. Journal of Microbiology* **80,** 433.

CUNLIFFE W. J., PERERA W. D. H., THACKRAY P., WILLIAMS M. & WILLIAMS S. M. (1976) Pilosebaceous duct physiology III—observations on the number and size of pilosebaceous ducts in acne vulgaris. *British Journal of Dermatology* **95,** 153.

EVANS C. A., SMITH W. H., JOHNSON E. A. & GIBLETT E. R. (1950) Bacterial flora of the normal skin. *Journal of Investigative Dermatology* **15,** 305.

FULTON J. E., McGINLEY K., LEYDEN J. & MARPLES R. R. (1968) Gram-negative folliculitis in acne vulgaris. *Archives of Dermatology* **97,** 348.

HILL L. R. (1976) International Committee on Systematic Bacteriology Subcommittee on the Taxonomy of Staphylococci and micrococci. *International Journal of Systematic Bacteriology* **26,** 332.

HOLLAND K. T., ROBERTS C. D., CUNLIFFE W. J. & WILLIAMS M. (1974) A technique for sampling microorganisms from the pilosebaceous ducts. *Journal of Applied Bacteriology* **37,** 289.

HOLLAND K. T., ROBERTS C. D. & CUNLIFFE W. J. (1977) Acne vulgaris: An investigation into the number of anaerobic diphtheroids and members of the Micrococcaceae in normal and acne skin. *British Journal of Dermatology* **96,** 623.

IZUMI A. K., MARPLES R. R. & KLIGMAN A. M. (1970) Bacteriology of acne comedones. *Archives of Dermatology* **102,** 397.

KELLUM R. E. (1966) Isolation of human sebaceous glands. *Archives of Dermatology* **93,** 610.

KLIGMAN A. M. (1974) An overview of acne. *Journal of Investigative Dermatology* **62,** 268.

KLOOS W. E., TORNABENE T. G. & SCHLEIFER K. H. (1974) Isolation and Characterisation of micrococci from Human skin including 2 new species: *Micrococcus lylae* and *Micrococcus kristinae. International Journal of Systematic Bacteriology* **24,** 79.

LEDERBERG J. & LEDERBERG E. M. (1952) Replica plating and indirect selection of bacterial mutants. *Journal of Bacteriology* **63,** 399.

MARKS R. & DAWBER R. P. R. (1971) Skin surface biopsy, an improved technique for the examination of the horny layer. *British Journal of Dermatology* **84,** 117.

MARPLES R. R. & IZUMI A. K. (1970) Bacteriology of pustular acne. *Journal of Investigative Dermatology* **54,** 252.

MARPLES R. R., LEYDEN J. L., STEWART R. N., MILLS O. H. & KLIGMAN A. M. (1974) The skin microflora in acne vulgaris. *Journal of Investigative Dermatology* **62,** 37.

MARPLES R. R. (1974) The microflora of the face and acne lesions. *Journal of Investigative Dermatology* **62,** 326.

MARPLES R. R. & McGINLEY K. J. (1974) *Corynebacterium acnes* and other anaerobic dipththeroids from human skin. *Journal of Medical Microbiology* **7,** 349.

PILLSBURY D. M., SHELLEY W. B. & KLIGMAN A. M. (1965) *Dermatology,* p. 1331. W. B. Saunders, Philadelphia.

PUHVEL S. M., REISNER R. M. & AMIRIAN D. (1975) Quantification of bacteria in isolated pilosebaceous follicles in normal skin. *Journal of Investigative Dermatology* **65,** 525.

REIBEL C., GROSSHAMS E., MINCK R. & BASSET A. (1967) Bacteriologie de la peau saine. *Bulletin Societe Dermatologie Syphiliographie* **74,** 308.

ROBERTS C. D. (1975) *The role of bacteria in acne vulgaris.* PhD Thesis (Leeds).

SCHLEIFER K. H. KLOOS W. E. (1975) Characterisation of staphylococci from Human skin. 1. Amended description of *S. epidermidis* and *S. saprophyticus* and descriptions of 3 new species: *S. cohnii, S. haemolyticus* and *S. xylosus. International Journal of Systematic Bacteriology* **25,** 50.

SHALITA A. R. & ROSENTHAL S. A. (1972) Tetracycline resistant staphylococci in acne vulgaris. *Acta Dermato-Venereologica* **52,** 64.

SHIFRINE M. & MARR A. G. (1963) The requirements of fatty acids by *Pityrosporum ovale. Journal of General Microbiology* **32,** 263.

SMITH M. A. & WATERWORTH P. M. (1961) The bacteriology of acne vulgaris in relation to its treatment with antibiotics. *British Journal of Dermatology* **73,** 152.

STRINGER M. F. & MARPLES R. R. (1976) Ultrasonic methods for sampling human skin microorganisms. *British Journal of Dermatology* **94,** 551.

ULRICH J. A. (1964) Techniques of skin sampling for microbial contaminants. *Health and Laboratory Science* **1,** 133.

UPDERGRAFF D. M. (1964) A cultural method of quantitatively studying the microorganisms in the skin. *Journal of Investigative Dermatology* **43,** 129.

VAN ABBE N. J. (1964) The investigation of dandruff. *Journal of the Society of Cosmetic Chemists* **18,** 629.

VERDON P. E. (1961) Efficiency tests on a series of common skin antiseptics under ward conditions. *Journal of Clinical Pathology* **14,** 91.

WILCOXON F. (1945) Individual comparisons by ranking methods. *Biometric Bulletin* **1,** 80.

WILLIAMS M., CUNLIFFE W. J. & GOULD D. (1974) Pilosebaceous duct physiology. I—Effect of hydration on pilosebaceous duct orifice. *British Journal of Dermatology* **90,** 1.

WILLIAMSON P. & KLIGMAN A. M. (1965) A new method for the quantative investigation of cutaneous bacteria. *Journal of Investigative Dermatology* **45,** 498.

3

Technique of patch tests

C. D. CALNAN

The big four therapeutically unsolved skin problems for the general practitioner or dermatologist are acne, warts, psoriasis and eczema/dermatitis. (A majority of dermatologists now use the words eczema and dermatitis interchangeably, and they will be so used here).

Eczema is best regarded as a pathological change in the skin like cirrhosis or a tuberculoid granuloma. And, like a granuloma, it can be produced by various agents and mechanisms. But the only well studied mechanism is cell-mediated immunity. Hence every case of eczema should be regarded as cell-mediated immunity to a contact allergen until proved otherwise. The appropriate investigation for this purpose is the patch test.

A patch test is not an attempt to reproduce a contact dermatitis in miniature. It is a biological test designed to detect the presence or absence of delayed type hypersensitivity or cell-mediated immunity to a specific contact allergen.

MATERIALS

Allergens

The haptenic allergen is normally available in liquid or solid form, rarely gaseous. Some allergens are suitable for testing undiluted—pure, neat or 'as is'. Many require dilution to a suitable concentration to avoid irritant or false positive reactions. Only pure substances should be used if possible; otherwise the source and degree of purity should be known. They must be made up freshly or kept in a stable state, to avoid oxidation, polymerization, photochemical, molecular or other change, or changes in concentration from evaporation of solvent. They must not react or become contaminated with any part of the container, such as rubber or metal caps. The best form at present is a mixture with yellow soft paraffin (petrolatum), kept in an all-polypropylene syringe, and stored in the dark.

Allergens can be made up as mixtures with substances such as metal salts, rubber chemicals, dyes and groups of medicaments—antihistamines, antibiotics, local anaesthetics, preservatives and so on. When a positive reaction is obtained, each ingredient should be tested separately.

Concentration

The ideal concentration of an allergen is high enough to detect the weakest degree of sensitivity, but low enough to avoid an irritant reaction. With a few allergens this is 100%. With most allergens it varies between 0.01 and 30%, with an average of 1–5%; there is no absolutely correct figure, only one which is found appropriate for the majority of patients. For some it will be too low and for others too high. Hence, one must, on occasion, vary the concentration to decide whether or not a particular patient is allergic to the allergen in question. The usual concentrations and ranges can be found in standard dermatological texts.

It is rarely necessary to use a dilution higher than 20%, for a substance which cannot be applied undiluted. There is evidence that positive reactions may actually diminish with higher concentrations, probably because of the physicochemical state of the material in petrolatum.

Diluents

Petrolatum is the best diluent, because it is the most stable and unreactive. Water and organic solvents will slowly evaporate and alter concentrations, but are often the most readily available. Olive oil, castor oil or liquid paraffin are useful for some allergens but they tend to spread on the skin surface. Suitable organic solvents are methyl ethyl ketone, acetone and ethyl acetate. When they are put on the cellulose patch a few minutes should be allowed for the organic solvent to evaporate before it is applied to the skin.

Containers

All-polypropylene syringes (without a rubber plunger) are best for petrolatum. Glass drop-bottles can be used for liquids, preferably all-glass or with a plastic cap. Fixed quantity delivery bottles have been designed but are more expensive.

Solids

If the suspected allergen is in a solid form it may need to be prepared for testing. Thin materials such as textiles, paper and leaves of plants are applied as a small piece (at least 0.5 cm^2) taking care that each of differing parts of a garment, shoe or other compound article is tested. In general, there is no difference in the allergenicity of petals and leaves of flowers. All timbers should be applied as sawdust, using a water moistened patch to pick up the powder. Other solid objects should be scraped, grated or powdered in the same way as finely as possible, making sure that adequate amounts are used. Thick materials like rubber, leather or plastic should be fragmented into small pieces or very thin slices for application, avoiding sharp spicules which are liable to produce pressure effects.

Extraction of allergens

Some allergens are present in solid materials in very small amounts or firmly bound; for example, the dyes and finishes in textile. In use the allergen is leached out by prolonged contact, heat and sweat on the skin surface. If a test with the material is negative, the allergens may be extracted and concentrated with solvents (water, acetone, alcohol etc).

Patches

Absolutely pure and non-irritant and non-allergenic materials are essential. Suitable patches are the Al-test (Imeco, Astra AB) and Fintchamber. The former consists of a pure cellulose paper disc (diameter 0.5 cm) attached by heat without adhesive to aluminium foil square (1 × 1 cm) and supplied in rolls of 1000 patches. The latter is an aluminium disc with a flange round the edge. It does have a number of advantages.

Many other types of conventional patch with a cellulose or lint disc, cellophane cover and adhesive tape are available in different countries. Potentially reacting substances may be present in these, for example, chromium ions in the cellulose discs, adhesives between the disc and cellophane, and plasticizers in the cellophane.

Various types of cup or container have been used for tests with volatile liquids. They are strapped to a forearm for 24–48 hours. They are like an unspillable ink bottle; the vapour is concentrated and enabled to penetrate the skin. It may be useful for potentially dangerous materials.

Adhesive tape

The function of adhesive tape is not only to keep the tests in place, but also to provide some degree of occlusion, with resultant hydration of the horny layer and, therefore, better penetration. Closed patches are better detectors of sensitivity than open tests for this reason. The more occlusive the tape, however, the greater is the risk of tape reactions. The less occlusive the tape the more sensitivities will be missed, and the more frequently will they fall off. The only present alternative is to find the best compromise between the two disadvantages.

If the patient is known or suspected to be sensitive to colophony-based tape, an acrylic-based or plastic-based tape can be used.

Many varieties of tape are available in different countries. The usual ones are zinc oxide tapes with a colophony resin adhesive. They appear to vary in composition since some produce more reactions than others.

Testing a new substance

One frequently needs to test patients with a substance for which no correct concentration is available in reference books. Its solubility should be tested first in the range of diluents—water, oil or organic solvent. If none is found suitable, petrolatum must be used although this is time consuming for a material which may not be used again. It saves time to make up a range of concentrations: 0.01, 0.1, 1.0, 2, 5, 10, 20%. One may start with 1.0%. If it is positive, apply 0.1 and 0.01%. If it is negative, apply 2 and 5%; if they are negative, apply 10 and 20% and the pure material as an open test. If any of these dilutions are positive, then carry out the procedures for differentiating between allergic and irritant reactions (see p.45).

Compounds and fractions

Sometimes a patch test with a compound material such as a medicament, cosmetic or industrial preparation gives a positive reaction (and satisfies the criteria for evidence of allergy); each of the ingredients are then tested in suitable dilution but none is positive. The whole material must be applied at the same time to confirm that the patient is still reacting to it. Each ingredient must be applied, not necessarily in the concentration used in the material, but in a high enough concentration to detect allergy. The explanation is obscure. An analagous phenomenon is said to occur with reagins. The constituents may interreact with one another to produce an allergen; or there may be a summation effect of two or more allergens, each of which is unable to produce a reaction alone.

Patch test dispenser

The time required for testing patients with standard series of allergens can be shortened considerably by the use of a patch test dispenser, of the type designed by Hjorth *et al* (1970). It consists of racks of five allergen syringes which can be made to deliver at the same time the correct amount of allergen on rows of five patches. They are only suitable for use with the Al-test strip patches.

METHODS

The test procedures for contact allergens are the open and closed patch test, and the intradermal test. Various methods of preparation or prior treatment of the skin, such as washing with soap or cleanser, disinfecting, degreasing, scarification, tape stripping or other minor injury, have been advocated. There is no strong evidence that they are necessary for ordinary clinical testing, and I believe they are contraindicated since they introduce a further variable in assessing results. The only preparation which may be necessary is shaving in very hirsute patients, and I normally use a dry safety razor.

Open patch tests

The degree of sensitivity of open tests is much less than closed tests because of the lesser penetration of allergen. It is normally used:

a As a safety measure when testing a potentially potent dermatitic agent.

b When testing a known irritant which may also be a sensitizer.

c For organic solvents.

d If there is a risk of systemic effects from absorption.

e To confirm allergy to a substance which has given an unexpected positive reaction.

Open tests are normally applied to the flexor surface of the forearm, but the trunk, limbs or head may also be used. The manufacturers of a para-phenylenediamine hair dye recommend a test over the mastoid process, but any site is suitable. Knee and elbow flexures, axillae, groins and sides of the neck should not be used. These areas have a non-specific increased sensitivity and may give false positive results. Similarly a site such as the wrist, which is subjected to repeated trauma from clothing or in other ways should not be used.

The test material is applied over an area of about 1 cm². With fluids or with water, oil or organic solvents if used, care must be taken to ensure that the material does not spread widely. A glass or Perspex ring can be used; avoid pressure on the ring which will concentrate the fluid at the edges. Organic solvents and oils spread readily over a wide area in the surface lipid film and may obscure results. The test surface should be kept horizontal until the solvent has evaporated. A light non-occlusive dressing cover may be applied if necessary. Semisolids may be gently rubbed in. Sometimes more than one application is desirable at intervals to ensure adequate penetration.

Intradermal tests

Most contact allergens which produce a positive patch test will also give a tuberculin type reaction if injected intradermally. Since many of them are not water soluble, and may be locally irritant, it is not normally practical to use intradermal tests. Solutions should be sterile. The usual dose is 0.05 ml and the concentration used is the same or weaker than that used for patch tests. Controls must be done to exclude false positive reactions. Rarely there is a disparity between patch and intradermal tests.

Closed patch tests

The allergen is applied on a patch which is held in position with adhesive tape and the reaction read after 48 hours. The detailed methods used by different physicians may vary greatly from one to another. However, attempts are now being made to standardize them. With a biologic test this is essential if tests are to be compared and evaluated correctly and quantitatively.

Test sites

The areas normally used are the back, the outer upper arm and the thigh; less commonly the flexor aspect of the forearms and abdomen, but almost any area may need to be used. Both the front and back of the trunk are often needed for tests on small children. Since contact allergy is never localized, although claims for its existence have been made in the past, there is no justification for using areas adjacent to or the actual sites of the dermatitis. Comparative studies show that a higher proportion of positives are obtained on the back than on the arms or thighs, and on the extensor aspects rather than the flexor aspects of the limbs. This is almost certainly due to the effect of pressure on the back during sleep.

The presence of eczema, acne, large scars or other gross lesions may make some sites unsuitable, since they interfere with either the adhesion or interpretation of the tests.

Time of testing

The presence or recent presence of eczema may make the whole skin non-specifically hyperreactive—so-called status eczematicus, in which false positive reactions may be obtained. This has been shown in tests with turpentine; 6% of patients without eczema were positive and 20% with eczema were positive. However, this is a very variable phenomenon. Many patients with active eczema may be tested and no false reactions are obtained. And there is a risk at that time of precipitating a widespread flare-up of eczema. For these reasons it is advisable to wait several weeks or more before testing. The possibility of the patient being unreactive in a state of tolerance is very rare.

Time of application

The usual time for tests to be left on is 48 hours, but some physicians use 24 hours only. However, some allergies (eg neomycin) may be missed if 24 hours is used. Longer periods of 3, 4 or 5 days are advocated occasionally but I have no evidence of their advantage. There is no great disadvantage to using 3 days. For many years I have applied patches on Mondays, Wednesdays and Fridays; so that the Friday tests are removed on Mondays—after 3 days.

The application of tests

Each patient is first asked if he or she is allergic or sensitive to plaster (adhesive tape). If the answer is yes, an acrylic-based tape is used. The test sites are inspected to see if they are free of eczema, acne or large scars from burns, trauma or surgery and if they require shaving.

Tests may be applied singly or in vertical or horizontal strips. I now use vertical strips of five tests, arranged in two pairs on each side of the midline. The area over the vertebral column should be avoided. Tests should not be applied too close together, leaving at least 2 cm between each, because of the risk of spread of allergen or of severe reactions from one to another.

The margin of adhesive tape to secure the tests need not be more than 0.5

cm. Cross strips of tape may be applied if necessary, but I rarely need to use them.

Quantity of allergen

Patch tests are normally done to determine whether or not a patient is sensitive to an allergen, but are not quantitative measures. However, if comparisons are to be made and the procedure standardized, the amount of allergen applied should be controlled when possible. Petrolatum mixtures are applied in a strip equal to the diameter of the cellulose disc (1.0 cm). Two drops (0.25 ml) of liquids are used. With powders and grated solid materials it is not possible to give exact quantities, but they should be liberal. With plant leaves, textiles or paper, 0.5 cm^2 is usual.

Skin markers and recording

The precise sites of each patch must be marked and recorded, especially to identify late reactions. Most skin pencils are not indelible enough for the particular conditions and tend to soil the patient's clothes. Two useful markers are dihydroxyacetone (Epstein 1969) and fluorescein (Park 1970). Each test should be recorded with a number and the site of application noted on a body diagram. This is especially necessary for recording very late reactions.

Instructions to patients

The procedure and purpose of the tests should be explained to each patient. After they have been applied the patient is told he will need to return after 2–3 and 4–5 days. He should avoid wetting the test areas. If the patches loosen they may be secured with further application of adhesive tape. If irritation from the patches is too severe, the patient should use his discretion in removing one or more or all of them. This may be because of an excessive reaction either to the adhesive tape or to an allergen. Sometimes, the patient will remove the patches unnecessarily, no reaction being found on examination; he will then need to have them reapplied and be reassured as to the normal sensation of having patches on the skin for 48 hours.

Removal of patches

It is preferable for the patches to be removed by the doctor or nurse/technician, rather than by the patient's relative or friend. The advantage is that the doctor can see which tests, if any, have become lost or misplaced, and note tape reactions or any unexpected findings. Patients are sometimes asked to remove their own tests about 1 hour before seeing the doctor, so that some 'trauma of removal' erythema may subside, and any positive tests will have time to develop to a maximum. The disadvantages of this are that the location of positive reactions may not be correctly recorded, lost patches may not be noted, the patient may wrongly interpret the reactions himself, and he may be unnecessarily alarmed by what he sees before he can be reassured by the doctor.

Provided that excessively hirsute test sites have been shaved, each strip of adhesive tape can be removed by pulling off with minimal discomfort. If necessary an organic solvent such as an ether/methanol mixture or acetone can be used to loosen the adhesive mass. Unabsorbed allergen and adherent remnants of tape are then wiped off with a similar solvent. Solid materials such as pieces of leather, rubber, paper, leaves and so on can readily become misplaced or be lost; it is advisable to check that they are still present on the test patches. The results are then read and recorded. They are often easier to read if the patient can wait up to 30 minutes after removal of the adhesive tape.

Photopatch tests (see also Chapter 6)

An increasing number of allergens are now regarded as potential causes of 'photocontact' dermatitis. Patch tests with them may only be positive after the test site is additionally exposed to ultraviolet light. Examples are sulphonamides, phenothiazine derivatives, halogenated salicylanilides and some related germicidal agents.

The activating wavelengths are always of longer wavelength than the normal sunburn spectrum (290–315 nm), and the quantum of energy required is variable. Ordinary therapeutic ultraviolet lamps are therefore inadequate. A suitable exposure is provided by so-called 'black light' lamps, and the exposure time is normally 30 minutes.

To provide adequate controls the phototest patches should be applied in triplicate. They should all be covered with black cloth in addition to the normal adhesive tape. After 2 days the first row is removed and read; the third row is removed and irradiated and recovered with black cloth; at 4 days, the second and third rows are removed and read.

RESULTS

The first problem is to decide what constitutes a positive result, and then to decide whether or not it is an immunologic reaction. Finally, one may quantitate the degree of sensitivity.

Morphology

A positive reaction does not need to simulate the morphologic appearance or severity of the clinical dermatitis. It may consist of four elements—redness, oedema, papules/vesicles/pustules, and bullae; less frequently, especially in irritant reactions, there is epidermal necrolysis and necrosis with erosions or ulceration. Each of these elements may be present alone or in any combination. Hence the appearance of a positive reaction is extremely variable.

The minimal positive reaction is erythema only, but it is unwise to accept this as a positive reaction unless it is consistent and reproducible and accompanied by even minimal oedema. Oedema or palpable elevation is a most important element of a positive reaction, whether or not papules and vesicles are seen. At the time of removal of patches it may be suppressed by the pressure indentation of the cellulose disc or of a piece of solid material such as leather or rubber. It will usually disappear within 30 minutes of removal.

The presence of papules and pustules alone often represents non-specific irritation reactions of pilosebaceous follicles or sweat duct openings, but they may accompany redness, oedema and vesicles. However, they may be found in allergic reactions. Vesicles may be of varying sizes and few or very numerous. Erythema and oedema is usually, but not always present. Bullae, usually flaccid, may be present alone or surrounded by vesicles with redness and oedema.

Epidermal necrolysis or soap-detergent effect is a macerated, wrinkled, horny layer which is readily detached. It may also be produced by organic solvents such as kerosene and petrol. It is usually followed by desquamation. Erosions and ulcers represent more severe cell damage and necrosis.

A positive patch test, like any area of dermatitis, is a dynamic process and the precise appearance may evolve and change within hours. Hence, examination of the reaction at intervals of an hour or more (which is easier in hospitalized patients) may be valuable.

Many variations may be seen. The positive reaction may spread beyond the cellulose disc or under the tape, or produce a wide red flare. It may be unevenly concentrated at the periphery of the disc, producing an edge effect (Fisher 1973). This happens most frequently with solids and with solvents and is usually an irritant rather than allergic reaction.

Recording

Many different notations have been used. The most usually advocated is that of Urbach and Gottlieb but is probably not so widely used.

+ = erythema only

++ = erythema, oedema and papules

+++ = erythema, oedema, many papules and vesicles

++++ = large confluent blisters

Many physicians use a simple positive (+) and negative (−) recording; others have up to eight or more gradations of positive reaction. This is not justified because the wide range of variables prevent such records being an accurate, reproducible quantitation of the immunologic reaction.

In an attempt to compromise the following is advocated by Wilkinson *et al* (1790):

NT = not tested

− = negative reaction

?+ = doubtful reaction

+ = weak (non-vesicular) reaction

++ = strong (oedematous or vesicular) reaction

+++ = extreme reaction (bullous or erosive)

Every patch should be read and recorded at the time of removal (first reading) and again after a further 2–3 days (second reading). Sometimes the tests will be read again after 7 days or more. The time of the readings should be recorded as the number of days after application as follows:

D1 = 24 hours (especially for phototests)

D2 = 48 hours (most tests)

D3 = 72 hours (usually Friday to Monday)

D4 = 96 hours (most tests)

D5 = 120 hours (48 hours after 72-hour reading)

D7 = 1 week

Allergic and irritant reactions

The chief difficulty in reading the results of patch tests is the differentiation of allergic and non-allergic reactions. In typical results with redness, oedema and vesicles, or with a necrotic erosion it is easy enough. But frequently the results are not typical, especially when testing new or little used substances. Irritants can produce almost identical morphological results to allergens, and so one cannot depend on appearances alone for distinguishing an immunologic reaction from an irritant effect. The distinction depends partly on the view that the allergic state is a sustained and persistent one. The following points will be helpful:

The chemical nature of the test substance, and its known or suspected role as an allergen or irritant. Substances like face powders, articles of clothing, topical medicaments and large polymers do not usually cause irritant reactions. Similarly, substances like mineral oils, metallic oxides, detergents and large polymers are not usually allergenic. An unexpected reaction should always raise one's suspicion and be critically evaluated.

Repetition of tests. The easiest and first procedure is to repeat it, either at once or after an interval. Allergic reactions are almost always reproducible, while irritant reactions are variable—sometimes they simply cannot be reproduced, and one must conclude that the original reaction was a false positive. However, some substances may still on repetition give a positive result, which is not allergic. The problem is illustrated by the following case (Calnan 1957):

A girl, aged 19 with fair skin and blue eyes, had a recurrent dermatitis of the face for 2 years; no previous history of eczema. Her brother had atopic eczema, asthma and hay fever, and her sister had asthma and hay fever. She had used Nivea cream, a face powder and a face cream containing stearic acid and nine other constituents. Patch tests results were:

19.3.1956	Nivea cream	—
	Face cream	++
	Face powder	—
27.4.1956	Stearic acid 100%	++
	Nine other constituents	—

16.7.1956	Stearic acid 100%	+
	Stearic acid 50%	−
	Stearic acid 25%	−
10.9.1956	Stearic acid 100%	−
	Face cream	−

A subsequent usage test was negative, and so it was concluded that the patient had not been allergic to the stearic acid in the face cream.

The effect of dilution. The test substance is taken and diluted further to 50, 10, 5 and 1% of the original and retested. Allergens give a graduated diminishing response, whereas irritants often give an irregular or sharply reduced response (see Table 3.1) (Calnan 1957). This, however, may not be conclusive since some irritants (eg quaternary ammonium compounds) may give such a graduated response.

Table 3.1 Results with varying dilutions of a test substance to differentiate allergens from irritants

Substance concentration (%)	Results		
100	+ + + +	+ + + +	+ + + +
50	+ + +	−	−
10	+ +	−	+
1	+	−	−
	Allergen	Irritant	Irritant

Focal flare-up of dermatitis. Not infrequently a positive patch test will evoke a flare-up of the patient's dermatitis at the sites originally affected. When this occurs, it may be used as evidence that the test substance was the allergen responsible for the original dermatitis. Although this is often a correct conclusion it is not necessarily so; the mechanism can be non-specific and sometimes a focal flare-up of this type can be evoked by a strong irritant test reaction.

Controls. Tests on control subjects are most useful, but they have certain pitfalls. A single control test is not adequate. At least ten should normally be done, and preferably fifty. Weak irritants, which are likely to be the source of most difficulty in differentiating allergic and irritant reactions, may not produce a positive test in more than a small proportion of control subjects (for example, only 1 or 2 out of 10). Eczema patients, when used as controls, will also be more sensitive detectors of irritants than normal healthy and presumably not eczema-prone subjects. Furthermore, when a small number of reactions with such irritants are obtained in controls, they are often not reproducible. For example, if control subjects number 2, 5, 11, 17 and 19 are positive out of 25 tested, on retesting a month later subjects number 5, 9, 14, 19, 21 and 22 may react. This inconsistency is a feature of irritants, when using standard patch test procedures.

False positive reactions

Gross toxic reactions with superficial necrosis, a single large bulla or a wrinkled 'soap' reaction are easily recognized. They usually have relatively little oedema associated with them. The difficulty occurs when a non-immunologic reaction imitates an immunologic one to a greater or lesser extent. Although most of them are found at the 48-hour reading some do not appear until the second or 96-hour reading. The main causes of false positive reactions are:

The patient is in status eczematicus. This is a theoretical state of temporary eczematous hyperreactivity of the skin. It is impossible to define just how active or widespread the eczema has to be to influence a patch test. The variation is enormous, and the 'status' may persist for some time after the eczema has healed. But many patients with extensive eczema are tested and no positive reactions at all obtained, even when maximal concentrations of allergens are used. Furthermore, often only one or a few but not all the tests applied will give a false reaction.

Adjacent to a very strongly positive reaction. Such a strong reaction, whether allergic or toxic, may produce a kind of local status eczematicus, so that one or more tests adjacent to it are also positive. When tested separately at a distant site they are negative.

Severe adhesive tape reactions. It is often difficult to read the results of tests in these circumstances, which probably also create a kind of local status eczematicus. If the tests are repeated with another tape and they are negative, one concludes that the original tests were false. The kind of substances most likely to give false positive reactions in a hyperreactive skin state are those potential irritants tested in maximal or near-irritant concentrations—for example, nickel, chromate, cobalt and mercury salts, formalin and turpentine.

Contamination of a patch with another allergen to which the patient is sensitive. This is most common with plant allergens, such as primula and poison ivy, from finger contact. One may often be able to detect it by the fact that the corner areas of adhesive tape (which have been handled) show the same reaction. It may also occur if excessive amounts of allergen dissolved in organic solvents or oil are applied; they spread easily in the patient's surface lipid film and so may contaminate other patches.

Pressure effects. Solid objects, such as large pieces of wood, metal, plastic or hard rubber exert such pressure under a closed patch that a wide variety of false reactions are produced. They vary from redness only, to oedema, pustules, and large bullae. The reaction is often most prominent around the edges. It is also very localized and does not show a widely spreading redness and oedema. Fisher (1973) has illustrated this well by tests in which a patient's denture is strapped on to the arm.

Artefacts. Rarely a patient may for various motives 'interfere' with his patch tests. The commonest form this takes is for him to complain of itching and grossly excoriate the test sites, claiming that he is allergic to the test material. The absence of localized oedema is often helpful in distinguishing this, but various subterfuges may have to be used to obtain a correct result. We have seen one patient who produced pustular and necrotic reactions at the sites of a medicament and a piece of rubber. The appearances suggested that phenol had been applied by the patient to several sites.

False negative reactions

A false negative patch test should be regarded as important as a false negative Wassermann reaction; the patient is left with his disease undiagnosed.

The main causes are:

Inadequate concentration of allergen. The figures given in standard texts for suitable concentrations are based on extensive experience, but they cannot be comprehensive. While 2.5% of nickel sulphate will detect most cases of nickel sensitivity a small proportion will only react to 5 or even 10%. Concentrations appreciably below 2% will not detect all cases of sensitivity to mercaptobenzthiazole. One per cent may be inadequate concentration for a perfume which is a mixture of a large number of potential allergens.

Inadequate penetration. There are now known to be many examples of inadequate penetration through normal skin by allergens at a concentration which has caused dermatitis. Examples are neomycin, eosin, ethylenediamine and lanolin alcohols. The test concentration may have to be increased more than tenfold.

Solid materials. When an allergen is present in a solid material, a small piece of which is in contact with skin test site, insufficient allergen may diffuse out of the material to produce a reaction. In such cases, the material must be cut, powdered or sliced in order to present a large surface area at the test site.

Failure to leach out. Even after 48 hours contact not enough allergen may be leached out. This occurs especially with articles of clothing, footwear and so on.

Inadequate quantity. For various reasons too little test material may have been applied.

Local sensitivity. All the skin area is potentially reactive in contact dermatitis, but penetration by the allergen is more effective at some sites than others. Because of poor penetration a patch test may be negative on the forearm, but positive on the back.

COMPLICATIONS

The list of possible complications from patch tests is a long one; most are of minor importance, while others are more serious. They are as follows:

1 Exacerbation of the patient's dermatitis.
2 Spread of dermatitis and generalization.
3 Spread of dermatitis from the patch test site.
4 A focal flare-up of a previously patch tested site.
5 Active sensitization.
6 Hyperpigmentation of the site.
7 Hypopigmentation of the site.
8 Ulceration and scarring.
9 Keloid formation.
10 Systemic effects from absorption.

Perhaps the most important is active sensitization. This is the induction of cell mediated immunity by the application of the patch test. It is often indicated by a test site becoming positive 10–14 days after application. It can usually be verified by retesting, in which case a positive reaction is produced at 48 hours.

CONTACT URTICARIA

Although it has long been recognized that low molecular weight allergens can produce type I as well as type IV allergy (of Gell and Coombs), there has been a recent increase in interest in type I reactions, the condition being termed contact urticaria.

Examples of such allergens are paraphenylenediamine, formaldehyde and diethyltoluamide and some systemically administered drugs. The reactions may be separate or combined. A number of food allergens producing IgE antibody in atopic persons can induce contact urticaria followed by dermatitis. This is particularly important in housewives, cooks, chefs and other food preparers. The most frequent are fish allergens.

In such cases a small piece of the suspected food is placed in contact with the skin under a patch and removed after 20 minutes, when an urticarial weal may be observed.

REFERENCES

CALNAN C. D. (1957) Studies in contact dermatitis. *Transactions of the St John's Hospital Dermatological Society* **39,** 20.

EPSTEIN E. (1969) Contact Dermatitis Newsletter p.25.

FISHER A. A. (1973) *Contact Dermatitis.* 2nd edn. Lea & Febiger, Philadelphia.

HJORTH N., TROLLE-HASSEN C. & WILKINSON D. S. (1970) Time-saving patch test antigen dispenser. *Archives of Dermatology* **102,** 300.

PARK R. (1970) Contact Dermatitis Newsletter p.91.

PIRILA V. (1975) Chamber test versus patch tests for epicutaneous testing. *Contact Dermatitis* **1,** 48.

WILKINSON D. S., FREGERT S., MAGNUSSON B., BANDMANN H. J., CALNAN C. D., CRONIN E., HJORTH N., MAIBACH H. J., MALTEN K. E., MENEGHINI C. L. & PIRILA V. (1970) Terminology of contact dermatitis. *Acta Dermato-Venereologica* **50,** 287.

4

In vitro tests of lymphocyte function

R. M. MACKIE

In the past decade several *in vitro* assays of lymphocyte function have been developed and can be used in studies where it is considered important to assess whether or not a normal cell-mediated immune response is present *in vivo*. The exact significance of *in vitro* abnormalities is not always clear in relation to the patient's disease state, and although it is tempting to regard any recorded abnormalities of cell-mediated immunity (CMI) as causative, they may well be the consequence of chronic disease, or indeed incidental findings unrelated to the disease under investigation.

There are, however, two dermatological situations in which the relationship of CMI changes to disease are reasonably clearly defined; in leprosy the work of Turk and his colleagues showed CMI depression in patients with the lepromatous form of the disease, with little detectable immunological abnormality in those with the tuberculoid form (Turk & Bryceson 1971).

Similarly, in chronic muccutaneous candidiasis a variety of *in vitro* tests of CMI have consistently demonstrated specific non-reactivity of the host to candida antigen (Kirkpatrick *et al* 1971).

In many other disease states *in vitro* tests of CMI show depression but the relationship of this to the stage or severity of the disease is not yet so clear. There are reports of CMI abnormalities in systemic lupus erythematosus and mycosis fungoides and by sequential testing of patients it should be possible to relate these observed abnormalities to disease severity (Hughes *et al* 1975; MacKie *et al* 1976).

An important distinction which must be made is that between specific and non-specific depression of CMI. Specific changes are related to only one antigen, generally that considered pathogenetic in the disease process under study, whereas non-specific changes relate to a lack of response to a wide variety of antigenic substances. Even this division is not adequate as in the area of specific CMI depression it may be noted that one or two tests of CMI are consistently negative and others positive. An excellent example of this is the chronic mucocutaneous candidiasis situation, where some patients' lymphocytes consistently fail to produce migration inhibition factor (MIF) on exposure to candida, but undergo brisk lymphocyte transformation. The opposite situation of positive MIF production but negative candida mediated lymphocyte transformation is also recorded, and it would therefore appear that

50

defects in lymphocyte recognition or processing of the antigen may be incomplete.

In the sections which follow describing techniques used in CMI assessment, a selection of tests are described. This is a rapidly changing field and the selection has been based on tests which are currently widely used; it is likely that some of those chosen will be superseded by more sophisticated methodology, and certainly new modifications of each technique are constantly being suggested. The aim therefore is to outline each method in such a way that the basic technique could be established by an isolated investigator with little or no access to academic departments of immunology. Once firmly established, minor modifications can easily be introduced, and regular perusal of such periodicals as the *Journal of Immunological Methods* is recommended.

For investigators who do have access to immunological expertise, close collaboration is strongly advised. Setting up of any of the techniques described can take at least 3 months, and collection of adequate normal control subjects in order to establish a normal range for the test as performed in your own laboratory can be very time-consuming. None of these methods is as yet so well standardized that an established normal range from another laboratory can be accepted in your own investigation. Likewise, no test of this nature is infallible and therefore if a worthwhile study of CMI is to be performed the establishment of at least two and preferably more of these techniques is highly desirable.

It therefore follows that a realistic amount of time must be allowed for a worthwhile study. Most of the methods require incubation of cells overnight or longer and it is suggested that at least 3 or 4 half-days weekly need to be set aside for a study of this kind.

SKIN TESTING

This is currently the only *in vivo* method of assessing CMI. It is a difficult test to standardize completely, and in any situation where repeated tests on the same subject are carried out the possibility of sensitization by skin test substances used must be borne in mind.

Specific skin testing can be directed towards any putative antigen; purified protein derivative of tuberculin, candida antigen and chromium bound to protein are three examples of specific antigens. In such situations, however, the reactivity of the general population is not constant; BCG immunization of infants in the neonatal period in Britain has resulted in a population of children and young adults virtually all of whom are skin test positive, but in older adults this is by no means the case.

The most useful manner, therefore, to use specific skin testing is in a situation where *in vitro* responses to the same antigen are also undergoing study; brisk *in vitro* lymphocyte transformation and MIF production on exposure to candida but a negative candida skin test might suggest some end point failure of antigen recognition, lack of activation of skin reactive factor, or blocking substances in the patient's serum.

Non-specific skin testing can be subdivided into two separate sections; those testing the patient's ability to form a response to a new antigen, and those testing an immunological memory of antigens the patient is likely to have encountered in the past. The problem with this latter group is lack of adequate knowledge of antigenic exposure or definition of a 'normal' response.

Sensitization to a new antigen and subsequent testing is a frequently employed method of screening a group of patients for gross CMI disorder. The substances used most frequently are dinitrochlorobenzene (DNCB) and the closely related substance dinitrofluorobenzene (DNFB), picrylchloride, and keyhole limpet haemocyanin (KLH). All are chosen on the basis of their ability to stimulate a brisk delayed hypersensitivity reaction in 95% of the normal population, and the infrequency with which any are encountered in a normal environment. A positive reaction to a neoantigen of this type is to be anticipated in all but relatively severe states of CMI depression. Ideally a primary irritant such as croton oil should be applied at the same time as the neoantigen challenge to ensure that any negative response is a true failure of development of delayed hypersensitivity and not of the inflammatory response. The choice of neoantigen will depend on local availability. DNCB has been the most widely used, but Turk & Waters (1969) have shown that DNCB sensitization is a relatively weak stimulus of CMI by comparison with picrylchloride in patients with lepromatous leprosy. KLH has more recently become available, and at present high cost and limited availability restrict its use.

The operator handling these neoantigens must take care not to sensitize himself to the substances and gloves should be used invariably.

Methodology: specific and recall antigens

Appropriate antigens (0.1 ml) are injected intradermally into the ventral surface of the forearm. Suitable negative control solutions should be used, and a space of at least 4 cm should be left between the sites of multiple tests. The injected site should be ringed with indelible felt-tipped pen, and the result read at 48 hours. No topical steroid should be applied to the site for 14 days prior to the test, or during its execution.

A positive test is an area of erythema or induration 5 mm or more in diameter.

Suggested battery for 'memory testing' in UK
PPD 1/1000 dilution
Candida (Bencard DHS)
T. Rubrum (Bencard)
Mumps (Eli Lily)
Streptokinase—streptodornase (Lederle) 10 and 2.5 units.
This last substance may give a very strong positive reaction.
DNCB sensitization: Purified DNCB (BDH)
Sentizing dose 2000 µg DNCB in acetone (0.1 ml)

Applied to upper arm. After drying naturally area is covered with vaccination dressing for 24 hours.

Simultaneously apply a challenge dose of DNCB to the opposite arm to allow for the possibility of prior sensitization. An adequate challenge dose is 50 µg DNCB in 0.1 ml acetone. Dry in air, cover, and read at 48 hours.

If the challenge dose at this time is negative, allow a period of at least 14 days to elapse before a further challenge. Careful observation of the sensitization site will often reveal a spontaneous flare at 7–10 days after primary sensitization. This is due to sensitized lymphocytes reacting with minute amounts of allergen remaining in the skin. The second challenge dose is again 50 µg DNCB in 0.1 ml acetone and is also read at 48 hours. A positive reaction is indicated by erythema and induration of 5 mm or more, but frequently a much stronger reaction with frank vesiculation is seen. Keeping the challenge dose to 50 µg should, however, prevent gross ulceration which has been reported in the past with higher challenge doses.

If it is considered necessary to test the integrity of the inflammatory response simultaneously 0.04 ml of a 10% croton oil solution should be applied to the forearm, allowed to dry, covered and read at 48 hours. A positive result is an area of vesicles, sometimes with additional pustules, of 10 mm in diameter or more. This can be a painful process and should not be undertaken lightly.

LYMPHOCYTE TRANSFORMATION

This method of assessing lymphocyte function dates from the report of Nowell (1960); an extract of the kidney bean, phytohaemagglutinin (PHA) when added to cultures of human peripheral blood resulted in the appearance within these cultures of large blast-like cells. This report was rapidly confirmed and the blast-like cells were identified as small lymphocytes.

Other plant lectins were then found to have similar non-specific stimulant qualities when incubated with cultured lymphocytes; pokeweed mitogen (PWM) and concanavalin A (con A) are two additional widely used stimulants, although PHA remains the most commonly used (Hirschorn 1965).

Following the identification of subpopulations of lymphocytes, analysis of the effects of non-specific mitogens on these subgroups suggested that PHA was primarily a T lymphocyte stimulant, that PWM stimulated both B lymphocytes and a subpopulation of T cells, and that con A stimulated predominantly a subpopulation of T lymphocytes (Janossy & Greaves 1971).

In PHA mediated lymphocyte transformation the majority of T lymphocytes are involved and it may therefore be used as a guide to T cell population in the assessment of immune deficiency states, or during therapeutic immunosuppression.

Following on the observations of non-specific lymphocyte stimulation by mitogens or activators were the reports from Hirschhorn *et al* (1963) and Pearmain *et al* (1963) that lymphocytes from individuals showing positive *in vivo* skin tests to tuberculin were stimulated *in vitro* the addition of tuberculin to cultures, but that this phenomenon was not observed in cultures from skin test negative individuals. This phenomenon of specific antigen mediated lymphocyte stimulation is seen with a variety of antigens, but there are significant differences between specific and non-specific lymphocyte stimulation, as in the former situation the majority of T lymphocytes are involved, whereas in the latter only the minute proportion of the T lymphocyte population which is sensitized to the antigen in question will be stimulated, although there may be some recruitment of non-sensitized cells. Antigen-mediated lymphocyte stimulation is therefore a slower process and a longer period of culture is required, usually 120 hours by comparison with 72 hours for PHA stimulated cultures. At the end of this period the cultures should be examined morphologically for the presence of blast-like cells and the degree of stimulation quantitated by measuring the incorporation of labelled thymidine into newly synthesized DNA.

Method for lymphocyte transformation test
Lymphocyte separation

For this a Ficoll-Triosil gradient is used. The specific gravity of the Ficoll-Triosil mixture should lie between 1.076 and 1.078. A 9% Ficoll solution in distilled water, and a 34% Triosil mixture are prepared separately. They are combined as required in the ratio of 2.4 volumes of Ficoll to one of Triosil. Both solutions should be freshly prepared weekly and stored at 4°C. Freshly drawn venous blood is treated with preservative-free heparin (20 units/ml blood), and is layered over the Ficoll Hypaque mixture. Three volumes of FH mixture are required for each two volumes of blood.

This mixture is spun at 400 *g* for 30 minutes. After this period of time the lymphocyte-rich layer will be seen to lie below the heparinized plasma, and can be removed by pipette.

The lymphocytes are then washed twice in Eagle's Minimal Essential Medium (MEM) with glutamine, penicillin and streptomycin (10 minutes each at 400 *g*).

Establishment of lymphocyte cultures

The lymphocyte count must be checked and the concentration adjusted to 5×10^5 lymphocytes/ml. A smear should also be made for morphological assessment of lymphocyte purity. The lymphocytes are resuspended in Eagle's MEM with additional 10% of heat inactivated fetal calf serum and 2% Hepes buffer (if obtainable pooled AB serum should be used in place of fetal calf serum).

Lymphocyte suspension (1 ml) is placed in each culture tube. All tubes should be set up in triplicate. Appropriate quantities of chosen mitogens or antigens are added to each culture tube. If adequate numbers of lymphocytes can be obtained, at least three concentrations of each mitogen or antigen should be used so that a dose-response curve can be obtained.

The tubes are incubated at 37°C in an atmosphere of 5–10% CO_2 for 48 hours. One tube is used at this stage for slide preparation for morphological confirmation of the presence of blast cells.

Labelling and harvesting

After C^{14} thymidine is added (50 μl containing 0.1 μCi in 0.1 ml) with a micrometer syringe, the tubes should be left for 4 hours for labelling to take place. The content of each tube is then drained on to a filter disc, and placed over a vacuum extractor. The disc is flooded with 10% trichloracetic acid in water, and the procedure is repeated using alcohol. The discs are dried in an oven (56°C), and then each disc is placed in a counting vial and 5 ml of a suitable scintillation fluid is added before counting in a scintillation-counter for 10 minutes.

The following should always be included:

1   Lymphocytes with no mitogen or label to give the background count.
2   Lymphocytes with label but no mitogen to give the spontaneous count.

Results are commonly expressed as counts/minute/10^6 lymphocytes. It should be remembered to correct the results for the lymphocyte percentage purity of the cultured population.

MACROPHAGE MIGRATION INHIBITION AND LEUCOCYTE MIGRATION INHIBITION

These two tests utilize the properties of a lymphokine, one of the members of a soluble dialysable group of substances produced by interaction of lymphocyte and antigen. The lymphokine in question is migration inhibition factor (MIF), and its use as an *in vitro* measure of delayed hypersensitivity was first advocated by George and Vaughan (1962). The original observation on which

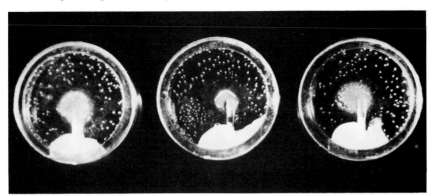

Fig. 4.1   Microculture chambers showing in the outer two chambers control lymphocytes with no inhibition of migration. In the central well, however, antigen has been added and migration inhibition has taken place. The area migrated by the leucocytes is therefore seen to be very much less than the control areas.

their system was based came from Rich and Lewis (1932) who noted that explants of spleens and lymph nodes from tuberculin sensitive animals grew out poorly in the presence of tuberculin, whereas those from animals not previously sensitized to tuberculin grew out very much better.

The original *in vitro* test, macrophage migration inhibition, was based on collection from guinea pigs of peritoneal exudate cells induced by oil injection. Of these cells, 70% had the morphological appearance of macrophages. These peritoneal exudate cells were then packed into capillary tubes open at one end and allowed to migrate from this end into surrounding media containing PPD. Migration covered a relatively large fan-shaped area when the exudate cells were from guinea pigs skin test negative to PPD, but a very much less extensive area when the peritoneal exudate was obtained from PPD positive animals (see Fig. 4.1).

This basic model was then developed by David, who reported that if peritoneal exudate cells from non-sensitized animals were admixed in the capillary tube with lymphocytes from a sensitized subject, inhibition of migration into medium containing the appropriate antigen still took place (David *et al* 1964).

This test is still in use, but collection of guinea pig macrophages can be a tedious and messy task, and therefore an adaptation of the technique using human peripheral blood leucocytes as the migrating cell population was developed by Bendixen and Søborg (1969); this method utilizes the same principle of packing cells into capillary tubes and measuring migration of these cells into tissue culture medium with and without added antigen but only human leucocytes are used with no admixed animal cells. Good correlation between inhibition of migration, presumed also to be the consequence of MIF production, and skin test reactivity was reported in the case of brucella antigen, but a less clear-cut situation obtained when PPD was used as antigen. Since the original report, however, satisfactory use of the test as a measure of delayed hypersensitivity has been reported in many test systems using as antigen tuberculin (Clausen & Søborg 1969; Federlin *et al* 1971), transplantation antigens (Falk *et al* 1970), tumour associated antigens (Andersen *et al* 1970; MacKie *et al* 1972) and chromium (Thulin & Zachariae 1972).

The advantages of the test are that it is relatively simple and reproducible, requiring no expensive equipment. However, it must be borne in mind that there are situations where MIF production does not parallel activity in the lymphocyte transformation system and therefore results should be interpreted with caution. Many modifications of the system exist, and the following details are those of the original methods, with brief details appended of some of the modifications.

Macrophage migration inhibition

Sterile liquid paraffin (20–30 ml) is injected intraperitoneally into guinea pigs. After 72 hours the animals are sacrificed and the peritoneal cavity irrigated with Hank's balanced salt solution (pH 7.2). The cell yield from this procedure is very variable, and can be most disappointing, but the predominant cell type should be the macrophage, and this can be confirmed by phase contrast microscopy; the oil droplets in the macrophage cytoplasm will be clearly visualized. The yield from several guinea pigs will probably be required and is washed two or three times in Hank's medium by centrifugation at 400 *g* for 10 minutes. The resulting cell pellet is then resuspended in twenty volumes of Eagle's MEM.

A cell count and check of cell viability by trypan blue exclusion should be made at this stage. A further wash by centrifugation at 250–300 *g* for 3 minutes is carried out, and the cells resuspended in Eagle's MEM with additional inactivated serum; a concentration of 10–15% is usual, and in this system normal heat inactivated guinea pig serum is suitable.

The cell suspension is then drawn into capillary tubes with dimensions of 1.0–1.2 mm internal diameter and length 7–10 cm. These are stoppered with inert clay at the lower end and placed in a test tube. Centrifuge at 500 *g* for 5 minutes, when a cell button will have formed adjacent to the clay stopper. Cut the glass tube at the cell–medium interface, and place the button in a disposable tissue culture planchette, holding it in place by fixing the closed end in a mount of silicone grease.

The planchette is then filled with Eagle's MEM to which appropriate concentrations of the test antigen are added, closed with a coverslip and incubated at 37°C in air. In all tests planchettes should be prepared containing MEM but no antigen and various concentrations of antigen must be used to allow for preparation of a dose response curve. At least four planchettes should be prepared for each antigen concentration.

After 3–6 hours fanwise migration of the cells from the open end of the tube will be observed. In a positive test this will be minimal or absent, but in the control tubes with no antigen this may cover a considerable area.

The test is read at 18–24 hours. The areas migrated by the macrophages are projected on to a camera lucida and outlined. This is then quantitated either by weighing the area of paper covered by the migration, or by using a planimeter to measure this area in arbitrary units.

The area migrated by the cells in the presence of antigen is compared with the area migrated without antigen, and thus the migration index (MI) is obtained. Migration indices of 0.80 or less are considered indicative of a positive test.

Occasionally enhancement rather than inhibition of migration in the presence of antigen is observed. The significance of enhanced migration is not clearly established but Bendixen has observed this phenomenon in situations where very weak sensitization to brucella antigen was present (Bendixen & Søborg 1969).

Macrophage migration inhibition using human lymphocytes

Human peripheral blood is treated with preservative-free heparin (20 units heparin/ml blood).

Lymphocytes are then separated as described above (see p.34) and the lymphocyte-rich population suspended in Eagle's MEM with 10% heat inactivated fetal calf serum to give a cell concentration of 5×10^5 cells/ml. Antigen is added to the culture tubes in the appropriate concentrations and the cells cultured for 48 hours at 37°C in an atmosphere of 5% CO_2.

The supernatant from these tubes is then added to the tissue culture planchettes in which capillary tubes containing guinea pig macrophages have been placed.

In a positive test, MIF will be present in the supernatant and therefore migration inhibition will be observed.

Incubation time, measurement of area and calculation of results are as described above (see p.57).

Leucocyte migration inhibition

This test utilizes only human blood with no involvement of guinea pig macrophages. It is therefore simpler to perform and results are available within 24 hours of venepuncture. The classic Bendixen and Søborg technique is described in detail below, but useful variations include those of MacKie *et al* (1972) involving preincubation of the leucocyte population with antigen before packing cells into the capillary tubes, and that of Clausen and Søborg (1969) involving migration of the leucocyte population under an agarose gel.

Classic method (Bendixen & Søborg 1969)

Freshly drawn human peripheral blood is heparinized (20 units preservative-free heparin/ml blood) and is allowed to sediment naturally at 37°C for 1–2 hours. The leucocyte-rich suspension is then withdrawn from the red cells and centrifuged at 400 *g* for 10 minutes. The resultant cell pellet is then washed twice in phosphate-buffered saline pH 7.4 (200 *g* for 10 minutes).

The cells are then resuspended to give a concentration of 10^8 cells/ml in Eagle's MEM with 10% heat inactivated serum added. This suspension is then drawn into capillary tubes, sealed at one end with clay and spun at 50 *g* for 5 minutes. The tubes are then cut at the cell–fluid interface, and the method from this point is as for macrophage migration (see p.57).

MEASUREMENT OF ROSETTE FORMING LYMPHOCYTES

This method, currently widely used, is one used to distinguish between T lymphocytes of thymic origin and B lymphocytes derived from a non-thymic site, as yet unidentified in the human. T lymphocytes possess the unique property of spontaneously forming rosettes (E rosettes), with unsensitized washed sheep red blood cells. The precise nature of the receptor sites involved in this reaction has not been clearly defined, but it is a useful and simple method of counting T lymphocytes.

It is, however, a method where minor differences in technique can change the numbers of rosetting cells, and it is therefore essential to stick consistently to one method and to establish a control range for your laboratory by this method.

By contrast, B lymphocytes have a variety of cell surface receptors not identified on T lymphocytes. Their property of synthesizing and excreting specific antibody can be utilized as, by the use of fluorescein-conjugated antisera, B lymphocytes can be identified by membrane immunofluorescence. A receptor for the Fc component of immunoglobulin is also present on the surface of the B lymphocyte; macrophages also possess this Fc receptor and therefore macrophage contamination of a lymphocyte population will influence results obtained by utilization of this receptor. A third method of enumerating B lymphocytes is to utilize the surface receptor specific for complement components; sheep red cells coated with an antisheep-cell antibody plus complement are prepared to form an Erthrocyte-Antibody-Complement (EAC) and the lymphocytes in a given population forming EAC rosettes using this technique taken as B lymphocytes. Once again macrophage contamination will influence results.

This field of immunological technique is undergoing rapid expansion and at present methods of pretreating lymphocytes with neuraminidase and other enzymes to reveal other receptor sites on the lymphocyte and surface are being developed. Hopefully this will allow further subclassification of lymphocytes but for current technical information on these modifications the reader is referred to the journals dealing with this topic.

E rosette method for T lymphocytes

Lymphocytes are separated from heparinized blood as described in the section on lymphocyte transformation. They are suspended in Eagle's MEM at a concentration of 4×10^6 lymphocytes/ml; 0.25 ml aliquots of this suspension are then mixed with 0.25 ml of a 1% solution of fresh sheep red cells and allowed to stand for 15–20 minutes at 37°C. They are then pelleted and incubated for a further 24 hours at 4°C; at this temperature rosetting capacity of the lymphocytes is maximal. The cells are then gently resuspended and the number of lymphocytes forming rosettes counted. Three or more sheep red cells adherent to a lymphocyte are considered a 'rosette', and a minimum of 400 lymphocytes should be counted. A haemocytometer is used for rosette counting.

EAC method for B lymphocytes

Lymphocytes are separated as previously described. Rabbit antisheep erythrocyte antibodies are prepared by immunizing rabbits with boiled sheep erythrocyte stroma. High affinity antibodies will be obtained and can be separated by gel filtration on Sephadex G 200 columns into IgM and IgG fractions. The concentration of antibody used to treat sheep erythrocytes is chosen to produce maximum haemolysis in the presence of guinea pig complement at 37°C.

Then 0.25 ml aliquots of lymphocyte suspension (4×10^6/ml) are admixed with 0.25 ml of a 1% solution of sheep erythrocytes freshly coated with rabbit antisheep erythrocyte haemolysin and a source of complement. Normal human plasma is the most commonly used source. After 15–20 minutes incubation at 37°C the number of rosette-forming lymphocytes (three or more adherent erythrocytes) are counted using a haemocytometer. Again, a total of 400 lymphocytes should be counted.

LYMPHOCYTE CYTOTOXICITY

This test is based on the early studies of Medawar on allograft rejection and tumour immunity. Significant manifestations of both these events are target cell destruction and this can be passively transferred with lymphocytes but not with serum. Since these initial studies much work has been devoted to elucidating the exact mechanism of cell destruction in this situation and at the present time several methods have been proved to be active and several others are considered theoretically possible. Four established methods of action are firstly, cytotoxicity of sensitized lymphocytes for target cells bearing membrane-associated antigen, secondly, sensitization of lymphocytes by non-specific antigens or mitogens to exert cytotoxicity on target cells unrelated to the stimulating antigen or mitogen, thirdly, the induction of normal lymphoid cells to cause destruction of target cells in the presence of specific antitarget cell antibodies, and fourthly, lysis of target cells coated with complement components by normal lymphocytes.

It is apparent, therefore, that this is a complex system and there are situations where specific cytotoxicity may be measured and also situations where non-specific killing of target cells may occur. This problem makes building up of an adequate control series extremely difficult as lymphocytes from healthy donors may exert unexpected non-specific cytotoxicity on the target cells. Sequential studies on lymphocytes from a healthy individual may also show considerable variation in cytotoxicity, and minor viral infection may temporarily increase target cell killing.

Measurement of target cell death may be morphological by making cell counts. This is the simplest variation but does not identify cells which have been rendered incapable of division. Isotope incorporation is also used and ^{51}Cr is widely employed; this binds to cell membranes and is released into the surrounding culture medium with membrane disruption; some spontaneous release from normal healthy membranes will also take place.

After ^{3}H-labelled proline has been incubated with target cells, its release into the medium is taken as indicating cell destruction, but this method presupposes actual cell dissolution which may not always accompany cell death. The incorporation of ^{125}I-labelled iododeoxuridine into nuclear DNA of target cells is also used, and allows large number of samples to be used although it clearly cannot allow differentiation between a few active cells and a larger number of less rapidly metabolizing cells.

An alternative method of utilizing this technique is to add serum to the target cell-lymphocyte system to assess the ability of the serum to block a cytotoxic interaction. There are several situations in tumour immunology where serum has been found capable of this activity and it is currently considered that in different stages of tumour growth this serum blocking factor may be either free antigen or antibody or antigen-antibody complexes.

The most difficult problem in this group of methods at the present time is the distinguishing of specific from non-specific cytotoxicity, and until cell separation studies clearly establish the cells responsible for killing in different situations it is a method which can yield results which are at times difficult to interpret.

Microcytotoxicity method

Target cells for this assay can be from fresh tissue or from established culture lines. They should be prepared to give an individual cell suspension of $10^4–10^5$ cells/ml, and suspended in tissue culture medium (Eagle's MEM) with the addition of 10–20% heat inactivated serum. Fetal calf serum is frequently used.

Disposable microtest tissue culture plates are used (see Fig. 4.2). One hundred target cells (10 µl of suspension) should be delivered into each well using a dispensing syringe (Eppendorf type). The plates are then placed in an

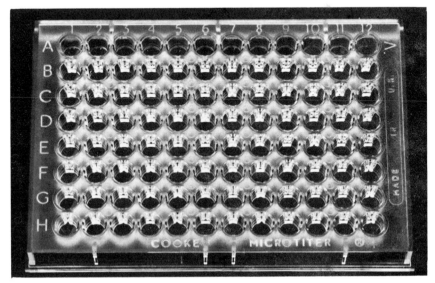

Fig. 4.2 A microcytotoxicity plate showing the multiple wells for seeding of target cells and subsequent addition of chosen lymphocytes.

atmosphere of 5% CO_2 at 37°C for 24 hours to permit adhesion of target cells. After this time invert the plate to remove non-adherent cells, and refill the wells with medium and additional serum. Check the cell count in a small number of wells so that the appropriate ratio of effector to target cells can be calculated. This ratio can be adjusted for the system under study. A realistic figure would be 50 or 100 lymphocytes per target cell but some workers use higher ratios up to 200 or even 1000 lymphocytes per target cell, and others reduce this ratio as low as 20 lymphocytes per target cell. Adequate numbers of wells must be used in each situation to allow statistical evaluation of results and for this at least twelve wells must be prepared for each lymphocyte concentration. In addition, at least twelve wells must have no additional lymphocytes added to the target cells.

The plates are reincubated at 37°C in 5% CO_2 for a further 48 hours, and then gently rinsed in medium, fixed in alcohol and stained with Giemsa's stain. The number of target cells remaining in each well are now counted and the percentage cytotoxicity calculated as follows:

Mean number of target cells after incubation in medium alone or with control lymphocytes.	—	Mean number of target cells after incubation with test lymphocytes.

$$\frac{}{\text{Mean number of target cells after incubation in medium alone or with control lymphocytes.}}$$

A problem with this method is that in the wells with test lymphocytes some target cell death may be due to exhaustion of medium by the larger number of cells, and therefore a further series of wells with control lymphocytes in the same numbers as test lymphocytes should ideally be used. However, the problem already discussed of non-specific cytotoxicity of supposedly normal control lymphocytes may make the target cell killing in these wells as great as, or in extreme cases, even greater than the test situations (de Vries & Rumke 1973).

The other control which should if possible be used is control target cells of histogenetically similar type to the test target cells. Thus if fibroblasts in patients with systemic sclerosis are under study, normal fibroblast target cells from a healthy donor should also be used in this situation.

If the system is used to assay the ability of serum to block a cytotoxic interaction, a suitable ratio of lymphocytes to target cells should first be established by adding varying numbers of lymphocytes to the plates, and thereafter the ratio kept constant while the volume of serum added to the test wells is varied.

^{51}Cr release assay

If the chosen target cells are a cell line, they are treated with Trypsin EDTA solution to give a cell suspension. These cells are washed in phosphatebuffered saline and 10^6 cells labelled by incubation with 150 μCi Na_2 ^{51}Cr O_4

(Amersham) for 30 minutes at 37°C. The cells are then washed three times and suspended in Eagle's MEM with 10% heat inactivated fetal calf serum. The final concentration should be 10^5 cells/ml.

Aliquots of 10^4 cells (0.1 ml) are prepared in quadruplicate in test tubes and the appropriate number of aggressor lymphocytes added (5×10^5 for a ratio of fifty lymphocytes per target cell). If quantities permit, a dose response curve should be established. Incubate the tubes for 8 hours at 37°C in 5% CO_2. The radioactive output in each tube is then measured in a scintillation-counter and the results expressed as per cent specific ^{51}CR release. As in the microcytotoxicity test, control lymphocytes should be used against test target cells and control target cells against test lymphocytes (Brunner 1968).

Residual ^3H proline method

Target cells are labelled in proline free Eagle's MEM for 24 hours with 50 µCi ^3H proline (500 mCi/mmol) per 2.5 ml volume of cells containing 10^7 cells.

After this time the cells are washed and 5000 cells per well delivered to a microtiter plate; after 24 hours to allow cell adherence, the medium is changed and the appropriate number of lymphocytes delivered to each plate. The plates should be incubated at 37°C in 5% CO_2 for 48 hours.

The lymphocytes and target cells are then harvested using a dispensing pipette (Eppendorf type). Adherent residual target cells are harvested after the addition of 0.25% trypsin to the wells. Each well is then washed twice with phosphate-buffered saline.

The cell suspensions are then filtered on Millipore glass filters. A Millipore Sampling Manifold will simplify this. They are then precipitated in the filter with 5% trichloracetate, the filter disc dried, and counted in counting fluid in a scintillation-counter.

Results are expressed as:

$$\frac{(\text{counts per minute medium control} - \text{counts per minute test sample}) \times 100}{\text{counts per minute medium control}}$$

Each cell concentration should be prepared in quadruplicate and for every situation a similar number of control wells should be prepared (Bean *et al* 1973).

^{125}I iododeoxuridine incorporation into nuclear DNA

After the suspension of 10^6 chosen target cells in 5 ml Eagle's MEM they are placed in tissue culture flasks containing 100 µCi ^{125}I I-DU and incubated for 24 hours in 5% CO_2 at 37°C. Of these labelled target cells 10^3 are then delivered to each well of a microtest plate and incubated for a further 24 hours at 37°C in 5% CO_2 to allow adherence of cells. The medium in each well is then changed and appropriate numbers of test lymphocytes added to the wells. As in the other methods, some wells should contain target cells with no additional lymphocytes and some, if possible, target cells and control lymphocytes. After a further 18–24 hours incubation the plates are washed twice, aspirated dry and sprayed with plastic film. Individual wells are then separated from the plate with a band saw and residual radioactivity measured in a gamma counter for 4 minutes. A minimum of six test wells should be used for each situation.

Percentage cytotoxicity is assessd as in the previous methods (Fritze *et al* 1974).

THE MIXED LYMPHOCYTE REACTION

This test is used to identify antigenic differences between two lymphocyte populations. In the past it has most frequently been used for identifying major histocompatibility differences, in humans the HLA system. It can also be used for sequential studies in individuals with progressive diseases, such as malignancy or connective tissue disorders. If lymphocytes are taken from the patient at regular intervals and stored in a suitable system they can be used to identify changing antigenic recognition throughout the disease.

The usual method of performing this test is as a unidirectional test in which one lymphocyte population is treated with Mitomycin C to render it incapable of DNA synthesis, without affecting its antigenic properties. The two populations are then incubated together and DNA synthesis stimulated in the untreated population by the presence of the treated lymphocytes is measured by C^{14} or H^3 uptake.

Method

Lymphocytes are separated from freshly drawn heparinized blood as described under lymphocyte transformation. Alternatively, the blood can be defibrinated by agitation in a flat-bottomed flask containing glass beads. Once defibrination is complete the blood is mixed with 3% gelatine in the ratio of one part gelatine to three parts blood in a measuring cylinder and allowed to sediment for 1 hour at 37°C. The supernatant will then contain most of the lymphocytes with a few admixed red cells and granulocytes; this supernatant is washed twice and suspended in Eagle's MEM. Cell viability is checked by trypan blue exclusion and the concentration adjusted to 10^6 trypan blue unstained cells/ml medium containing 10% heat inactivated human AB serum.

Mitomycin C (50 µg) is then added to 2×10^6 lymphocytes (2 ml) of the population to be inactivated. After incubation at 37°C for 30 minutes they are centrifuged (200 *g*) and washed twice in medium. The concentration is then again adjusted to 10^6 lymphocytes/ml and 0.1 ml of each of the two lymphocyte preparations is added to the culture tube; this therefore contains 10^5 lymphocytes from each population.

Various combinations should be used:

Combination	Reason
1 R + Dm	Stimulation of responder by donor.
2 R + Rm	Non-specific activity of R.
3 Rm + Dm	Efficiency of inhibition by Mitomycin C.
4 R + PHA	Ability of responding cells to react.

R = Responding population.

Rm = Responding population treated with Mitomycin C.

D = Donor population used as stimulant to R.

Dm = Donor population treated with Mitomycin C.

All tubes should be prepared in quadruplicate. Incubation of the cultures then takes place at 37°C in 5% CO_2. Cultures 1 to 3 should be maintained for 5–7 days but culture 4 should be assayed at 3 days.

Four hours before termination of culture 0.1 µCi of ^{14}C thymidine in 0.1 ml (specific activity 25 µCi/µg) is added to the culture tubes. Thereafter harvesting is as described above (see p.55).

REFERENCES

ANDERSEN V., BJERRUM O., BENDIXEN G., SCHIODT T. & DISSING I. (1970) Effect of autologous mammary tumour extracts on humans leukocyte migration *in vitro*. *International Journal of Cancer* **5**, 357.

BEAN M. A., PEES H., ROSEN G. & OETTGEN H. F. (1973) Prelabelling target cells with $\frac{3}{8}$H proline as a method for studying lymphocyte cytotoxicity. *National Institute of Cancer—Monograph* **37**, 41.

BENDIXEN G. & SØBORG M. (1969) A leucocyte migration technique for *in vitro* detection of cellular (delayed types) hypersensitivity in man. *Danish Medical Bulletin* **16**, 1–6.

BRUNNER K. T. (1968) Quantitative assay of the lytic action of immune lymphoid cells on ^{51}Cr-labelled allogenic target cells *in vitro*. Inhibition by isoantibody and drugs. *Immunology* **14**, 181–196.

CLAUSEN J. E. & SØBORG M. (1969) *In vitro* detection of tuberculin hypersensitivity in man. *Acta Medica Scandinavica* **186**, 227.

DAVID J. R., AL ASKARI S., LAWRENCE H. S. & THOMAS L. (1964) Delayed hypersensitivity *in vivo*. The specificity of inhibition of cell migration by antigens. *Journal of Immunology* **93**, 264–273, 274–392, 393–402.

DE VRIES J. E. & RUMKE P. H. (1973) Immunological studies in melanoma patients treated with BCG. *British Journal of Cancer* **28**, suppl. 1, 97–102.

FALK R. E., THORSEY E., MOLLER E. & MOLLER G. (1970) *In vitro* assay of cell-mediated immunity. The inhibition of migration of sensitized human lymphocytes by HL-A antigens. *Clinical Experimental Immunology* **6**, 445.

FEDERLIN K., MAINI R. N., RUSSELL A. S. & DUMONDE D. C. (1971) A micromethod for peripheral leucocyte migration in tuberculin sensitivity. *Journal of Clinical Pathology* **24**, 533.

FRITZE D., KERN D. H. & PILCH Y. H. (1974) Quantitation of cytoxic antitumour antibody *in vitro*; a microassay using ^{175}I Iododeoxuridine as a tumour cell label. *Journal of the National Institute of Cancer* **53**, 1403.

GEORGE M. & VAUGHAN G. H. (1962) *In vitro* migration as a model for delayed hypersensitivity. *Proceedings of the Society of Experimental Biological Medicine* **11**, 2.

HIRSCHORN K., BACH F., KOLODNY R. L., FIRSCHEIM I. L. & HASHAM N. (1963) Immune response and mitosis of human peripheral blood lymphocytes *in vitro*. *Science* **142**, 1185.

HIRSCHORN K. (1965) The mitogenic effect of different substances in tissue culture. *Series Haematologica* **9**, 26.

HUGHES P., HOLT S. & ROWELL N. R. (1975) The modifying effect of autologous serum on leucocyte migration inhibition by liver antigens in SLE. *British Journal of Dermatology* **92**, 401–406.

JANOSSY G. & GREAVES M. F. (1971) Response of T & B lymphocytes to phytomitgens. *Clinical Experimental Immunology* **9**, 483–495.

KIRKPATRICK C. H., RICH R. R. & BENNETT J. E. (1971) Chronic mucutaneous candidiasis. Model building in cellular immunity. *Annals of Internal Medicine* **74**, 955–978.

MACKIE R. M., SPILG W. G. S., THOMAS C. E. & COCHRAN A. J. (1972) Cell-mediated immunity in patients with malignant melanoma. *British Journal of Dermatology* **87**, 523.

MACKIE R. M., DE SOUSA M., SLESS F. R. & COCHRAN R. (1976) Lymphocyte abnormalities in mycosis fungoides. *British Journal of Dermatology* **94**, 173–178.

NOWELL P. C. (1960) PHA: An initiator of mitosis in cultures of normal human lymphocytes. *Cancer Research* **20**, 562–564.

PEERMAIN G., LYCETTE R. R. & FITZGERALD P. H. (1963) Tuberculin induced mitosis in peripheral blood leucocytes. *Lancet* **i**, 637–638.

RICH A. & LEWIS M. (1932) The nature of allergy in tuberculosis as revealed by tissue culture studies. *Bulletin of Johns Hopkins Hospital* **50**, 115.

THULIN H. & ZACHARIAE H. (1972) The leucocyte migration test in chromium hypersensitivity. *Journal of Investigative Dermatology* **58**, 55.

TURK J. L. & WATERS M. F. R. (1969) Cell-mediated immunity in patients with leprosy. *Lancet* **ii**, 243.

TURK J. L. & BRYCESON A. D. M. (1971) Immunological phenomena in leprosy and related disorders. *Advances in Immunology* **13**, 209–266.

5

Detection of immune complexes

J. J. CREAM

In 1958 Dixon *et al* described an experimental animal model in which complexes of antigen and antibody formed in the blood, deposited in the vessels and gave rise to tissue damage. The immunopathological hallmarks of this type of disorder were established as an acute reaction in which could be found deposits of antigen, antibody, complement and fibrin, and evidence of activation of the serum complement sequence at a time when immune complexes could be demonstrated in the circulation. Since then many studies have shown that immune complexes are important in the pathogenesis of disease in man, but one problem has been the lack of simple methods for their detection. In the last few years more and more techniques have become available and the principal ones will be reviewed here.

DETECTION OF IMMUNE COMPLEXES IN TISSUES

In experimental immune complex disease, where the nature of the antigen and antibody are known, the use of radio-labelled antigen enables the site of deposition to be precisely determined, and this method is eminently suitable for quantitation.

For biopsies from man, labelled antisera can be used to detect the components of complexes. The most commonly employed labels are the fluorescent dyes—fluorescein isothiocyanate, rhodamine isothiocyanate and Lissamine rhodamine sulphonyl chloride. The degree of non-specific staining and the sensitivity depend on the type of fluorescent illumination employed. (Wilson & Dixon 1974; Johnson & Holborow 1973; Nairn 1969). An alternative label that can be used with an ordinary light microscope is the enzyme horseradish peroxidase, the site of its deposition being revealed by a coloured reaction product. (Andres *et al* 1973). For even greater resolution in the electron microscope, antisera can be labelled with electron dense materials. These include ferritin and the enzymes—peroxidase and cytochrome C—which can be rendered electron dense by subsequent histochemical reactions. (Andres *et al* 1973).

No matter what the method or equipment used, the final result will depend on the specifity of the antisera and many commercial antisera have proved unsatisfactory. The specifity of the antiserum can be shown by absorption with specific antigen or blocking with unlabelled antibody. Even where there is no doubt about the specificity of the antiserum the possibility of cross-reactions with other antigens has to be borne in mind. In grossly inflamed tissues it may not be easy to distinguish immune complex deposits from exuded serum protein. Antisera against albumin, transferrin and α_2-macroglobulin, proteins that do not take part in immune complex reactions, may help in interpretation. In the case of the strongly membrane bound complement component C3, specifically fixed C3 resists elution with 2 M NaCl (Lachmann 1973).

Negative results with immunohistochemical techniques are not necessarily significant. It has been shown that indubitable immune complex nephritis can occur without deposits demonstrable by immunofluorescence and this appears to be due to the fact that the deposits may be redissolved in the presence of excess antigen. (Germuth *et al* 1975). The components of complexes are cleared from the skin within 24–48 hours (Cream *et al* 1971) and so the timing of the biopsy is important. Suction (Copeman 1975) or injection of histamine (Braverman & Yen 1975) can be used to induce purpura as and where required, thus allowing the biopsy to be taken at a precise time. Negative results may also be obtained because the binding sites on the protein being sought are covered, and here elution prior to immunohistochemical staining may be revealing.

Deposits of antigen and antibody in the skin have been detected by these methods in various vasculitides (Parish 1971), immune complex cryoglobulinaemic vasculitis (Cream 1971) and meningococcal septicaemia (Greenwood *et al* 1973).

DETECTION OF IMMUNE COMPLEXES IN THE BLOOD

The methods can be divided into two groups—direct, in which the immune complexes can be concentrated or separated and visually identified and the indirect, in which the evidence for the presence of immune complexes is circumstantial.

Direct methods

Electron microscopy

Negative staining with phosphotungstic acid allows visualization of immune complexes on a grid, but a background of low molecular weight protein, such as is present in serum, interferes. However, the technique is applicable where the complexed material possesses a distinctive structure and is present in high titre in the serum. Hepatitis B antigen fulfils both these criteria since it has a distinctive morphology and can be present in titres as high as 10^{13} particles/ml (Almeida 1976). The relative concentrations of antigen and antibody can be ascertained by this technique (Almeida & Waterson 1969).

Precipitation techniques

Certain immune complexes can be precipitated out of solution by cooling, the first component of complement—Clq, rheumatoid factors or antiglobulins and polyethylene glycol.

The advantages of these methods are their simplicity and low cost, and, most importantly, they allow isolation of complexes for analysis of their components.

Precipitation by cooling—cryoglobulins. Two types of cryoglobulin occur in human sera—single component monoclonal immunoglobulins—as in myeloma, Waldenström's macroglobulinaemia or benign essential cryoglobulinaemia, and mixed component cryoglobulins consisting of at least two different immunoglobulins. One of the simplest ways of detecting certain antigen-antibody reactions, *in vitro,* is by precipitation. The amount of precipitate is often increased by cooling, so that the presence of mixed component cryoprecipitates in human sera aroused interest in the possibility that these were immune complexes. This has been confirmed by identification of antigen and antibody in cryoprecipitates (Cream 1976a). However, coprecipitation, that is non-specific, non-immune precipitation of two substances together can occur in the cold, giving rise, for example, to lipoprotein-immunoglobulin complexes (Linscott & Kane 1975). Thus, ideally, before concluding that a mixed cryoprecipitate is an immune complex, it is desirable to show that the antigen combining site on the antibody molecule—the Fab portion—is taking part in the reaction. Usually, insufficient antibody is obtained for this final proof, but in the case of IgG-IgM cryoglobulins it has been possible to show that the Fab portion of the IgM is reacting with its IgG antigen (Grey & Kohler 1973).

The demonstration of cryoglobulins is essentially a simple procedure. However, cryoglobulins may (a) precipitate rapidly at room temperature and be lost with the red cells, (b) only be present in small amounts, (c) remain suspended as floccules and be inapparent in a lipaemic serum and (d) not precipitate until 3 or 4 days have elapsed. Precautions are, therefore, necessary if cryoglobulinaemia is not to be missed. A quantitative method has been described in detail elsewhere (Cream 1972). Loss of a rapidly precipitating cryoglobulin can be prevented by using prewarmed syringes and collecting the blood in a 37°C hot room. Alternatively, a thermos flask containing water at 37°C can be used to transport blood between patient and laboratory. A warm centrifuge should be used to spin off the cells, or the blood can be allowed to stand at 37°C until the serum separates. The serum should be stored at 4°C for a minimum of 4 days. After centrifugation at 4°C, any precipitate is washed in large volumes of phosphate-buffered saline and redissolved in a suitable solvent, prior to estimation of total protein and immunoelectrophoresis or immunodiffusion. Increased turbidity of the serum with clearing in the warm does not necessarily indicate the presence of a cryoglobuli   and immunological identification of an immunoglobulin is essential. Phosphate-buffered saline is usually adequate to redissolve the precipitate, but other solvents have been assessed by Weisman and Zvaifler (1975). They obtained satisfactory results with twice normal (0.3 M) saline for solubilization followed by the addition of an equal volume of distilled water.

Small amounts of cryoglobulins may be found in normal sera, so that before the significance of cryoglobulinaemia can be assessed, the upper limit of normal should be established for each laboratory. In one study this was 80 μg/ml blood (Cream 1972). R. Penny (Personal communication 1975) noted a similar value—120 μg/ml.

Immune complex cryoglobulins have been detected in several disorders, notably infections, SLE, rheumatoid arthritis, renal diseases and tumours, although often, no cause is apparent (Cream 1976b). In a few instances, in patients with renal disease, it has been possible to identify the offending antigen in the circulating complexes. (McIntosh *et al* 1975; Ozawa *et al* 1975). In SLE, many autoantibodies are produced but it does not necessarily follow that they are all pathogenic. However, specific concentration of certain polynucleotide antibodies in the cryoprecipitates has been demonstrated and this provides information about which antigen-antibody systems are giving rise to circulating complexes (Winfield *et al* 1975). Identification of the antigen is not merely an academic exercise since one possible form of immunotherapy is administration of antigen (Soothill & Steward 1971; Wilson & Dixon 1971).

Clq precipitation. Clq—a subunit of C1, the first component of the complement sequence—is known to precipitate soluble immune complexes. It can be prepared from normal serum by precipitation with DNA (Agnello *et al* 1970) or, with better results, precipitation at low ionic strength in the presence of chelating agents (Yonemasu & Stroud 1971).

The precipitation reaction between Clq and the test sera is most conveniently demonstrated by diffusion in agarose (Agnello *et al* 1970). However, the test should only be regarded as a screening procedure, since Clq will precipitate materials other than immune complexes including aggregated γ-globulin, DNA, meningococcal group A polysaccharides and endotoxin lipopolysaccharides (Agnello *et al* 1971). Clq can be used in solution when the precipitates may be separated and analysed. Non-specifically aggregated γ-globulin precipitates both in solution and agarose and cannot be distinguished from immune complexes, but polyanions, such as DNA, can be differentiated since they are resistant to reduction and alkylation unlike γ-globulins.

In spite of these snags, Clq has been of value to screen for possible complexes in SLE (Agnello *et al* 1971) leprosy (Moran *et al* 1972; Rojas-Espinosa *et al* 1972) dermatitis herpetiformis (Mowbray *et al* 1973) and allergic vasculitis (Asghar *et al* 1975).

Precipitation by rheumatoid factors. Rheumatoid factors are antiglobulin antibodies that react with IgG. The specificities of rheumatoid factors vary but reactions are most readily demonstrated with altered IgG. Winchester *et al* (1971) noted that certain monoclonal rheumatoid factors would precipitate small complexes or aggregates of IgG either in free solution or agar. The choice of a suitable rheumatoid factor reagent involves screening for one that does not react with normal serum and the best reagents are likely to be found amongst patients with a lymphoproliferative disease giving rise to an IgM rheumatoid factor that does not form a cryoprecipitate. (Winchester & Agnello 1976). In general, these monoclonal rheumatoid factors show a greater tendency to react with complexes than do polyclonal rheumatoid factors isolated from sera of rheumatoid arthritis patients. Winchester *et al* (1971) found that monoclonal rheumatoid factors precipitated low molecular weight complexes, whereas Clq precipitated larger complexes and aggregates.

The technique can be carried out in agar gel or in free solution using microprecipitation curves for quantitation. Like the Clq test, large numbers of sera can be screened but non-specific IgG aggregates will give false positives.

Isolated monoclonal rheumatoid factor obtained from a single subject has the disadvantage that it must be regarded as a unique biological reagent and the type of complex precipitated will depend on the specificity of the rheumatoid factor. Clq can be prepared from blood of several subjects and problems of peculiar specificity therefore do not arise.

Precipitation by polyethylene glycol. Polyethylene glycol (PEG) (molecular weight 6000) is a water soluble polymer that precipitates plasma proteins according to their molecular size. Thus PEG in serum at a concentration of less than 5% leads to precipitation of high molecular weight proteins including macromolecular aggregates such as immune complexes. However, small amounts of monomeric IgG, IgM and other macromolecules are also precipitated and the amount of monomeric IgG precipitated is related to the total serum IgG concentration. The amount of protein precipitated cannot, therefore, be used to indicate the serum level of complexes, but the method does allow the complexes to be removed from the serum and concentrated prior to their further separation.

Analytical ultracentrifugation

High speed, ultracentrifugation of serum results in separation of the proteins according to their molecular weight. During the ultracentrifugal run the position and size of the various protein components can be recorded by optical methods and the presence of complexed material is indicated by protein peaks additional to those found in normal serum. The approximate molecular weight, and, therefore the possible constituents of the complexes, can be determined.

In rheumatoid arthritis, such studies have shown the presence of 22S IGG-IgM complexes in which IgM is the antiglobulin rheumatoid factor. IgG antiglobulins also occur and give rise to IgG-IgG complexes intermediate in size between 10S and 13S, sedimenting between the 7S IgG and 19S IgM peaks. These intermediate complexes appear to be characteristic of benign hyper-gammaglobulinaemic purpura of Waldenström (Kyle *et al* 1971; Capra *et al*

1971), but such complexes are not invariably associated with purpura in that they be symptomless, or, rarely, give rise to a hyperviscosity syndrome (Jasin *et al* 1970; Blaylock *et al* 1974). Hypergammaglobulinaemia and a positive latex test in a patient with vasculitis would indicate the need for analytical ultracentrifugation. An analytical ultracentrifuge is, however, costly and not usually readily accessible. The sensitivity is low, although with the newer machines and methods as little as 2% of aggregates can be detected (Stanworth & Johns 1976).

Preparative ultracentrifugation of serum on density gradients followed by fractionation and scanning for protein peaks is an alternative method that can be employed. Although it does permit isolation of the complexes, it is slow and only suitable for one sample at a time.

Column chromatography. Similar objections apply to this method limiting its use to the occasional serum. Isolation of the complexes is however possible. (Jasin *et al* 1970).

Binding of complexes by lymphoblastoid cells

The Raji cell, derived from a patient with Burkitt's lymphoma, is a lymphoblastoid cell with B cell characteristics. On its surface it has receptors for IgG and the activated complement components C3b and C3d. Theofilopoulos *et al* (1974) have developed a test in which the Raji cell is incubated with the serum and then the possible components of complexes are detected on the cell surface by immunofluorescent microscopy. Rabbit or mouse IgG attach to the cells only when complexed or aggregated, but human IgG will bind even in its unaggregated 7S form. When testing human sera it is, therefore, first necessary to block the IgG binding sites on the cell with normal serum, leaving exposed the sites for C3b and C3d. As a result, with human sera, the test will only detect complement-fixing complexes. The technique is very sensitive—as little as 200–300 ng aggregated human globulin or immune complexes per ml of serum can be detected. In experimental serum sickness, where the antigen is known, it has been possible, using fluorescent-labelled antibody, to demonstrate antigen on the surface of the Raji cell. Thus, the method is potentially of great value, since it may allow identification of antigen in complexes. The type of complex most readily bound by the Raji cell is one formed in moderate antigen excess.

Indirect methods

In contrast with the direct methods in which the complexes can be isolated or visualized the indirect tests provide, at best, only circumstantial evidence for the presence of circulating immune complexes.

Changes in serum complement

Many antibody molecules are capable of fixing complement when they aggregate or form antigen-antibody complexes. Thus, activation of the serum complement cascade provides evidence for a circulating immune complex pathogenesis. Such activation is indicated by a fall in total complement or complement component levels in the blood, or by the appearance of complement breakdown products. Activation may take place via two pathways—the classical, involving C1, C2 and C4, or the alternative, which utilizes properdin and factors A and B. Both pathways converge on C3, conversion of which from inactive to active form subsequently gives rise to labile complement components with various pathological properties. The classical pathway can be activated by complement-fixing subclasses of immunoglobulins—IgG1, IgG3 and most IgM molecules. Aggregates of various classes of immunoglobulin that fail to activate the classical pathway, IgA and IgG4, can activate the alternative pathway. However, complement activation is not a reliable indicator for the presence of immune complexes since as well as non-immune aggregates of immunoglobulin, some highly charged polyanions, DNA, polyinosinic acid and bacterial endotoxins will fix complement (Lachmann 1975).

Complement assays. It is possible to measure total haemolytic activity, CH_{50}, and functional assays are available for all the components of the classical pathway and for some of those of the alternative pathway. Specific antisera can now be prepared for many components, allowing quantitative assays to be simply performed by single radial immunodiffusion. Complement levels in serum depend on rates of production and breakdown, so that complement utilization may not be reflected by low levels if production is increased, and here turnover studies with radio-labelled C3 and C4 may be helpful.

Complement conversion. Activation of the complement pathway leads to the appearance of altered C3 (βIA) which can be distinguished from the unaltered form (βIC) because it has a different electrophoretic mobility. Qualitative (Soothill 1967) and quantitative assay methods (Versey *et al* 1973) are available. The altered form is also antigenic and elicits the production of an autoantibody—immunoconglutinin—which can be detected by its ability to aggregate complement-coated erythrocytes (Lachmann 1967).

Macromolecular binding of C3. The molecular weight of C3 is 200 000. The presence of C3 in serum fractions of much higher molecular weight could be interpreted as evidence that the serum contains circulating complexes to which complement has bound. The method has, however, been little used since it involves the slow process of column chromatography and false positive results would be given by non-specific complement-fixing aggregates (Soothill & Hendrickse 1967).

Binding methods of C1

Complement-fixing complexes present in serum will bind added C1—the first component of complement—and several techniques utilize this affinity for C1 as the basis for the detection of complexes.

Anticomplementary activity. If C1 is added to a serum containing complement-fixing complexes the C1 will bind to the complexes and no longer be available to a complement-requiring indicator system. A convenient system is provided by red cells coated with antibody and lysis will only occur in the presence of free C1.

In many circulating immune complex disorders C1, present in the blood, probably saturates the C1 binding sites on the complex. Where the blood level of C1 is markedly depressed, as for example in SLE, C1 binding sites will remain exposed, but in other conditions with more normal levels of C1, the extrinsic C1 added in the test will not bind to the immune complexes unless the patient's own C1 is destroyed by heating. This produces an additional complication in that heat aggregated γ-globulin fixes complement. Johnson *et al* (1975) have gone into these problems and recommended preliminary heating of serum for 60 minutes at 56°C in borosilicate glass bottles, with careful standardization of the method for baseline anticomplementary activity in normal sera. Anticomplementary activity increases with storage unless a −70°C deep freeze is used. The method is very sensitive and Johnson and Mowbray (1976) report that it will detect complexes in either antigen or antibody excess, but that IgM containing complexes are less well detected than those containing IgG.

The method has been used to screen for complexes in patients with cutaneous vasculitis, urticaria, nephritis and gluten-enteropathy (Cream 1973; Johnson *et al* 1975). In dermatitis herpetiformis, Mowbray *et al* (1973) were able to show, after fractionation of the serum by column chromatography, that the anticomplementary activity resided in fractions containing molecules between 8S and 10S—the size of IgG complexes.

125I-C1q binding test. Again, this test measures the ability of complexes to bind C1. An advantageous modification of the previous test is that the patient's C1 is removed from the binding sites on the complexes not by heating but by incubation with EDTA, calcium ions being required for C1 binding.

In a second step ^{125}I-C1q and 2.5% polyethylene glycol are added. Free C1q remains in solution whilst C1q bound to macromolecular complexes is precipitated by polyethylene glycol and the amount of radioactivity in the precipitate indicates the C1 binding activity in the serum.

In SLE, Zubler and Lambert (1976) have reported that 90% of patients had increased binding activity in the serum which correlated with disease activity anti-DNA antibody levels and depression of complement.

C1q binding in a solid phase radioassay. In this test C1q is immobilized on the surface of a plastic tube. Patient's serum is added to the tube and complement-fixing complexes are bound to the C1q. After washing, bound immunoglobulin can be measured by adding radio-labelled anti-IgG. (Hay *et al* 1976).

Inhibition of rheumatoid factor binding for altered immunoglobulin

The reaction between rheumatoid factor and altered IgG can be inhibited by immune complexes.

Two tests have been developed on this principle. Cambiaso *et al* (1976) have described an automated technique in which they used latex particles coated with human IgG and counted the agglutinated particles in an automatic platelet counter. They could detect down to 1 µg/ml of aggregated IgG but noted that all fresh normal sera gave positive results. This agglutinating activity in normals disappeared after 24 hours storage. Cowdery *et al* (1975) allowed IgM rheumatoid factor to bind to ^{125}I-labelled heat aggregated IgG and precipitated the IgM rheumatoid factor-IgG complex with anti-IgM. After centrifugation the amount of precipitate can be determined from the radioactivity in the sediment. The presence of immune complexes in a test serum prevents binding of the rheumatoid factor to the labelled aggregated IgG and results in lower radioactivity in the sediment. This test is very sensitive—it will detect 125 ng of immune complexes.

Both aggregated IgG and rheumatoid factor will interfere with these tests and the type of complex detected will depend on the specificity of the rheumatoid factor reagent. The one used by Cowdery *et al* (1975) reacted best with complexes in which antigen and antibody were present in near equivalent amounts.

Cell binding methods

Macrophages, platelets and certain lymphocytes may have receptors for immunoglobulins and complement on their surfaces and various tests have been devised to measure either binding of immune complexes or inhibition of binding of aggregated IgG immune complexes.

Radiobioassay for immune complexes using macrophages. Guinea pig peritoneal macrophages will take up aggregated human IgG and immune complexes. Thus, if radio-labelled aggregated IgG is added at the same time as the test serum, the inhibition of binding of radio-labelled aggregated IgG to the macrophages indicates the presence of immune complexes or aggregated IgG in the test serum (Mohammed *et al* 1976).

Inhibition of complement dependent lymphocyte rosette formation. A subpopulation of human B lymphocytes—the complement receptor lymphocytes —have on their surfaces receptors for activated C3. Such receptor sites can be demonstrated by adding red cells coated with antibody and complement when rosettes of the coated red cells form around the lymphocytes. Activated complement components C3b and C3d in the test solution will inhibit rosette formation. (Eden *et al* 1973). Sera from patients with Crohn's disease, lepromatous leprosy, mesangiocapillary glomerulonephritis, steroid-sensitive nephrotic syndrome, Henoch-Schönlein nephritis and acute poststreptococcal nephritis also inhibit rosette formation and this has been taken to indicate the presence of activated complement (Ezer & Hayward 1974; Smith *et al* 1975). The exact nature of the inhibiting factor is at present uncertain. However, there is evidence that it may be of high molecular weight, is heat stable and is not simply an antilymphocyte antibody (Hayward *et al* 1976). A major snag of this test is that it requires fresh human adenoid tissue.

K cell inhibition. When IgG aggregates or binds to free antigen or antigenic sites on a cell surface it undergoes an alteration in its molecular conformation.

Cytotoxic lymphocytes, or K cells, possess on their surfaces receptors for altered IgG, and will lyse cells coated with IgG antibody. Immune complexes containing IgG or altered IgG present in the suspension will compete for the receptor sites on the K cells and inhibit lysis of the target cell. MacLennan (1972) has developed a test in which a polyploid line of liver cells—Chang cells—are labelled with ^{51}Cr. When antiChang antibody and cytotoxic lymphocytes are added lysis occurs with release of ^{51}Cr. The presence of immune complexes or altered IgG blocks the receptors on the lymphocytes so that they do not combine with the antibody on the liver cell. As a result, lysis of the liver cell does not occur and there is no release of the radio-label. Jewell and MacLennan (1973) have noted inhibitory activity in the sera from patients with ulcerative colitis and Crohn's disease and have obtained evidence that the inhibiting factor is in serum fractions containing high molecular weight IgG. There is some evidence that this IgG is in the form of complexes rather than aggregated IgG. This test will only detect IgG containing complexes or aggregates, and sera that contain anti-K cell antibody will give false positive results.

Platelet aggregation test. A platelet aggregation technique for the detection of immune complexes has been developed by Myllyä (1973). It has proved to be a demanding test in that the platelets are prepared by repeated centrifugation of large amounts of fresh blood, and must be used within 2 days.

False positives results are given by aggregated γ-globulin and antiplatelet antibodies. The complexes that cause aggregation are those that sediment at approximately 19S and smaller complexes and complexes containing IgM cannot be detected (Penttinen 1976).

Most of these tests based on cellular reactions are elaborate and time-consuming. The results obtained will depend on the source of the cells, and therefore be subject to variation with consequent difficulties in standardization and interpretation. This is most evident in the case of the platelet aggregation test which many workers have found difficult technically as well as demanding in that it requires large volumes of fresh human donor blood. The source and possible variation of the cells are also potential problems in the lymphocyte rosette inhibition test which uses human adenoid tissue. Guinea pig peritoneal macrophages can be produced as required, but more satisfactory are cultured cells—such as the Chang liver cell—which can be assumed to be fairly uniform in their reactivities. All these cellular techniques will give false positive results because they will detect aggregated immunoglobulins as well as immune complexes, and antibodies directed against the cells will interfere. The Raji cell binding method was not dealt with in this section because the nature of the bound material can be identified on immunofluorescent microscopy and the Raji cell can be regarded as a means of concentrating complexes prior to their identification.

Table 5.1 summarizes the tests that have been used to detect circulating immune complexes and indicates their virtues or lack of them. At present a plethora of tests is becoming available, so much so that a new worker in this field is faced with a perplexing array. The World Health Organisation has

Table 5.1 Methods for detecting circulating complexes

Method	Type of complexes detected	False positive	Sensitivity	Isolation of complexes	Cost	Suitable for large numbers of samples
Direct						
Electron microscopy	—	—	low	yes	high	yes
Precipitation by cold	cold precipitating	coprecipitates	low	yes	low	yes
Precipitation by C1q	C1 binding	AGG and polyanions	—	yes	low	yes
Precipitation by rheumatoid factor	—	AGG	low	yes	low	yes
Analytical ultracentrifuge	—	AGG	low	*	high	no
Column chromatography	—	AGG	low	yes	low	no
Raji cell binding	—	AGG	high	yes	low	yes
Indirect						
Complement assays	complement activating	AGG	low	no	low	yes
Complement conversion β1C → β1A	complement activating	AGG and other C activators	low	no	low	yes
Immunoconglutinin	complement activating	} AGG and other C activators	low	no	low	yes
Macromolecular binding of C3	complement activating	AGG	—	no	low	no
C1 binding						
anticomplementary	C1 binding	AGG	high	no	low	yes
125I-C1q/PEG	C1 binding	AGG	high	no	low	yes
Solid phase radioassay	C1 binding	AGG	—	no	low	yes
Rheumatoid factor inhibition	—	AGG	high	no	low	yes
Cell binding						
Macrophage	—	AGG	high	no	low	yes
Lymphocyte rosette inhibition	C activating	AGG other C activators, and antilymphocyte antibody	—	no	low	yes
K cell inhibition	IgG only	AGG anti-K cell antibody	—	no	low	yes
Platelets	19S complexes not IgM	AGG antiplatelet antibody	high	no	low	yes

AGG = aggregated γ-globulin.   * = use preparative ultracentrifuge.

started a comparative interlaboratory study, but until the results are available it would seem advisable to use only those tests which are reliable and whose interpretation is straightforward. Since no single test will, as yet, detect all types of complex it is desirable, when screening for circulating complexes, to employ several methods and choice should be made firstly from the direct methods—electron microscopy, precipitation techniques, analytical ultracentrifugation and Raji cell binding, and secondly from the indirect methods—complement assays and C1 binding methods—in particular anticomplementary activity. The cellular techniques, with the exception of the Raji cell binding method, present many problems.

REFERENCES

ALMEIDA J. D. (1976) Electron microscopic observations on immune complexes. *Annals of Rheumatic Diseases* Vol. 36. (Supplement) Page 2.

ALMEIDA J. D. & WATERSON A. P. (1969) Immune complexes in hepatitis. *Lancet* ii, 983.

AGNELLO V., WINCHESTER R. J. & KUNKEL H. G. (1970) Precipitin reactions of the C1q component of complement with aggregated γ-globulin and immune complexes in gel diffusion. *Immunology* **19**, 909.

AGNELLO V., KOFFLER D., EISENBERG J. W., WINCHESTER R. J. & KUNKEL H. G. (1971) C1q precipitins in the sera of patients with systemic lupus erythematosus and other hypocomplementemic states: characterization of high and low molecular weight types. *Journal of Experimental Medicine* **134**, 228.

ANDRES G. A., HSU K. G. & SEEGAL B. C. (1973) Immunological techniques for the identification of antigens or antibodies by electron microscopy. In *Handbook of Experimental Immunology,* 2nd edn., vol. 2, ed. Weir D. M., p.341. Blackwell, Oxford.

ASGHER S. S., FABER W. R. & CORMANE R. H. (1975) C1q precipitin in the sera of patients with allergic vasculitis (Gougerot-Ruiter syndrome). *Journal of Investigative Dermatology* **64**, 113.

BLAYLOCK W. M., WALLER M. & NORMANSELL D. E. (1974) Sjögren's syndrome: Hyperviscosity and intermediate complexes. *Annals of Internal Medicine* **80**, 27.

BRAVERMAN I. M. & YEN A. (1975) Demonstration of immune complexes in spontaneous and histamine-induced lesions, and in normal skin of patients with leukocytoclastic angiitis. *Journal of Investigative Dermatology* **64**, 105.

CAPRA J. D., WINCHESTER R. J. & KUNKEL H. G. (1971) Hypergammaglobulinemic purpura. Studies on the unusual anti-γ-globulins characteristic of the sera of those patients. *Medicine (Baltimore)* **50**, 125.

CAMBIASO C. L., RICCOMI H. & MASSON P. L. (1976) Automated determination of immune complexes by their inhibitory effect on the agglutination of IgG-coated particles by rheumatoid factor or C1q. *Annals of Rheumatic Diseases* Vol. 36 (Supplement) Page 40.

COPEMAN P. W. M. (1975) Cutaneous angiitis. *Journal of the Royal College of Physicians of London* **9**, 103.

COWDERY J. S., TREADWELL P. E. & FRITZ R. B. (1975) A radioimmunoassay for human antigen-antibody complexes in clinical material. *Journal of Immunology* **114**, 5.

CREAM J. J. (1971) Immunofluorescent studies of the skin in cryoglobulinaemic vasculitis. *British Journal of Dermatology* **84**, 48.

CREAM J. J. (1972) Cryoglobulins in vasculitis. *Clinical and Experimental Immunology* **10**, 117.

CREAM J. J. (1973) Anticomplementary sera in cutaneous vasculitis. *British Journal of Dermatology* **89**, 555.

CREAM J. J. (1976a) Immune complexes in cryoprecipitates. *Annals of Rheumatic Diseases* Vol. 36 (supplement) Page 45.

CREAM J. J. (1976b) Clinical and immunological aspects of cutaneous vasculitis. *Quarterly Journal of Medicine* **45, (178)**, 255.

CREAM J. J., BRYCESON A. D. M. & RYDER G. (1971) Disappearance of immunoglobulin and complement from the Arthus reaction and its relevance to studies of vasculitis in man. *British Journal of Dermatology* **84**, 106.

DIXON F. J., VAZQUEZ J. J., WEIGLE W. O. & COCHRANE C. G. (1958) Pathogenesis of serum sickness. *A.M.A. Archives of Pathology* **65**, 18.

EDEN A., BIANCO C. & NUSSENZWEIG V. (1973) Mechanism of binding of soluble immune complexes. *Cellular Immunology* **7**, 459.

EZER G. & HAYWARD A. R. (1974) Inhibition of complement-dependent lymphocyte rosette formation: a possible test for activated complement products. *European Journal of Immunology* **4**, 148.

GERMUTH F. G., VALDES A. J., TAYLOR J. T., WISE O. L. & RODRIGUEZ E. (1975) Fatal immune complex glomerulonephritis without deposits. *Johns Hopkins Medical Journal* **136**, 189.

GREENWOOD B. M., WHITTLE H. C. & BRYCESON A. D. M. (1973) Allergic complications of meningococcal disease. II Immunological investigation. *British Medical Journal* **2**, 737.

GREY P. & KOHLER P. F. (1973) Cryoglobulin. *Seminars in Haematology* **10**, 87.

HAY F., NINEHAM L. J. & ROITT I. M. (1976) Detection of immune complexes by a solid phase radioassay. *Annals of Rheumatic Diseases* Vol. 36. (Supplement) page 31.

HAYWARD A. R., EZER G. & SMITH M. D. (1976) Inhibition of complement-dependent lymphocyte rosette formation. *Annals of Rheumatic Diseases* Vol. 36. (Supplement) Page 21.

JASIN H. E., LOSPALLUTO J. & ZIFF M. (1970) Rheumatoid hyperviscosity syndrome. *American Journal of Medicine* **49**, 484.

JEWELL D. P. & MACLENNAN I. C. M. (1973) Circulating immune complexes in inflammatory bowel disease. *Clinical and Experimental Immunology* **14**, 219.

JOHNSON A. H., MOWBRAY J. F. & PORTER K. A. (1975) Detection of circulating immune complexes in pathological human sera. *Lancet* **i**, 762.

JOHNSON A. H. & MOWBRAY J. F. (1976) Detection of immune complexes by the anticomplementary method. *Annals of Rheumatic Diseases* Vol. 36. (Supplement) Page 17.

JOHNSON G. D. & HOLBOROW E. J. (1973) Immunofluorescence. In *Handbook of Experimental Immunology,* 2nd edn., vol. 1, ed. Weir D. M., p.18.1. Blackwell, Oxford.

KYLE R. A., GLEISH G. J., BAYRD E. D. & VAUGHAN J. H. (1971) Benign hypergammaglobulinemic purpura of Waldenström. *Medicine (Baltimore)* **50**, 113.

LACHMANN P. J. (1967) Conglutinins and immunoconglutinins. *Advances in Immunology* **6**, 480.

LACHMANN P. J. (1973) Complement Technology. In *Handbook of Experimental Immunology,* 2nd edn., vol. 1, ed. Weir, D. M. p.5.1. Blackwell, Oxford.

LACHMANN P. J. (1975) In *Clinical Aspects of Immunology,* 3rd edn., eds. Gell P. G. H., Coombs R. R. A. & Lachmann P. J., p.323. Blackwell, Oxford.

LINSCOTT W. D. & KANE J. P. (1975) The complement system in cryoglobulinaemia. Interaction with immunoglobulin and lipoproteins. *Clinical and Experimental Immunology* **21**, 510.

MCINTOSH R. M., GRISWOLD R. W., CHERNAK W. B., WILLIAMS G., STRAUSS J., KAUFMAN D. B., KOSS M. N., MCINTOSH J. R., COHEN R. & WEIL R. (1975) Cryoglobulins III: further studies on the nature, incidence, clinical diagnostic, prognostic, and immunopathologic significance of cryoproteins in renal disease. *Quarterly Journal of Medicine, N.S.* **34**, 285.

MACLENNAN I. C. (1972) Competition for receptors for immunoglobulin on cytotoxic lymphocytes. *Clinical and Experimental Immunology* **10**, 275.

MOHAMMED I., THOMPSON B. & HOLBOROW E. J. (1976) Radiobioassay for immune complexes using macrophages. *Annals of Rheumatic Diseases* Vol. 36. (Supplement) Page 49.

MORAN C. J., RYDER, G., TURK J. L. & WATERS M. F. R. (1972) Evidence for circulating immune complexes in lepromatous leprosy. *Lancet* ii, 572.

MOWBRAY J. F., HOFFBRAND A. V., HOLBOROW E. J., SEAH P. P. & FRY L. (1973) Circulating immune complexes in dermatitis herpetiformis. *Lancet* i, 400.

MYLLYLÄ G. (1973) Aggregation of human blood platelets by immune complexes in the sedimentation pattern test. *Scandinavian Journal of Haematology* supplementum 19.

NAIRN R. C. (1969) *Fluorescent protein tracing* 3rd edn. Livingstone, Edinburgh.

OZAWA T., PLUSS R., LACHER J., BOEDECKER E., GUGGENHEIM S., HAMMOND W. & MCINTOSH R. (1975) Endogenous immune complex nephropathy associated with malignancy, I. Studies on the nature and immunopathogenic significance of glomerular bound antigen and antibody, isolation and characterization of tumour specific antigen and antibody and circulating immune complexes. *Quarterly Journal of Medicine, N.S.* **34**, 523.

PARISH W. E. (1971) Studies on vasculitis: I. Immunoglobulins, βIC, C-reactive protein, and bacterial antigens in cutaneous vasculitis lesions. *Clinical Allergy* I, 97.

PENTTINEN K. (1976) Platelet aggregation test. *Annals of Rheumatic Diseases* Vol. 36. (Supplement) Page 45.

ROJAS-ESPINOSA O., MENDEZ-NAVARRETE I. & ESTRADA-PARRA S. (1972) Presence of C1q-reactive immune complexes in patients with leprosy. *Clinical and Experimental Immunology* **12**, 215.

SMITH M. D., BARRATT T. M., HAYWARD A. R. & SOOTHILL J. F. (1975) The inhibition of complement-dependent lymphocyte rosette formation by the sera of children with steroid-sensitive nephrotic syndrome and other renal diseases. *Clinical and Experimental Immunology* **21**, 236.

SOOTHILL J. F. (1967) Altered complement component C¹3A (βIC−βIA) in patients with glomerulonephritis. *Clinical and Experimental Immunology* **2**, 83.

SOOTHILL J. F. & HENDRICKSE R. G. (1967) Some immunological studies of the nephrotic syndrome in Nigerian children. *Lancet* ii, 6291.

SOOTHILL J. F. (1967) Altered complement component C¹3A (βIC−βIA) in patients with heterogeneity of antibody affinity. *Clinical and Experimental Immunology* **9**, 193.

STANWORTH D. R. & JOHNS P. (1976) Ultracentrifugation studies for detection of complexes. *Annals of Rheumatic Diseases*, Vol. 36 (Supplement) Page 12.

THEOFILOPOULOS A. N., WILSON C. B., BOKISCH V. A. & DIXON F. J. (1974) Binding of soluble immune complexes to human lymphoblastoid cells. II. Use of Raji cells to detect circulating immune complexes in animal and human sera. *Journal of Experimental Medicine* **140**, 1230.

VERSEY J. M., HOBBS J. R. & HOLT P. J. (1973) Complement metabolism in rheumatoid arthritis. I. Longitudinal studies. *Annals of Rheumatic Diseases* **32**, 557.

WEISMAN M. & ZVAIFLER N. (1975) Cryoimmunoglobulinemia in rheumatoid arthritis. *Journal of Clinical Investigation* **56**, 725.

WILSON C. B. & DIXON F. J. (1971) Quantitation of acute and chronic serum sickness in the rabbit. *Journal of Experimental Medicine* **134**, 7s.

WILSON C. B. & DIXON F. J. (1974) Diagnosis of immunopathologic renal disease. *Kidney International* **5**, 389.

WINCHESTER R. J., KUNKEL H. G. & AGNELLO V. (1971) Occurrence of γ-globulin complexes in serum and joint fluid of rheumatoid arthritis patients: use of monoclonal rheumatoid factors as reagents for their demonstration. *Journal of Experimental Medicine* **134**, 286s.

WINCHESTER R. J. & AGNELLO V. (1976) Precipitin tests for immune complexes. *Annals of Rheumatic Diseases* Vol. 36 (Supplement) Page 35.

WINFIELD J. B., KOFFLER D. & KUNKEL H. G. (1975) Specific concentration of polynucleotide immune complexes in the cryoprecipitates of patients with systemic lupus erythematosus. *Journal of Clinical Investigation* **56**, 563.

YONEMASU K. & STROUD R. M. (1971) C1q: Rapid purification method for preparation of monospecific antisera for biochemical studies. *Journal of Immunology* **106**, 304.

ZUBLER R. & LAMBERT P. H. (1976) The ¹²⁵I-C1q binding test for detection of immune complexes. *Annals of Rheumatic Diseases*, Vol. 36. (Supplement) Page 27.

6

Investigation of the photodermatoses

W. FRAIN-BELL

It is no longer possible to diagnose the photodermatoses simply by detecting a reaction of the skin which appears to be precipitated or aggravated by exposure to sunshine. The use, in the past, of such limited criteria has led to a lack of appreciation of the frequency of photosensitivity and of the variability of its presentation. It is only since the construction of suitable irradiation equipment and the development of investigative techniques capable of confirming or otherwise the presence of photosensitivity that the field of clinical photobiology has become more clearly defined.

It is now recognized that photosensitivity reactions of the skin can result from exposure to wavelengths from the whole or any part of the u.v. and visible light spectrum. Thus, these responsible wavelengths can be present all the year round and therefore distinct seasonal summertime episodes may not always be apparent. The patient thus may not believe that light plays any part in his eruption and may succeed in convincing his doctor that this is so. Also, photosensitivity reactions of the skin will not necessarily remain confined to exposed sites, and some of the newer fabrics do allow penetration of the responsible wavelengths so that the skin under thin clothing may react as well.

The possibility of photosensitivity must therefore be considered in the diagnosis of any reaction of the skin whether restricted to exposed sites or not, and whether the element of light exposure is a factor that is obvious or not. Such a statement becomes more acceptable when it is remembered that the skin changes occurring in a photosensitivity response may be any of the following in combination or alone: erythema, with or without oedema; urticaria; morbilliform eruptions; eczematous rashes, 'lymphoma-like' conditions; vesicles, bullae; scaling and crusting; papular; necrosis, scarring and sclerodermatous states; pigmentation; hirsutes; lymphocytoma, and so on. Even relatively severe symptoms may occur such as those of burning and pain without significant morphological change as can be found in erythropoietic protoporphyria.

In addition to affection of the obvious exposed sites, eg face, neck, hands, there are certain distribution features which if present give added support to a provisional diagnosis of photosensitivity. For example, in the male these are involvement of the rim of the ears, the sides and the back of the neck and in particular the mastoid region; also the scalp when the reaction is maximal on or restricted to areas affected by a male pattern baldness. In the female, on the other hand, differences in hair style will result in a variation in the distribution of the eruption such as would occur from an alteration in the length of the forehead fringe or its asymmetry, or the affection of the exposed lower third of the ear.

There are also certain morphological changes which, when taken along with the distribution, suggest a specific photodermatosis. Examples include the red itchy uniform photosensitivity dermatitis reaction with the lichenification of its later chronic persistent light reaction phase and the associated 'lymphoma-like' lesions of its most photosensitive form, that of actinic reticuloid; the regular or broken line of brown pigmentation bordering the normal unaffected skin in the phototoxic reaction. The blisters, pigmentation, scars, and milia of the fragile hepatic porphyric skin; the minimal skin change of erythropoietic protoporphyria associated with the complaint of severe discomfort; the bizarre often linear bullae on a background of oedematous erythema of the psoralen containing plant photocontact reaction; the variable sized blisters and scars of hydroa vacciniforme and the lesions of the 'light prurigos', and so on. The group of rare inherited conditions exemplified by Blooms and Rothmund-Thomson (see Table 6.1) will demonstrate cutaneous and other features peculiar to each one and facilitate diagnosis in this way, as will the premature development of premalignant and malignant skin changes in xeroderma pigmentosum. However, there are pitfalls involved in making a clinical diagnosis of the photodermatoses, and it is for this reason that the various investigative techniques are required. Such procedures are used to confirm photosensitivity and define the responsible wavelengths (ie the action spectrum of the eruption); to diagnose a specific dermatosis; to obtain evidence for causal factors, treatable or otherwise; to rationalize treatment by relating it to the responsible wavelengths of u.v.r. and visible light and to other etiological factors.

TECHNIQUES USED IN THE INVESTIGATION OF THE PHOTODERMATOSES

Phototesting

Phototesting requires the availability of a light source capable of providing a spectral emission which as closely as possible simulates the solar spectrum. The one of choice is probably that of the xenon arc. The energy output of this lamp must be such that its emitted spectrum can be divided up by the use of filters, prisms, or gratings, into bands of wavelengths of u.v.r. and visible light which can be varied in breadth appropriate to the type of photodermatosis under investigation. It is important that the chosen wavebands in the long u.v. (ie > 320 nm) and visible light (400 nm and above) are free from contamination with the shorter sunburn erythema producing wavelengths found between 290 and 320 nm, otherwise any assessment of photosensitivity with or without the

Table 6.1 The majority of the photodermatoses with reference to the information which can be obtained from phototesting and photopatch testing which will help in the diagnosis and the elucidation of responsible factors.

			Information obtained from photo-testing and photopatch testing
1. Rare inherited conditions	Blooms Rothmund-Thomson Hartnup Xeroderma pigmentosum	(I)	The definition of an action spectrum for erythema for comparison with that found in normal subjects
2. Precipitation or aggravation of a dermatosis	Atopic eczema Psoriasis Lichen planus Lupus erythematosus Pemphigus etc.	(I)	The definition of an action spectrum for erythema for comparison with that found in normal subjects
3. The idiopathic photo-dermatoses	Solar urticaria Polymorphic light eruption Summer prurigo Hydroa vacciniforme Photosensitivity dermatitis and actinic reticuloid syndrome	(I) (II) (III)	The definition of an action spectrum for erythema for comparison with that found in normal subjects The definition of an action spectrum for abnormal morphological responses Photopatch test evidence of photo-toxic reactions to bergapten, tar, etc., differing from that found in normal subjects
4. Due to a specific photoactive substance	Photocontact dermatitis Drug induced photo-sensitivity Porphyria Photosensitivity dermatitis and actinic reticuloid syndrome	(I) (II) (III) (IV)	The definition of an action spectrum for erythema for comparison with that found in normal subjects The definition of an action spectrum for abnormal morphological responses Photopatch test evidence of photo-toxic reactions to bergapten, tar, etc., differing from that found in normal subjects Photopatch test evidence of 'photoallergic' reactions to specific substances

definition of the action spectrum will be unreliable. Thus, the first essential feature of any phototesting equipment is the predictability of its waveband selection.

This selection of wavebands can be provided by the placing of optical glass filters between the subject's skin and the light source, choosing them so that you have a range of cut-off points (Turnbull *et al* 1967). This allows the investigator to say that the subject reacts abnormally or not to wavelengths above a certain point or between two points in the spectrum (see Fig. 6.1). To use this method to try to determine the extent of an action spectrum is however tedious and not always practicable. Also, the use of optical glass filters to

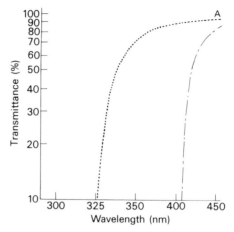

Fig. 6.1 ....WG 345 filter. - — - — - — - GG 420 filter. The use that can be made of optical filters to determine the wavelengths of u.v.r. or visible light to which the subject is reacting. For example, if a reaction of the skin is noted to irradiation which has been first passed through a Schott filter WG 345 (A) but no reaction when filter GG 420 is used would indicate that the responsible wavelengths lay between 325 and 400 nm, ie in the long u.v. part of the spectrum.

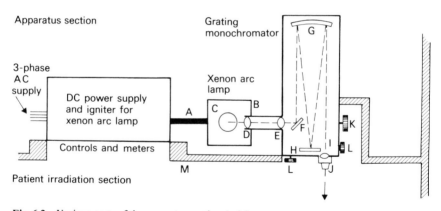

Fig. 6.2 Various parts of the apparatus section A–M.

    A = High tension cables
    B = Protective lamp housing
    C = 1600W xenon arc lamp
    D = Condenser lens
    E = Entrance slit and lens
    F = Plane entrance slit mirror
    G = Concave collimating mirror
    H = Diffraction grating
    I = Exit slit and lens
    J = Shutter, filter holder and nozzle
    K = Wavelength control
    L = Slit width controls
    M = Heat proof, light-tight partition

determine the irradiation spectrum is relatively crude and does not allow the controlled selection of a spectral band centred on a particular wavelength. However, the equipment recently described by Alsins *et al* (1975) appears to have avoided many of the disadvantages of this optical filter system. There is little doubt, however, that the selection of a range of wavebands is more easily achieved by using an irradiation monochromator and the type which makes use of a diffraction grating (Mackenzie & Frain-Bell 1974) rather than a prism (Magnus *et al* 1959) for separating the 'light' into its various wavebands is probably the 'best buy'. Although the ideal equipment has yet to be constructed where the purity of emission is guaranteed, the irradiation time short, and the predictability of the equipment assured, certain variations of the single monochromator have been described and extensively used (Sayre *et al* 1965; Knox *et al* 1967; Berger *et al* 1967; Cripps & Ramsay 1970).

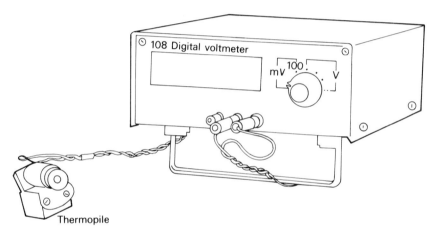

Fig. 6.3   The thermopile is attached to the grating monochromator at the exit slit (see Fig. 6.2J) and is coupled to a digital voltmeter. In this way the energy of the emitted u.v.r. or light can be estimated prior to irradiation of the skin.

The light source and the grating monochromator (see Figure 6.2) will require in addition equipment which when coupled to it will record the energy of u.v.r. or light emitted at the chosen wavebands (see Fig. 6.3). This irradiation monochromator equipment will also require checking from time to time to confirm the purity of the emitted wavelengths and to make sure that they do not contain significant amounts of wavelengths outside the chosen waveband. It is also important that the wavelength dial (see Fig. 6.2) is in fact choosing the correct wavebands and this should be checked weekly by making use of a mercury arc lamp source (see Fig. 6.4) of irradiation which is passed in the reverse direction through the monochromator system and the wavelength dial rotated to locate the mercury lines from 313 to 546 nm. For example, when the dial points to 313 nm a thin line appears on the fluorescent card located at 'N' (see Fig. 6.4) and if not the dial is altered accordingly. Monthly deterioration checks are required on the xenon arc lamp and the entrance and collimating

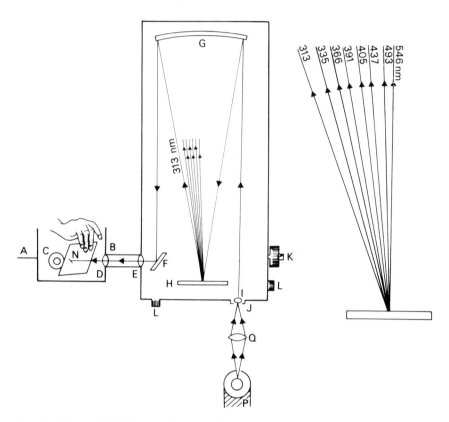

Fig. 6.4 The method of checking the calibration of the monochromator. When the wavelength control is set at any of the following wavelengths—313, 335, 366, 391, 405, 437, 493 and 546 nm—light only will be seen on the fluorescent card.

A = High tension cables (supply disconnected)
B = Protective lamp housing (open)
C = 1600W xenon arc lamp (lamp is turned off and protected with a safety cover)
D = Condensing lens
E = Entrance slit and lens
F = Plane entrance slit mirror
G = Concave collimating mirror
H = Diffraction grating
I = Exit slit and lens
J = Shutter, filter holder and nozzle
K = Wavelength control (set at 313 nm)
L = Slit width controls (set at 0.50 nm)
N = Fluorescent card
P = Mercury lamp
Q = Quartz lens

mirrors (see Fig. 6.2), recoating these mirrors when the output of the monochromator falls below an acceptable level. It has been the author's experience that a xenon arc lamp deteriorates fairly rapidly during the first 100 hours of use, eg around a 15–20% fall in output; thereafter for the next 300 hours or so the deterioration lessens to between 5 and 10%. The deterioration in output check should be carried out at a series of wavebands throughout the u.v.r. and visible light spectrum by means of a sensitive thermopile coupled to a digital voltmeter (see Fig. 6.3) or some other recording equipment.

There is no doubt that information regarding possible photosensitivity can be obtained simply by exposing the subject's skin to irradiation from a bank of fluorescent tubes, one bank being made up of those of the sunlamp type which concentrates the emission in the range of 270–370 nm peaking at 310 nm, and the other bank made up of long u.v.r. tubes emitting in the range of 300–400 nm peaking at 355 nm. Using such light sources, it is possible to say that the subject has a minimal response dose level for a single broad waveband (i.e. either 270–370 nm or 300–400 nm) which is different or not from that obtained in a group of normal non-photosensitive subjects, using the same equipment and technique. It goes without saying that it is of fundamental importance to have defined for the technique being used a range of minimal response doses in a group of normal subjects. Unfortunately, these simple techniques have not led, in the past, to reliable diagnosis of the photodermatoses and the advance in knowledge of photosensitivity dates from the appearance of the more sophisticated irradiation equipment already referred to.

Irrespective of the sophistication of the irradiation equipment, the principle is the same, that is to record the amount of energy required at a certain waveband to produce a minimal response, be it of erythema, urticaria, or what, at a specific time interval after irradiation (usually 7, 24, 48 hours, or later if required). A series of such minimal response doses for a range of wavebands constitutes the action spectrum of the eruption (see Fig. 6.5).

The definition of the action spectrum, be it for erythema or for erythematopapular, urticarial and other responses, is required to determine first of all whether photosensitivity is present and if so the responsible wavelengths. As a result, it is now appreciated that some patients for example with polymorphic light eruption will respond to wavelengths throughout the u.v.r. and visible light spectrum and not simply as first thought to the short u.v.r. from 290 to 320 nm; that the action spectrum in solar urticaria is very variable, the reaction occurring to band passes at various levels in the u.v.r. and visible light; that the action spectrum in hydroa vacciniforme is within normal limits as it is in some cases of summer prurigo, polymorphic light eruption, solar urticaria and so on; also that in those cases of psoriasis and lupus erythematosus where there is clinical evidence of light aggravation that this is often associated with an action spectrum for erythema which indicates some degree of photosensitivity to the sunburn wavelengths from 290 to 320 nm; that a suspected drug-induced photosensitivity is that much more likely if the action spectrum for erythema is abnormally present in the long u.v. (320–400 nm); that in the classical case of

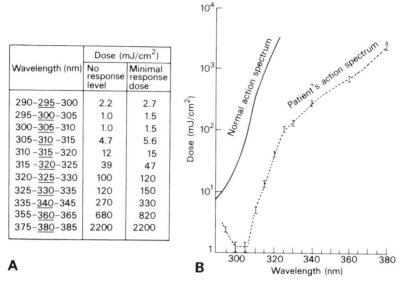

Wavelength (nm)	Dose (mJ/cm²)	
	No response level	Minimal response dose
290–<u>295</u>–300	2.2	2.7
295–<u>300</u>–305	1.0	1.5
300–<u>305</u>–310	1.0	1.5
305–<u>310</u>–315	4.7	5.6
310–<u>315</u>–320	12	15
315–<u>320</u>–325	39	47
320–<u>325</u>–330	100	120
325–<u>330</u>–335	120	150
335–<u>340</u>–345	270	330
355–<u>360</u>–365	680	820
375–<u>380</u>–385	2200	2200

Fig. 6.5   **A** lists the dose in mJ/cm² required to produce a minimal reaction of the skin in relationship to the dose at which no reaction could be detected, eg at the 295 nm peak the minimal response dose is 2.7 mJ/cm² and the no response level is at 2.2 mJ/cm². This data allows for the plotting of the action spectrum as illustrated in **B** the bars recording the range between the minimal response and no response levels. The action spectrum for the individual patient is drawn in comparison to that found in a group of normal subjects using the same technique (normal action spectrum).

xeroderma pigmentosum the erythema responses will be delayed and persistent with evidence of photosensitivity particularly in the short u.v. from 290 to 320 nm; that the single case of the Rothmund-Thomson syndrome investigated by the author, in which photosensitivity is considered to be a factor, showed no evidence of such on phototesting; and that the diagnosis of the porphyrias can sometimes be confirmed simply by the response to a single irradiation dose at 400 nm peak and so on and so on. Repeated action spectrum studies over the months and years also allows for the assessment of the progress of persistent light reaction and of the spread and broadening of the action spectrum to involve new wavelengths, which tend to occur in the most photosensitive subjects. Not only is the definition of the action spectrum of importance in diagnosis, but it is essential in the study of the natural history of the photodermatoses and in the choice of treatment and in the assessment of its efficacy.

Photopatch testing

A photosensitivity reaction may occur because of the arrival in the skin from an external or internal source of a photoactive substance which has the ability, on account of its structure, to absorb wavelengths of u.v.r. and/or visible light and thus to produce reactions some of which may make use of immunological pathways. The subsequent reaction will in most instances be that of either a 'phototoxic' or a 'photoallergic' type. The details of the photoallergic response are still uncertain but it is assumed that in the presence of light the hapten can join with protein to form a conjugate which triggers off an immunological response in the tissue. Alternatively, the light may act by producing a chemical change in the photoactive substance and then this new chemical triggers off a cell-mediated response similar to that occurring in non-light induced contact dermatitis. Some support for this so-called photoallergic reaction can be obtained from the use of the photopatch test. This test is a variant of the skin patch test and consists of the application to the skin, usually of the back, of the suspect substance in a concentration which is known not to produce a reaction in normal subjects whether with or without subsequent exposure to light. Two identical tests are applied for each substance, one of which is occluded and left for 48 hours before reading, whereas the other is removed after 24 hours and the site irradiated with u.v.r. or visible light, the dose used being that of a previously determined suberythema level. The light source most commonly used in photopatch testing is that of a single or a batch of long u.v.r. tubes emmitting in the range of 300–400 nm, peaking around 350–360 nm, and with a plain glass filter so as to remove the erythema producing wavelengths <320 nm. However, if the absorption spectrum of the test substance is outside the wavelength range of long u.v.r. tubes, eg in the visible light above 400 nm as occurs for example with certain dyes (Gardiner *et al* 1971), then other forms of irradiation equipment are required, for example the monochromator.

Using this technique a number of alternative results can be obtained which are illustrated in Fig. 6.6, using a known photosensitizing chemical quinoxaline-N-dioxide.

A			B		
Irradiated test sites			**Occluded non-irradiated test sites**		
A1 Concentration of quinoxaline			**B1** Concentration of quinoxaline		
1%	0.5%	0.1%	1%	0.5%	0.1%
A2 Preirradiated quinoxaline			**B2** Preirradiated quinoxaline		
A3 Purified photoproducts			**B3** Purified photoproducts		

Fig. 6.6 Quinoxaline refers to Quinoxaline-mono-*N*-oxide.

1 A positive reaction of equal intensity at A1 and B1 would indicate cell-mediated allergic sensitivity unrelated to light. The accuracy of this assessment depends on the complete exclusion of light from the unirradiated patch tests (B1). The interpretation of this result may be difficult since sometimes the irradiated site (A1) may produce a reaction greater than that seen in the non-irradiated covered site (B1). If this difference is marked then most probably both photoallergy of photocontact type and a cell-mediated allergic sensitivity of contact dermatitis type, are present.

2   A positive reaction at the irradiated sites (A1) only with a negative response at the non-irradiated site (B1) usually confirms 'photoallergy' and excludes routine contact dermatitis type of the cell-mediated allergic response except in the instance where the effect of light has been to change the chemical and the subsequent allergic reaction then occurs to the new chemical without any further irradiation. This possibility can be checked by irradiating the photoactive substance prior to its application to the skin when it will then produce a positive reaction without subsequent irradiation of the skin test site (see Fig. 6.6, A2 and B2).

3   Further information can be gained by including in the test series purified photoproducts of the parent substance (see Fig. 6.6, A3 and B3) and this will help to show whether in fact the parent substance alone is the culprit or whether it can be narrowed down to one or more chemicals produced following exposure to light (Zaynoun *et al* 1976).

Difficulty in interpretation can arise since some substances which are capable of producing photoallergic responses are also capable of producing phototoxic responses if applied to the skin in sufficient quantity and followed by appropriate amounts of irradiation. In most instances, however, if it has previously been shown that when using the same concentrations normal non-light sensitive subjects do not produce a reaction then it is unlikely that any positive response obtained is false, ie that the positive photopatch test reaction does in fact indicate a response peculiar to the individual being tested and is thus most likely of 'photoallergic' type. There is something 'special', however, about some individuals with photosensitivity, at certain stages of the reaction and particularly if the degree of photosensitivity is marked, whereby a positive photopatch test reaction may later be found to be negative. The explanation for this phenomenon is as yet unclear, and may account for the variation in photopatch test results in the photodermatoses.

It may well be that too much attention is paid to the study of the photoallergic reaction to the exclusion of the phototoxic one. It is important, therefore, to assess in subjects with a photosensitivity response their ability to produce phototoxic responses, eg to tar or oil of bergamot (bergapten—5-methoxy psoralen) and so on, and to compare this response with that known to occur in normal non-light sensitive subjects. This can be done using a range of concentrations as illustrated in Fig. 6.7. Most normal subjects will respond to oil of bergamot in a 2.5–5% concentration (bergapten conc. of 0.27 g in 100 ml of oil of bergamot) range when they are applied to the skin using the photopatch test technique and followed by irradiation with a suberythema dose

Concentration of oil of bergamot in pmf	0.25%	0.5%	1%	2.5%	5%
Percentage of positive reactions	0	10%	50%	90%	90%

Fig. 6.7   The frequency in normal subjects with which positive phototoxic erythema reactions occur to varying concentrations of oil of bergamot.

of long u.v.r. (eg a Philips black light fluorescent tube at a 10 cm distance emitting between 1000 and 1200 mJ/cm² over a period of 30 minutes which will not produce a reaction in the skin of normal non-photosensitive subjects). Thus a reaction to anything less than 1% concentration of oil of bergamot (see Fig. 6.7) suggests a greater phototoxic reaction potential than normal and this information may well be significant in the study of the individual case. Of course, each investigator will have to determine the range of responses in normal subjects for his own oil of bergamot sample since the quantity of the active phototoxic agent, bergapten, will vary from one sample to the next (Zaynoun *et al* 1977).

How then can these techniques of phototesting and photopatch testing be used in the diagnosis and assessment of the photodermatoses as listed in Table 6.1. The basic question of whether photosensitivity exists is answered by demonstrating by phototesting that the minimal skin response dose in the subject is less than that known to occur in normal non-light sensitive subjects. The definition of the full action spectrum will help to confirm the clinical diagnosis which has been based on history, morphology, distribution, and so on.

The correct use of the technique of photopatch testing will provide evidence of what is called for want of a better label 'photoallergy' and may show also that the subject has the ability to produce a 'phototoxic' reaction with greater facility than normal non-photosensitive controls. Until such time as it has been found possible to apply immunological tests to the study of the photodermatoses, much is to be gained by photopatch testing within the limits described.

The technique of phototesting with its definition of the responsible wavelengths of u.v.r. and visible light (the action spectrum) can also be used to assess the results of treatment, eg in the assessment of the effect of the administration of beta-carotene in erythropoietic protoporphyria and other photodermatoses. Perhaps, however, a more important application of this definition of the responsible wavelengths is that it allows for the selection of the appropriate protective light screening agent. It is a pointless exercise to apply to the skin for example para-aminobenzoic acid which is effective in the short u.v. wavelengths from 290 to 320 nm if the responsible wavelengths in the specific photodermatosis being treated are in fact from 320 nm upwards.

The treatment and care of patients with severe persistent light reaction, found particularly in the photosensitivity dermatitis and actinic reticuloid syndrome, is dependent for success on information obtained of the range of the responsible wavelengths of u.v.r. and visible light. This knowledge will help to justify the necessity for special light protection cubicles (Herd *et al* 1973) in dermatological inpatient units and highlights the continuing importance of minimizing skin exposure to these responsible wavelengths when the patient leaves hospital. The alternative of maintenance systemic steroid therapy and life in 'the dark' is not necessary.

Although this chapter is concerned particularly with the *in vivo* techniques used in the investigation of a human subject with a photodermatosis, it is necessary that these should not be considered in isolation. It is important that levels of porphyrins are estimated in all cases of photosensitivity not only in the urine but also in blood and faeces, in addition to a range of routine haematological and biochemical tests, the results of which will give guidance as to the adequate function of the various body systems relevant or otherwise to the photosensitivity skin response.

The study of cellular changes resulting from u.v. exposure in relationship to deficient repair mechanisms and the development of skin malignancies in patients with xeroderma pigmentosum and in normal subjects, is part of the continuing clinical and laboratory research in the photodermatoses. Also, the newer pharmacological techniques are starting to provide information of the fundamental processes occurring in the human skin following exposure to u.v.r. Immunological techniques related to the study of antigen-antibody interaction and to cell-mediated responses are particularly relevant to the group of idiopathic photodermatoses and the reaction to photoactive substances. A range of *in vitro* techniques are also available for the study of photoactive substances and in particular in the assessment of phototoxicity and the effect on the nucleus and other parts of the cell.

In conclusion, it cannot be overemphasized that a close liaison with a department of physics is essential so that the irradiation equipment used by the clinician in the investigation of the photodermatoses can be shown to be predictable and efficient. If the results of the irradiation of the skin cannot be relied on then any form of interpretation of them will remain suspect.

REFERENCES

ALSINS J., CLAESSON S., FISCHER T., & JUHLIN L. (1975) Development of high intensity narrow band lamps and studies of the irradiation effect on human skin. *Acta Dermato-Venereologica* **55,** 261.

BERGER D., URBACH F. & DAVIES R. (1967) The action spectrum of erythema induced by ultraviolet radiation. Preliminary report. In *XIII Congressus Internationalis Dermatologiae Munchen,* vol. 2, p. 1112 Springer-Verlag, Berlin.

CRIPPS D. J. & RAMSEY C. A. (1970) Ultraviolet action spectrum with a prism-grating monochromator. *British Journal of Dermatology* **82,** 584.

GARDINER J. S., DICKSON A., MACLEOD T. M. & FRAIN-BELL W. (1971) The investigation of photocontact dermatitis in a dye manufacturing process. *British Journal of Dermatology* **85,** 264.

HERD J., STURROCK I. & FRAIN-BELL W. (1973) The use of plastic material for the protection of patients with severe photodermatoses *British Journal of Dermatology* **88,** 283.

KNOX J. M., WARSHAWSKY J., LICHODZIEJEWSKI W. & FREEMAN R. G. (1967) Design of a high intensity monochromator. *Archives of Dermatology* **95,** 319.

MACKENZIE L. A. & FRAIN-BELL W. (1973) The construction and development of a grating monochromator and its application to the study of the reaction of the skin to light. *British Journal of Dermatology* **89,** 251.

MAGNUS I. A., PORTER A. D., McCREE K. J., MORELAND J. D. WRIGHT W. D. (1959) A monochromator. An apparatus for the investigation of the responses of the skin to ultra-violet, visible and near infra-red radiation. *British Journal of Dermatology* **71,** 261.

SAYRE R. M., STRAKA E. R., ANGLIN J. H. & EVERETT M. A. (1965) A high intensity ultraviolet monochromator. *Journal of Investigative Dermatology* **45**, 190.

TURNBULL B. C., FRAIN-BELL W. & MACKENZIE L. A. (1967) The development of xenon arc lamp equipment for the assessment of photosensitivity. *British Journal of Dermatology* **79**, 369.

ZAYNOUN S., JOHNSON B. E. & FRAIN-BELL W. (1976) The investigation of quindoxin photosensitivity. *Contact Dermatitis* **2**, 3430.

ZAYNOUN S., JOHNSON B. E. & FRAIN-BELL (1977) A study of oil of bergamot and its importance as a phototoxic agent. *British Journal of Dermatology* **96**, 475.

7

Identification of mediators of inflammation

M. W. GREAVES & A. KOBZA BLACK

In order to identify mediators we must not only demonstrate the presence of the mediator in inflamed skin, but we must show that it is the cause of the inflammatory changes. To do this we have to set up criteria analogous to those which have to be fulfilled in order to identify a specific microbial agent as the cause of an infection. These criteria ideally include:

1 The skin should be capable of forming or synthesizing the agent and be able to release it in response to an appropriate stimulus.

2 It should be absent or in low concentrations in its active form in healthy skin.

3 The agent should be able to reproduce at least some of the signs or symptoms of inflammation in concentrations in which it is found in inflammation.

4 Local tissue depletion of stores of the agent or its precursor should inhibit inflammation.

5 Specific antagonists or inhibitors of the agent or its formation should inhibit inflammation.

6 Antiinflammatory drugs should inhibit the formation, release or effects of the agent.

7 Inhibition of destruction of the agent should amplify its effect.

In this account we will not describe the methodology relating to each of these criteria systematically. Instead, we shall outline the different types of preliminary experiments one can do which may provide sufficiently encouraging data to make a more detailed programme seem worthwhile carrying out.

Two types of experiment can be performed. *Direct experiments* involve analysis of inflamed tissue or samples of inflammatory exudate by chemical or pharmacological methods. These methods can be either non-specific screening methods in which pharmacological activity is sought which is subsequently analysed or one can look for specific activity at the beginning. The weakness of this direct approach is that it only reveals the presence of an agent; it does not tell you that it is behaving as a mediator. However, within this limitation a positive result is of high validity.

In contrast, *indirect methods* which involve the use of other drugs as tools to reveal the presence of mediators depend for their validity on the specificity of these drugs, an assumption which is very often incorrect. However, indirect methods do have the advantage that they take the problem a step further than the direct methods, since they not only reveal the presence of the mediator but also provide supporting evidence for its role as a mediator.

DIRECT METHODS

Recovery of exudate

The first step is to obtain samples of inflammatory exudate for analysis. Biopsy of inflamed skin has the drawback of scarring and the tissue injury involved will itself generate mediators on a massive scale. An alternative method that has been used with some success is a skin perfusion technique (see Fig. 7.1). The problem with it is that you are diluting the very material you are trying to recover. It is also only semiquantitative since the concentration of any activity recovered depends amongst other things on tissue diffusion and on uptake by lymphatic and blood vasculature. Nevertheless, we obtained highly specific

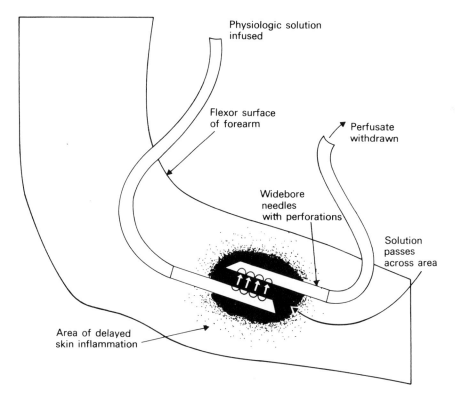

Fig. 7.1 Schematic representation of skin perfusion technique. Two wide bore needles with holes drilled into the sides of the shaft, are inserted in parallel 1 cm apart immediately subdermally. Sterile Tyrode solution is inserted through one needle and recovered through the other by applying gentle suction. The perfused skin is confined by applying elastic bands proximal and distal to the perfused area to prevent diffusion.

findings with this technique including prostaglandin activity in delayed inflammation from a number of different causes, as well as histamine in immediate wheal and flare reactions (Greaves *et al* 1971; Greaves & Sondergaard 1970).

Because of the drawbacks of this method we are now examining an alternative technique in which we obtain mechanically-induced blister fluid from inflamed skin. We have been examining suction blister fluid from normal skin and comparing it with similar fluid obtained from inflamed skin. Fluid from inflamed skin (essentially an undiluted sample of inflammatory exudate) contains specific pharmacological activity. In contrast, there is little or no activity in fluid obtained from normal skin. Our results indicate that this method may be of great value in investigation of mediators of inflammatory skin disease.

A third approach which we are exploring is examination of blood from veins draining inflamed skin. The assumption is that mediators released in inflammatory exudate will find their way into the blood plasma. There is, however, bound to be some loss due to tissue enzyme degradation, blood enzyme degradation, and dilution by blood.

Analysis of the perfusate

It is possible to apply to the exudate specific tests for individual known mediators. However, there is then the risk that pharmacological agents hitherto unsuspected may be missed. Probably a more satisfactory procedure is to screen the exudate for pharmacological activity and then break this activity down into its component parts by successively identifying and eliminating known mediators. Ideally the screening method ought to test for pro-inflammatory activity of one type or another. This could be done by using increased vascular permeability as an indication of pharmacological activity. The difficulty is that although it is quite easy to identify and quantitate permeability producing agents in skin by means of dye leakage in animal skin (Harada *et al* 1971), the method is performed *in vivo* and this makes analysis by use of antagonists imprecise since they have to be administered to the whole animal. However, testing for vasoactivity by the *in vivo* dye method in rats is probably a useful procedure as a preliminary to the systematic analysis described below.

The method most widely used is to test the exudate for smooth muscle contracting activity *in vitro* on the basis that most known vasoactive agents are also smooth muscle contracting agents. The technique we use is called cascade superfusion (Gaddum 1953; Vane 1964). It makes use of the fact that smooth muscle preparations from different organs and species have distinctive and specific responses to different pharmacological agents. Several different isolated organ preparations are mounted in series and bathed in physiological solution. The exudate is cascaded over the preparations and the identity of agents in the exudate established by observation of characteristic responses of the preparation and by use of suitable specific antagonists. The use of this procedure is illustrated by the examination of exudate obtained from delayed

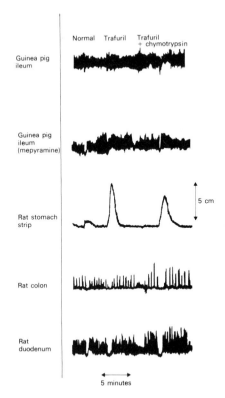

Normal   Trafuril   Trafuril
+ chymotrypsin

Guinea pig
ileum

Guinea pig
ileum
(mepyramine)

Rat stomach
strip

5 cm

Rat colon

Rat
duodenum

5 minutes

Fig. 7.2   Pharmacological activity in inflammatory exudate obtained from delayed human skin inflammation due to application of Trafuril (tetrahydrofurfuryl nicotinate). Cascade superfusion technique. All exudates applied in 1 : 5 dilution Trafuril + Chymotrypsin prior to assay. Note the reduced response of the rat stomach strip to Trafuril after incubation with Chymotrypsin.

inflammation in skin due to application of tetrahydrofurfuryl nicotinate (Trafuril) (see Fig. 7.2). The exudate contracted both the rat stomach and duodenum preparations and suggested that prostaglandin activity was present. That this combination of responses was not due to adrenaline acetyl choline, histamine or serotonin is indicated by the failure of the specific antagonists propranolol, phentolamine, atropine, mepyramine or methysergide to inhibit the responses. That kinin activity was also present was suggested by the ability of the exudate to relax the rat duodenum and by reduction in the contractile responses by incubation of the blister fluid with chymotrypsin. Having obtained clues to the identity of the unknown mediator the next step is to carry out specific extraction and identification procedures for known mediators. References to appropriate methods are given in Table 7.1.

Before discussing individual mediators it is worth making some general points. Bioassay is still probably the most satisfactory way of identifying pharmacological activity because it measures biological activity. It can be made highly sensitive if combined with a specific physical separation procedure, eg chromatography. It can also be made highly accurate and specific by using parallel quantitative assay as described by Chang and Gaddum (1953). In this technique the unknown activity, eg histamine-like activity, is tested against standard histamine solutions using several different isolated organ prepara-

Table 7.1 Methods for identification of some vasoactive agents

Agent	Methods	References
Histamine	Bioassay	Schild (1942)
	Spectrophotofluorometry	Oates *et al* (1962)
Catecholamines	Bioassay	Gaddum *et al* (1949)
Serotonin	Spectrophotofluorometry	Crawford and Rudd (1962)
Bradykinin	Bioassay	Edery (1968)
		Ferreira and Vane (1967)
	Radioimmunoassay	Goodfriend and Ball (1969)
Prostaglandins	Thin layer chromatography	Green and Samuelsson (1964)
	and bioassay	Greaves *et al* (1971)
	Radioimmunoassay	Caldwell *et al* (1971)
	Radio gas chromatography	Hensby (1975)
	Gas chromatography/	
	mass spectrometry	

tions. If the same quantitative result is achieved using each preparation, accurate identification can be assumed.

A more recent development in pharmacological assay is the use of radioimmunoassay. Radioimmunoassay is extremely useful because it enables rapid assay of a large number of samples. It has at least two important drawbacks. It measures immunoreactivity and not biological activity and thus its validity must be confirmed by appropriate bioassay. Furthermore, cross reaction with chemically similar agents is very hard to exclude.

Histamine

The standard method for identification of histamine in solutions is by bioassay using a strip of terminal guinea pig ileum in an organ bath. Dose related contraction in the presence of atropine (to exclude acetylcholine activity) followed by inhibition of this activity by the antihistamine mepyramine confirms the presence of histamine. This method reliably and reproducibly detects concentrations in the 1.0–2.5 ng/ml range. The problem with this method arises when there is other smooth muscle contracting activity in the solution which is neither due to histamine nor to any other agent for which there is a specific antagonist. Cases in point are prostaglandin or bradykinin activity. There are no specific antagonists of either of these agents. Thus in a solution with enough prostaglandin or bradykinin activity to mask the histamine activity the histamine may go unrecognized.

One can get round this by extracting or removing the non-histamine activity. One way is to use the fact that histamine is acid stable even after boiling in concentrated hydrochloric acid to remove other agents. Another more satisfactory method is to use the fact that conjugates of histamine with the fluorophore orthophthalaldehyde enables fluorometric assay with an excitation wavelength of 360 nm and an emission wavelength of 450 nm. This method does involve a preliminary extraction procedure to eliminate non-histamine fluorescent material which interferes with the assay. The method is not normally accurate in detecting concentrations of histamine less than 10 ng/ml.

Bradykinin

Bradykinin can be identified by bioassay using the isolated rat uterus and rat duodenum preparations mounted in a single organ bath (Greaves & Sondergaard 1970). Bradykinin contracts the rat uterus but relaxes the duodenum. The assay has to be carried out in the presence of an alpha-adrenergic blocking agent such as phentolamine since noradrenaline and adrenaline cause a similar response. Confirmatory evidence of the presence of bradykinin in the solution can be obtained by carrying out the assay in the presence of chymotrypsin which enhances the response of the guinea pig ileum to bradykinin. Radioimmunoassay techniques for bradykinin have recently been proposed (Goodfriend & Bull 1969) but these are still in the early stages of development. The results will have to be carefully validated using the biological methods described above.

Serotonin (5 hydroxytryptamine)

Serotonin is normally detected fluorometrically after first extracting the serotonin to eliminate interfering fluorescent materials. Serotonin fluoresces at 540 nm following activation at 295 nm. The lower limit of reliable detection has been about 10–20 ng/ml.

Prostaglandins

Prostaglandins consist of a group of twenty carbon fatty acids whose estimation is complicated by the fact that the prostaglandin subclasses have diverse pharmacological actions even though the prostaglandins are extremely closely related chemically. There is increasing evidence that in many tissues or organs the endoperoxide prostaglandin precursors or their recently identified derivatives, the thromboxanes may possess a more central biological role then the better known prostaglandins E and F.

Three methods are normally used for identification of prostaglandin activity: combined extraction chromatography and bioassay; radioimmunoassay; and combined gas chromatography and mass spectrometry.

Combined extraction chromatography and bioassay has been widely used. Polar acidic prostaglandin activity is extracted by a suitable lipid solvent (ethyl acetate or petroleum ether) at low pH. The extracted prostaglandin activity is separated by thin layer chromatography using suitable solvent systems, into the subclasses (E_1, E_2, $F_{1\alpha}$ and $F_{2\alpha}$). The zones of the chromatoplate corresponding to simultaneously developed standard prostaglandins are then eluted and the eluates subjected to bioassay using an isolated rat uterus preparation and standard prostaglandin E_1. Most workers in this field would accept this procedure as adequate for identification of prostaglandin activity although some purists would insist on calling acidic lipid activity defined in this way 'prostaglandin-like' activity. The rat uterus preparation is extremely sensitive to the major subclasses of prostaglandin and can accurately measure concentrations as low as 1 ng/ml of E_1. Other equally sensitive organs include the chick rectum and the rat stomach fundus strip. One trap for the unwary in the bioassay of prostaglandins is the tendency for stimulated smooth muscle preparations to synthesise intrinsic prostaglandin activity during contraction, which brings about spuriously high values. This should be prevented by routinely including indomethacin (an inhibitor of prostaglandin biosynthesis) in the perfusion or superfusion fluid.

Radioimmunoassay has been widely used in the identification and assay of prostaglandins. I have already mentioned possible pitfalls in the procedure. The radioassay of prostaglandin F is well established and materials for it are now available in kit form. Radioassay of prostaglandin E is still in the experimental stage. It is worth stressing that in many biological and pathological situations where prostaglandins are being studied the ratio E:F may be crucial in the regulatory role of the prostaglandin system, since prostaglandin E and prostaglandin F frequently have opposing actions. Thus it may be misleading to measure either in isolation. A further point to remember is that there may be crossreactivity between inhibitory activity in the radioimmunoassay due to prostaglandin $F_{2\alpha}$ and other closely related lipids, including possibly prosatglandin D_2.

Combined gas chromatography and mass spectroscopy (GCMS) has the advantage that it will identify all prostaglandin subtypes and their congeners, present in the solution or exudate studied, but it does not reveal which of these are biologically inactive. After preliminary gas chromatographic preparation the prostaglandin molecule is fragmented in the mass spectrometer to yield characteristic ionized fragments whose mass is determined. The method can be made quantitative using deuterated standard prostaglandins and multiple ion detection. It is a highly accurate identification method, but is very cumbersome and there are few centres where the apparatus is available. The realization that precursor byproducts and metabolites of prostaglandin biosynthesis may turn out to be as important or more important than the classical prostaglandin classes makes data on biological material obtained by GCMS increasingly valuable relative to the other methods.

INDIRECT METHODS

Indirect methods for identification of mediators not only provide evidence of identity but also may enable tentative conclusions to be drawn about the role of the mediator. However, the specificity of these methods is usually not absolute and no complete reliance can be placed on positive or negative results.

Pharmacological antagonists

Ability of an antihistamine like mepyramine to block an event in the skin usually is taken as evidence that the event is triggered by histamine. However the capacity of mepyramine to block histamine responses depends on the affinity of this drug for histamine receptors relative to non-histamine receptors. That it also has a significant affinity for acetyl choline receptors is evident because of its well known atropine-like action in causing dryness of the mouth. Thus mepyramine's selectivity is only relative. There are now known to be two types of histamine receptor, the H_1 and H_2 receptors (Black *et al* 1972). H_1 receptors are found in the lungs, nasal mucosa and gut and are blocked by conventional antihistamines such as mepyramine and phenergan. H_2 receptors are found in the acid secreting glands of the stomach, the heart and peripheral arteries. They are not blocked by conventional antihistamines but by H_2 antagonists including metiamide and burimamide. Since skin blood vessels contain both receptors it is important to use both classes of antagonists in the investigation of skin inflammation by this means. In the practical use of antagonists to identify mediators in skin inflammation it is important to establish that adequate amounts of the antagonist are reaching the test site. This can best be done by comparing the effect of the antagonist simultaneously on both the inflammatory response under investigation and on an approximately equal response to intradermal injection of the corresponding agonist.

There is insufficient space to go into details concerning the complex subject of quantitation of wheals and flares in the skin. For wheals ideally one should measure in three dimensions using a silicone rubber impression. Alternatively, the area including pseudopodia can be measured using either squared paper or tracing paper and a planimeter. The duration of onset and regression may be just as important to measure as the maximum size. Regional difference greatly influence wheal size, wheals on the extensor surface of the forearm being smaller than on the flexor surface.

Receptor antiserum

Drug receptor specific antisera have been described (Berti *et al* 1974). Cholinergic receptor-rich fractions have been obtained from the electric organs of Torpedo marmorata. An antiserum raised in rabbits has potent specific anticholinergic activity, reversible by anticholinesterase. The development of other drug specific antisera could revolutionize therapeutics in the future, as well as providing valuable research tools.

Inhibition of formation

Although of relatively low specificity the ability of indomethacin to inhibit prostaglandin biosynthesis is frequently used in an attempt to implicate prostaglandins in physiological or pathological events. However, indomethacin has several independent effects including inhibition of polymorphonuclear migration which make results difficult to interpret.

Tissue depletion experiments

Agents which deplete tissues of mediators can be used to implicate the mediator in a given response. For example, studies of histamine concentrations in injected skin were used to implicate local histamine release in the whealing response to prostaglandin E (Sondergaard & Greaves 1971). We found significant reduction of histamine concentrations in PGE-injected thigh skin. An alternative approach is to deplete skin of histamine with compound 48/80 and show that this histamine depleted skin no longer responds by whealing following intradermal PGE_1 injection. It is important to take into account the possibility that compound 48/80 may deplete the skin of other agents besides histamine including possibly slow reacting substance of anaphylaxis (SRS-A).

In summary, indirect methods clearly have a useful role to play in the identification of mediators especially as preliminary studies. They should be followed up by more detailed analysis by direct techniques.

REFERENCES

BERTI F., CLEMENTI F., CONTI-TRONCONI B. & OMINI C. (1974) Pharmacological properties of a cholinergic receptor antiserum. *British Journal of Pharmacology* **52,** 408.

BLACK J. W., DUNCAN W. A. M., DURANT C. J., GANELLIN C. R. & PARSONS E. M. (1972) Definition and antagonism of histamine H_2 receptors. *Nature* **236,** 385.

CALDWELL B. V., BURSTEIN S., BROCK W. A. & SPEROFF L. (1971) Radioimmunassay of the F prostaglandins. *Journal of Clinical Endocrinology* **33,** 171.

CHANG H. O. & GADDUM J. H. (1933) Choline esterase in tissue extracts. *Journal of Physiology* **79,** 255.

CRAWFORD N. & RUDD B. T. (1962) A spectrophotofluorimetric method for the determination of serotonin (5 hydroxytryptamine) in plasma. *Clinica Chimica Acta* **7,** 114.

EDERY H. (1968) New test for biological identification of bradykinin. *Nature* **217,** 70.

FERRIERA S. H. & VANE J. R. (1967) The detection and estimation of bradykinin in circulating blood. *British Journal of Pharmacology* **29,** 367.

GADDUM J. H. (1953) The technique of superfusion. *British Journal of Pharmacology* **8,** 321.

GADDUM J. H., PEART W. S. & VOGT M. (1949) The estimation of adrenaline and allied substances in blood. *Journal of Physiology* **108,** 467.

GOODFRIEND T. L. & BALL D. L. (1969) Radioimmunassay of bradykinin: Chemical modification to enable use of radioactive iodine. *Journal of Laboratory and Clinical Medicine* **73,** 501.

GREAVES M. W. & SONDERGAARD J. (1970) Urticaria pigmentosa and factitious urticaria: Direct evidence for release of histamine and other smooth muscle contracting agents in dermographic skin. *Archives of Dermatology* **101,** 418.

GREAVES M. W., SONDERGAARD J. S. & McDONALD-GIBSON W. (1971) Recovery of prostaglandins in human cutaneous inflammation. *British Medical Journal* **2,** 258.

GREEN K. & SAMUELSSON B. (1964) Prostaglandins and related factors. XIX. Thin layer chromatography of prostaglandins. *Journal of Lipid Research* **5,** 117.

HARADA M., TAKEGUCHI M., FUKAO T. & KATAGIRI C. (1971) A simple method for quantitative extraction of dye extravasated into the skin. *Journal of Pharmacy and Pharmacology* **23,** 218.

HENSBY C. (1975) Distribution studies on the reduction of prostaglandin E_2 to prostaglandin $F_{2\alpha}$ by tissue homogenates. *Biochimica and Biophysica Acta* **409,** 225.

OATES J. A., MARSH E. & SJOERDESMA A. (1962) Studies on histamine in human urine using a fluometric method of assay. *Clinica Chimica Acta* **7,** 488.

SCHILD H. O. (1942) A method of conducting a biological assay on a preparation giving repeated graded responses illustrated by the estimation of histamine. *Journal of Physiology* **101,** 115.

SONDERGAARD J. & GREAVES M. W. (1971) Prostaglandin E$_1$. Effect in human cutaneous vasculature and skin histamine. *British Journal of Dermatology* **84,** 424.

VANE J. R. (1964) The use of isolated organs for detecting active substances in the circulating blood. *British Journal of Pharmacology* **23,** 360.

Genetic techniques in dermatology

P. S. HARPER

The hereditary nature of many disorders of the skin, and of some of its normal properties, has been well recognized since long before the principles of Mendelian inheritance became generally accepted. Charles Darwin (1875) was almost certainly describing the X-linked anhidrotic ectodermal dysplasia when recording the 'toothless men of Sind', while the inheritance of skin pigmentation had received much discussion based on the descendants of interracial marriages. With the rediscovery by Bateson and others of Mendel's neglected work, and the equally fundamental recognition by Archibald Garrod (1908) of the concept of 'inborn errors of metabolism', the way was open for both accurate documentation of the pattern of heredity in individual disorders (epitomized by the monograph of Cockayne 1933) and, more gradually, for the elucidation of the precise biochemical nature of the underlying defect. Today the descriptive aspects and the types of inheritance are for the most part well established, but only in a minority of disorders do we have more than a fragmentary knowledge of the molecular processes involved. This Chapter outlines some of the different forms of genetic investigation that may prove fruitful in investigating the molecular basis of hereditary skin disease. None is exclusively or even predominantly the tool of the geneticist, but when used in conjunction with other techniques the genetic approach has already shown itself of value in the accurate definition and separation of the fundamental biochemical basis of these disorders.

The basic patterns of inheritance

Simple Mendelian inheritance, whether autosomal dominant, autosomal recessive or X-linked recessive, gives characteristic pedigree patterns which mostly need no description here. Some of the less common types may, however, be overlooked or mistaken, as the following examples show (see Fig. 8.1):

X-linked dominant inheritance, eg keratosis follicularis spinula decalvans (see Fig. 8.1 B). This can be easily mistaken for autosomal dominant inheritance, but the offspring of affected males provide the distinction—all sons are unaffected, all daughters affected.

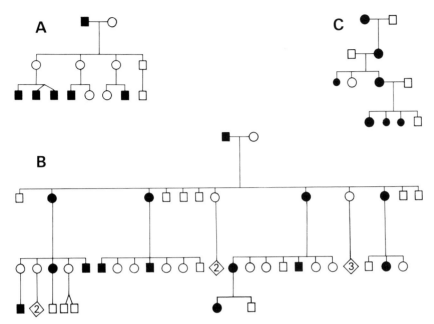

Fig. 8.1 X-linkage in inherited skin disorders; A, X-linked recessive inheritance (X-linked ichthyosis) (after Miller 1973); B, X-linked dominant inheritance (keratosis follicularis spinulosa decalvans) (after Jonkers 1950; Waardenburg 1963); C, X-linked dominant inheritance lethal in the male (focal dermal hypoplasia) (after Goltz *et al* 1962).

X-linked dominant inheritance, lethal in the male, e.g. focal dermal hypoplasia (see Fig. 8.1 C) incontinentia pigmenti. Here the disorder is generally seen in females alone, but there is an altered male: female ratio (1:2) of live births, and an excess of spontaneous abortions presumed, though not so far proven to represent the hemizygous affected males.

Sex limited inheritance: here the expression of a major autosomal gene is influenced by sex; eg early baldness, inherited in many families as an autosomal dominant trait, is usually expressed only in the male. In contrast to X-linkage, transmission is seen from male to male.

Y-linked inheritance: in addition to its primary role in determination of gonadal sex, the Y-chromosome is known to carry genes influencing stature and histocompatibility status. No major genes have conclusively been shown to be Y-linked in man, but the only two possibilities have both been dermatological; transmission in Y-linked inheritance must be strictly along the male line of descent. The first, ichthyosis hystrix gravior in the Lambert family, 'the porcupine men', was for many years considered to be an example of Y-linkage, but was shown not to have solely male to male transmission when reinvestigated by Penrose and Stern (1958); the second, the occurrence of hairy pinnae (Dronmraju 1965) is also under doubt both because of variable expression in the male and as possibly being secondarily influenced by hormonal factors in the female.

Turning from the single gene to quantitative or 'polygenic' inheritance, the skin provides two of the clearest examples of genes with additive effect. Skin colour in the offspring of interracial marriages was the first human character to which the principles of polygenic inheritance were applied (Davenport 1913); the original hypothesis of two loci has required expansion to the involvement of at least five loci (Stern 1970) producing a range of phenotypes which appear continuous in a population, but which may give a sharply discontinuous distribution within a single family. The problems of accurate measurement and of environmental influences are discussed by Harrison (1973). The inheritance of dermal ridge patterns (Holt 1968) follows almost exactly that predicted for a characteristic controlled by a large number of genes and a negligible environmental component; the correlation coefficient between identical twins is +0.95, while that for both non-identical twins and for sibs is +0.49. Study of dermatoglyphic abnormalities has so far proved of more value in chromosomal disorders and limb abnormalities than in primary disorders of skin (Miller 1973).

In general, few of the common normal variations are determined by single major genes, a possible exception being red hair, which when strictly defined follows autosomal recessive inheritance in some families.

The Lyon hypothesis

Many X-linked characters show an unusual patchy mode of expression in the heterozygous female, a phenomenon originally studied by Lyon (1961) in the genes controlling coat-colour in mice and other mammals, but subsequently found to be of almost universal application in human X-linked traits as well. In early embryonic life one of the two X-chromosomes of female cells becomes inactivated becoming visible as the sex chromatin or Barr body. For a female heterozygous for an X-linked trait all descendants of a particular cell will show the same X-chromosome inactivated and thus such a female is essentially a mosaic, with small patches of tissue showing of action of the different X-chromosomes. This patchy distribution is seen most clearly in the variegated pattern of coat colour in animals heterozygous for X-linked colour genes, but it is also shown in human females heterozygous for disorders such as ocular albinism, where the fundi show patchy depigmentation, and in skin disorders such as anhidrotic ectodermal dysplasia, where the heterozygote may show patchy reduction in sweat glands (Verbov 1970) dermatoglyphic changes (Verbov 1972) and minor dental abnormalities. It also explains the generally greater variability seen in females heterozygous for X-linked as opposed to autosomal recessive disorders, since some females will by chance have an abnormally high proportion of their cells with the abnormal X-chromosome active, while others will have a relatively low proportion. This creates practical problems in the detection of carriers for such important X-linked disorders as haemophilia and Duchenne muscular dystrophy.

Direct biochemical confirmation of X-chromosome inactivation in the human female has now been obtained for several loci. Cultured cells have been cloned from females heterozygous for glucose-6-phosphate dehydrogenase electrophoretic variants (Davidson *et al* 1963) and for the X-linked Hurler (type II) mucopolysaccharidosis (Danes & Bearn 1966). In each case separate clones of normal and abnormal cells could be obtained, each breeding true— confirming both the existence and the permanence in cell culture of X-inactivation. The only X-linked locus in man that does not appear to be subject to X-inactivation is that controlling the Xg blood groups. (Ducos *et al* 1971)

Mapping of the genes

Only within the past decade has the human gene map become a reality. Previously chromosomal assignment was possible only for X-linked genes, and there was no information as to which of the 22 pairs of autosomes a particular gene might be located on. The combined use of a number of techniques has changed this situation:

1   The recognition of numerous simply inherited and polymorphic blood group, serum protein and red cell enzyme systems, which can be used as marker loci to test for genetic linkage both with other markers and with inherited disorders (Giblett 1969). Thus the nail-patella syndrome shows linkage with the ABO blood-group system (Renwick & Lawler 1955) and the enzyme adenylate kinase (Schleuterman *et al* 1969).

2   Developments in cytogenetic technique. The new fluorescent and Giemsa banding techniques, unlike the older Orcein staining of chromosomes, allow each chromosome to be distinguished with confidence. The fluorescent method, developed originally by Caspersson on plant material, makes use of the banded pattern of fluorescence shown under u.v. light after staining with quinacrine mustard and related substances (Caspersson *et al* 1970). The Giemsa methods, which have largely replaced the fluorescent methods on account of their simplicity, produce a similar pattern of transverse banding when Giemsa stain is used following partial denaturation with trypsin. Although the precise mechanism underlying the banding is not understood, the banding pattern is constant and specific for each chromosome and forms the basis of the current international classification of the human karyotype (Paris Conference 1971). In addition to the accurate recognition of individual chromosomes it is possible to show minor rearrangements and variations in morphology which are often harmless and which show simple Mendelian inheritance. Deletion of a small chromosome segment may give rise to anomalous inheritance of a marker located in that segment. In this way the genetic marker acid phosphatase was located on chromosome 2 (Ferguson-Smith *et al* 1973), along with the MN blood group system and the form of sclerotylosis described by Huriez *et al* (1968) which was already known to be closely linked to the MN system.

3   Cell hybridization. The discovery that hybrid cells could be induced between different cell strains and even different species (Harris & Watkins 1965; Ephrussi 1972) has had a profound impact on cell biology. Cell fusion may occur spontaneously at a low frequency in tissue culture, but can be increased considerably by such agents as Sendai virus, while the use of selective

nutrient media which permit growth of hybrid cells but not of either parent strain enhances the detection of such hybrid cell lines as do occur (Littlefield 1966). The chromosomes of the hybrid cells are usually enclosed within a single nuclear envelope, undergo synchronous division of both chromosome complements, and in general, show a remarkable degree of normal cell function while continuing to produce enzymes and other cell products characteristic of the parental cells. Aspects of cell hybridization concerning neoplasia will be discussed later, but the application of the technique in chromosome mapping arises from the orderly and sequential loss of human chromosomes from the hybrid cell line during continued cell divisions. When the loss of a particular chromosome can be correlated with loss of a specific human enzyme, one can infer that the enzyme is normally born on that chromosome or part of that chromosome. In this way the gene for thymidine kinase was localized to chromosome 17 in man (Migeon & Miller 1968) and numerous other human enzymes have since been assigned by a similar approach (Ruddle & Chen 1973). Partial loss of a chromosome can be used for more precise localization of a gene: α-galactosidase, the enzyme deficient in Fabry's disease has been located on a particular region of the short arm of the X-chromosome, (Pearson *et al* 1974) X-linkage already being known from pedigree data.

It is likely that known linkages will soon be sufficiently numerous and close to allow their use as predictors of disease, as can already be done to a limited extent for the disorder myotonic dystrophy (Harper 1974). Details of the rapidly evolving human gene map are given in the National Foundation symposia on the subject (Bergsma 1974) and in McKusick's invaluable catalogue, *Mendelian Inheritance in Man* (1975).

The cultured skin fibroblast in inherited metabolic disease

Our knowledge of the biochemical basis of many inherited metabolic disorders, some involving the skin but others without dermatological aspects, has been greatly increased by the discovery that the cultured skin fibroblast expresses the majority of enzymes which are responsible for inborn errors of metabolism, in addition to these enzymes involved in collagen synthesis which are most directly related to its special function. In particular all the known lysosomal enzymes are expressed in the cultured fibroblast, as are most enzymes of amino-acid, lipid and carbohydrate metabolism, and some more specialized systems, such as the enzymes of haem biosynthesis. There are notable exceptions, such as phenylketonuria and alkaptonuria, in which the relevant enzymes (phenylalanine hydroxylase and homogentisic acid oxidase) are confined to the liver, and it cannot be assumed that an enzyme present in intact skin is similarly present in the cultured fibroblast. Thus histidase, the enzyme deficient in histidinaemia, is confined to epithelial cells and is absent in the cultured fibroblast (Barnhisel *et al* 1970); conversely cystathionine synthetase, deficient in homocystinuria, is not found at significant concentrations in intact skin but is present in the cultured fibroblast (Uhlendorf & Mudd 1968).

Probably the best example of the application of cell culture techniques to this field has been the work of Neufeld and her colleagues on the mucopolysaccharidoses. Here cultured skin fibroblasts from affected individuals show mucopolysaccharide accumulation which can be measured by incorporation of inorganic S^{35} sulphate. Neufield and Cantz (1971) found that cells grown together from patients with different forms of mucopolysaccharidosis showed normal S^{35} uptake—the cells had corrected each other presumably as a result of each cell line possessing a factor lacked by the other. No correction was shown between most cell lines from patients with the same clinical type of mucopolysaccharidosis, confirming that both were lacking in the same factor. Extension of this work not only confirmed the biochemical specificity of the main types of mucopolysaccharidosis already delineated, but showed that in some instances heterogeneity existed within each group, eg in type III (Sanfilippo syndrome) where two types were demonstrated on the basis of correction studies and were later confirmed to have a different enzymatic basis despite producing an identical clinical syndrome. Conversely two types of mucopolysaccharidosis thought on clinical grounds to be distinct (Hurler, type I and Scheie, type V) were shown by cell culture studies to show no crosscorrection and were later shown to have deficiency of the same enzyme, α-L-iduronidase (Bach *et al* 1972).

In many groups of inherited dermatological disorder heterogeneity remains unproven at a biochemical level, despite clinical, histological and genetic evidence of its existence. The ichthyoses, the group of palmo-plantar hyperkeratoses and the epidermolysis bullosa group, are cases in point, and with increasing biochemical knowledge genetic heterogeneity has become the rule rather than the exception. In the absence of a clear biochemical basis it is essential that the genetic evidence from pedigree patterns and linkage analysis is taken into account. Thus, in any investigation on ichthyosis it would be most unwise to combine data from patients with the autosomal dominant form with data from those showing X-linked transmission, since the existence of two distinct genetic loci clearly implies a different molecular basis for each, even though we remain ignorant of their nature.

The extensive experience available from studying the cultured fibroblast has so far not been matched by culture of epidermal cells, but the development of techniques allowing culture of pure epidermal cell lines in experimental animals should allow a similar approach to normal and diseased human epidermis (Flaxman & Harper 1975). It is likely that such an approach will prove as fruitful in the study of genetic epidermal disorders as the fibroblast has been in the study of more generalized metabolic conditions. It is noteworthy that the great majority of disorders whose metabolic basis is understood are recessively inherited; the acute porphyrias are among the very few dominantly inherited conditions that have been found to have an enzymatic basis (Sassa *et al* 1975); deficiency of a serum complement inhibitory protein is responsible for hereditary angio-oedema (Donaldson & Evans 1963), while an abnormality in a structural protein (keratin) has been reported in the

Clouston type of ectodermal dysplasia (Gold & Scriver 1971). For most dominantly inherited disorders of the skin, as for other systems, we have little or no information regarding the primary biochemical defect.

Prenatal diagnosis in inherited dermatological disorders

For many untreatable genetic disorders, particularly those involving severe mental or physical handicap, diagnosis *in utero,* followed by termination of an affected pregnancy has become a valuable technique in allowing families to reproduce without running the high risk of having an affected child. Since most skin disorders are not lethal, this approach is perhaps generally less appropriate than in, for example, the inherited neurological degenerations of infancy, but already several conditions exist where prenatal diagnosis has a valuable role. Metabolic disorders detectable prenatally by use of the cultured amniotic cell include Fabry's disease (α-galactosidase; Brady *et al* 1971), congenital erythropoietic porphyria (uroporphyrinogen cosynthetase; Romeo *et al* 1970) and xeroderma pigmentosum (endonuclease; Ramsey *et al* 1974). Another group of disorders which may prove recognizable *in utero* is that characterized by areas of skin defect present at birth, as for example focal dermal hypoplasia. Following the discovery of raised α-fetoprotein levels in association with open neural tube defects (Brock & Sutcliffe 1972; Brock 1976), it has become realized that other defects allowing transudation of fetal fluid into the amniotic cavity may show similar high levels, possibly including skin defects such as the above, though no cases have as yet been identified.

Population genetic studies

Inherited skin disorders provide especially suitable examples for the study of the population basis of the transmission and distribution of the abnormal genes, owing to the fact that many of the defects are conspicuous, readily traced in previous generations and often relatively trivial and thus interfering little with reproduction. A classical example is seen in porphyria variegata, studied by Dean (1963) in South Africa. Prior to the introduction of modern anaesthetics and hypnotics this autosomal dominant disorder did not have serious effects in most individuals, and Dean was able to trace all known cases to a single common ancestor originating from Holland in the late seventeenth century. This is an example of the 'founder effect', by which a gene of no particular selective advantage can multiply to a much greater extent than usual, when present in a rapidly expanding population derived from a small number of founding members.

A similar example is seen in the high incidence of the Ellis van Creveld type of ectodermal dysplasia in the Amish communities of Pennsylvania. McKusick *et al* (1964) were able to record more instances in this localized community than had previously been recognized in the entire world literature, and all cases showed common descent from a single founding immigrant from Switzerland in the mid eighteenth century. The Ellis van Creveld syndrome, unlike porphyria variegata, is inherited as an autosomal recessive disorder, and thus the founding member was not himself affected, but a heterozygous carrier. The subsequent frequent occurrence of the disease in homozygous state many generations later is the result not only of the expansion of the population, but of the strict inbreeding practised by the community.

Many small and isolated communities show a high incidence of particular autosomal recessive disorders, resulting from the combined or separate effects of consanguinity, founder effect, and genetic drift. Albinism is a striking example in several such populations, including the San Blas Indians of Panama and certain West African tribes, and conditions occurring in this way provide a valuable record of the genetic structure and origin of the population in question, as well as causing local problems of prevention and control. It is rare that such situations are the direct result of natural selection, in contrast to disorders such as sickle cell disease, where relative resistance of the heterozygote to malarial infection is the major factor in maintaining the frequency of the HbS gene in populations where falciparum malaria is or has been endemic.

Genetic factors in skin cancer

Much previous work on neoplasia affecting the skin and other organs has been concerned with search for extrinsic factors possibly involved in carcinogenesis, and some of these, such as irradiation and chemicals such as benzpyrene, have undoubted importance as causative factors. More recently, emphasis has shifted to the role of intrinsic factors, such as immunological deficiencies, spontaneous somatic mutation and the normal repair processes of the genetic material, and it is now realized that not only may these intrinsic processes play a fundamental part in the causation of neoplasia, but that some of the external factors already recognized may act by disturbance of these intrinsic processes. Burnet (1974) gives a stimulating review of this field.

The skin offers some special advantages for study of the molecular basis of neoplasia. Firstly there exists an unusual number of neoplasms involving skin which show simple Mendelian inheritance, and in which a single basic molecular defect is thus likely to be acting. These are listed in Table 1. It can be seen that while in some, such as the basal cell naevus syndrome, the regular development of skin cancer is an integral part of the disorder, in others, such as the form of palmo-plantar hyperkeratosis (tylosis) with oesophageal cancer, the skin abnormality is more a marker for the development of cancer elsewhere (Howel-Evans *et al* 1958; Harper *et al* 1970). As yet we have no information on why in a small number of families oesophageal cancer occurs in all individuals bearing the abnormal gene while in most families with tylosis there is absolutely no association with visceral malignancy.

A particularly intriguing phenomenon is the occurrence as the result of a single autosomal dominant gene of multiple selfhealing epitheliomas with a histological appearance remarkably similar to the virally-induced keratoacanthoma (Ferguson-Smith *et al* 1971). No viral cause has been implicated in

Table 8.1 Mendelian heredity and neoplasia

A	Neoplasms of skin showing Mendelian inheritance.	Inheritance
	Basal cell naevus syndrome.	AD
	Multiple self healing epithelioma.	AD
	Cylindromatosis.	AD
	Neurofibromatosis.	AD
	Steatocystoma multiplex.	AD
B	Mendelian disorders involving skin, associated with a high incidence of neoplasia.	
	Xeroderma pigmentosum.	AR
	Ataxia telangiectasia.	AR
	Bloom's syndrome.	AR
	Fanconi's anaemia.	AR
	Chediak Higashi syndrome.	AR
	Palmo-plantar hyperkeratosis (tylosis) with oesophageal cancer.	AD
	Pachyonychia congenita.	AD
	Dyskeratosis congenita.	XR

AD = autosomal dominant; AR = autosomal recessive; XR = X-linked recessive

the genetic disorder, but is seems clear that the tissue reaction resulting in these individuals from an intrinsic genetic defect is likely to be closely related to the tissue response seen more commonly in relation to the extrinsic viral factor in keratoacanthoma.

In few of these genetically determined neoplasms has the molecular basis been investigated in detail. No chromosomal abnormality has been found in either the individuals with tylosis and oesophageal cancer or those with selfhealing epithelioma, nor has any immunological abnormality been established in most of the single gene cancers involving skin. Much more information is, however, becoming available on the group of autosomal recessively inherited disorders characterized by a high incidence of neoplasia, and including xeroderma pigmentosum, Bloom's syndrome and ataxia telangiectasia. Xeroderma pigmentosum is the most thoroughly studied of this group, and has been responsible for a major advance in our knowledge of the molecular processes involved in neoplasia, as well as demonstrating that the processes involved in mutation and its repair are essentially the same in man as in microorganisms. The work of Cleaver (1968) was the first to show that skin fibroblasts from patients with xeroderma pigmentosum failed to show the normal response of DNA synthesis following exposure to ultraviolet light as measured autoradiographically by uptake of tritiated thymidine. Subsequent work (Cleaver 1973) has shown that the specific step involved is the excision of a DNA strand involved in a thymine dimer, normally performed by an endonuclease, and that the accumulation of genetic errors resulting from the persistence of such dimers is likely to be directly related to the occurrence of malignancies in light exposed areas that is the hallmark of this disorder. The abnormality can be detected in infancy before skin lesions appear, and prenatally in early pregnancy by use of cultured amniotic cells (Ramsey *et al* 1974).

The discovery of a specific DNA repair defect in xeroderma pigmentosum has led to intense interest in the possibility of other disorders being the result of similar repair failures, as well as to analysis of the normal repair processes of human cells. Although the evidence remains fragmentary, it is sufficient to indicate that a family of inborn errors of metabolism relating to these processes probably exists, with tendency to neoplasia, premature ageing and photosensitivity as major clinical features. Disorders under investigation at present include progeria, Cockayne's syndrome, porokeratosis of Mibelli and Werner's syndrome. There is already clear evidence that xeroderma pigmentosum itself is heterogeneous, since some cases fail to show the expected excision repair defect (Cleaver 1972). An abnormality of the related repair stage of photoreactivation has been reported in such variants (Sutherland & Oliver 1975). Crosscorrection studies on cultured cells analogous to those already described for the mucopolysaccharidoses have shown that at least four groups exist between which crosscorrection of the metabolic defect occurs, suggesting different enzymatic steps deficient for each group (Robbins *et al* 1974). Heterogeneity is also evident at a clinical level since in some families mental subnormality and other neurological problems are associated with the skin disorder (De Sanctis-Cacchione syndrome).

Further evidence of the involvement of DNA repair processes in neoplasia comes from studies on other recessively inherited disorders showing a high incidence of lymphoid tumours and leukaemias, and including ataxia telangiectasia, Bloom's syndrome and Fanconi's anaemia (German 1973). All show a high incidence of chromosomal breaks and rearrangements in both white blood cells and fibroblasts, with the emergence of specific abnormal clones of cells which may be precursors of actual malignancies. In ataxia telangiectasia a specific region of chromosome 14 appears to be consistently involved in such clones (Oxford *et al* 1975) and both cultured cells and the whole patient show an unusual degree of radiosensitivity. The chromosome abnormalities are not seen at birth but steadily increase with age, suggesting an underlying chromosal instability, though as yet no specific defect of DNA repair has been found.

The cytogenetic studies on ataxia telangiectasia and related disorders raise for the first time the possibility of identification of specific genetic loci or chromosomal regions which may be particularly concerned with the development of cancer, or in the protective mechanisms which normally act in preventing it. Further exploration of this area has been made possible by the application of cell hybridization studies as mentioned above. Many cell cultures possess some of the features of malignancy, including aneuploid chromosome complement and unrestrained and indefinite cell growth, and it has been shown that hybridization may reverse such changes under certain circumstances (Ephrussi 1972). Study of hybrids containing a limited number of human chromosomes gives the opportunity of identifying those which play a key role in these processes.

The clonal origin of tumours has been the subject of debate for many years, and has recently been studied by applying the principle of X-chromosome inactivation already discussed. Tumours occurring in females heterozygous for glucose-6-phosphate dehydrogenase variants have been analysed electrophoretically to determine whether one or both variants are present in the tumour cells (Beutler *et al* 1967). In the case of epidermal carcinoma of the cervix, Bowen's disease of the vulva and chronic myeloid leukaemia only one variant was found in the tumour tissue, supporting a unicentric origin from a single cell line (Smith *et al* 1971); in other tumours such as hepatoma and adenocarcinoma of breast and colon, both types were consistently present, supporting a multicentric origin. Wider study of skin tumours by this approach will be of considerable interest, though consideration must be given to the possibility of reactivation of the second X-chromosome occurring in tumour cells (Straub *et al* 1969).

REFERENCES

BACH G., FRIEDMAN R., WEISSMANN B. & NEUFELD E. F. (1972) The defect in the Hurler and Scheie syndromes: deficiency of a α-L-iduronidase. *Proceedings of the National Academy of Science USA* **69,** 2048.

BARNHISEL M. L., PRIEST R. E. & PRIEST J. H. (1970) Histidase function in human epithelial cells. *Journal of Cell Physiology* **76,** 7.

BERGSMA D. (1974) *Human Gene Mapping.* National Foundation, New York.

BEUTLER E., COLLINS Z. & IRWIN L. E. (1967) Value of genetic variants of glucose-6-phosphate dehydrogenase in tracing the origin of malignant tumours. *New England Journal of Medicine* **276,** 398.

BRADY R. D., UHLENDORF B. W. & JACOBSON C. B. (1971) Fabry's disease: antenatal detection. *Science* **172,** 174.

BROCK G. J. H. & SUTCLIFFE R. G. (1972) Alpha-fetoprotein in the antenatal diagnosis of anencephaly and spina bifida. *Lancet* **ii,** 197.

BROCK D. J. H. (1976) Prenatal diagnosis—chemical methods. *British Medical Bulletin* **32,** 16.

BURNET F. M. (1974) *Intrinsic Mutagenesis.* Medical and Technical Publishing Co., Lancaster.

CASPERSON T., ZECH L., JOHANSSON C. & MODEST E. J. (1970) Identification of human chromosomes by DNA binding fluorescent agents. *Chromosoma* **30,** 215.

CLEAVER J. E. (1968) Defective repair replication of DNA in xeroderma pigmentosum. *Nature* **218,** 652.

CLEAVER J. E. (1972) Xeroderma pigmentosum: variants with normal DNA repair and normal sensitivity to ultraviolet light. *Journal of Investigative Dermatology* **58,** 124.

CLEAVER J. E. (1973) Xeroderma pigmentosum—progress and regress. *Journal of Investigative Dermatology* **60,** 374.

COCKAYNE E. A. (1933) *Inherited Abnormalities of the Skin and its Appendages.* Oxford University Press, London.

DANES B. S. & BEARN A. G. (1966) Hurler's syndrome. A genetic study in cell culture. *Journal of Experimental Medicine* **123,** 1.

DARWIN C. (1875) *The Evolution of Animals and Plants under Domestication.* John Murray, London.

DAVENPORT C. B. (1913) *Heredity of Skin Color in Negro-White Crosses.* Carnegie Institute, Washington D.C.

DAVIDSON R. G., NITOWSKY H. M. & CHILDS B. (1963) Demonstration of two populations of cells in the human female heterozygous for glucose-6-phosphate dehydrogenase variants. *Proceedings of the National Academy of Science,* **50,** 481.

DEAN G. (1963) *The Porphyrias. A Story of Inheritance and Environment.* Lippincott, Philadelphia.

DONALDSON V. H. & EVANS R. R. (1963) A biochemical abnormality in hereditary angioneurotic oedema. Absence of serum inhibitor of $C^1$1-esterase. *American Journal of Medicine* **35,** 37.

DRONMRAJU K. (1965) The function of the Y chromosome in man, animals and plants. *Advanced Genetics* **13,** 227.

DUCOS J., MORTY Y., SANGER R. & RACE R. R. (1971) Xg and X chromosome inactivation. *Lancet* **ii,** 219.

EPHRUSSI B. (1972) *Hybridization of Somatic Cells.* Princeton University Press, New Jersey.

FERGUSON-SMITH M. A., WALLACE D. C., JAMES Z. H. & RENWICK J. H. (1971) Multiple self-healing squamous epithelioma. *Birth defects original article series* **7,** 157.

FERGUSON-SMITH M. A., NEWMAN B. F., ELLIS P. M., THOMSON D. M. G. & RILEY I. D. (1973) Assignment by deletion of human red cell acid phosphatase gene locus to the short arm of chromosome 2. *Nature New Biology* **243,** 271.

FLAXMAN B. A. & HARPER R. A. (1975) Primary cell culture for biochemical studies of human keratinocytes. *British Journal Dermatology* **92,** 305.

GARROD A. E. (1908) Inborn errors of metabolism. Croonian lectures. *Lancet* **ii,** 1.

GERMAN J. (1973) Genetic disorders associated with chromosomal instability and cancer. *Journal of Investigative Dermatology* **60,** 427.

GIBLETT E. R. (1969) *Genetic Markers in Human Blood.* Blackwell, Oxford.

GOLD R. J. M. & SCRIVER C. R. (1971) The characterisation of hereditary abnormalities of Keratin: Clouston's ectodermal dysplasia. *Birth defects original article series* **7,** 91.

GOLTZ R. W., PETERSON W. C., GORLIN R. J. & RAVITZ H. G. (1962) Focal Dermal Hypoplasia. *Archives of Dermatology* **86,** 708.

HARPER P. S., HARPER R. M. J. & HOWEL-EVANS A. W. (1970) Carcinoma of the oesophagus with tylosis. *Quarterly Journal of Medicine* **39,** 317.

HARPER P. S. (1974) Myotonic dystrophy: some genetic problems. *Birth defects original articles series* **10,** 120.

HARRIS H. & WATKINS J. F. (1965) Hybrid cells derived from mouse and man: artificial heterokaryons of mammalian cells from different species. *Nature* **205,** 640.

HARRISON G. A. (1973) Differences in human pigmentation: measurement, geographic variation and causes. *Journal of Investigative Dermatology* **60,** 418.

HOLT S. (1968) *The Genetics of Dermal Ridges.* Thomas, Springfield.

HOWEL-EVANS A. W., MCCONNELL R. B., CLARKE C. A. & SHEPPARD P. M. (1958) Carcinoma of the oesophagus with keratosis palmaris et plantaris (tylosis): a study of two families. *Quarterly Journal of Medicine* **27,** 413.

HURIEZ C., DEMINATTI M., AGACHE P. & MENNÉCIER M. (1968) Une génodysplasie non encore individualisée. *Semaine des Hopitaux de Paris* **44,** 481.

JONKERS G. H. (1950) Hyperkeratosis follicularis and corneal degeneration. *Ophthalmologica* **120,** 365.

LITTLEFIELD J. (1966) The use of drug resistant markers to study the hybridisation of mouse fibroblasts. *Experimental Cell Research* **41,** 190.

LYON M. (1961) Gene action in the X chromosome of the mouse (Mus musculus L.). *Nature* **190,** 372.

MCKUSKICK V. A., EGELAND J. A., ELDRIDGE R. & KRUSEN D. E. (1964) Dwarfism in the Amish, the Ellis van Creveld syndrome. *Bulletin of Johns Hopkins Hospital* **115,** 306.

MCKUSICK V. A. (1975) *Mendelian Inheritance in Man.* Johns Hopkins University Press, Baltimore.

MIGEON B. R. & MILLER C. S. (1968) Human-mouse somatic cell hybrids with single human chromosome (group E): link with thymidine kinase activity. *Science* **162,** 1005.

MILLER J. R. (1973) Dermatoglyphics. *Journal of Investigative Dermatology* **60**, 435.

NEUFELD E. F. & CANTZ M. J. (1971) Corrective factors for inborn errors of mucopoly-saccharide metabolism. *Annals of the New York Academy of Science* **179**, 580.

OXFORD J. M., HARNDEN D. G., PARRINGTON J. M. & DELHARTY J. D. A. (1975) Specific chromosome aberrations in ataxia telangiectasia. *Journal of Medical Genetics* **12**, 251.

PARIS CONFERENCE (1971) Standardisation in human cytogenetics. *Birth defects original article series* **8**, 7.

PEARSON P. L., VAN DER LINDEN G. & HAGEMEIJER A. (1974) In *Human Gene Mapping,* ed. Bergsma D. National Foundation, New York.

PENROSE L. S. & STERN C. (1958) Reconsideration of the Lambert pedigree (ichthyosis hystrix gravior). *Annals of Human Genetics* **22**, 258.

RAMSEY C. A., COLTART T. M., BLUNT S., RAMSEY S. & GIANELLI F. (1974) Prenatal diagnosis of xeroderma pigmentosum. *Lancet* **ii**, 1109.

RENWICK J. H. & LAWLER S. D. (1955) Genetical linkage between the ABO and nail-patella loci. *Annals of Human Genetics* **19**, 312.

ROBBINS J. H., KRAEMER K. H., LUTZNER M. A., FESTOFF B. W. & COON H. G. (1974) Xeroderma pigmentosum: an inherited disease with sun sensitivity, multiple cutaneous neoplasms and abnormal DNA repair. *Annals of Internal Medicine* **80**, 221.

ROMEO G., KABACK M. M. & LEVIN E. Y. (1970) Uroporphyrinogen 3 cosynthetase activity in fibroblasts from patients with congenital erythropoietic porphyria. *Biochemical Genetics* **4**, 659.

RUDDLE F. H. & CHEN T. R. (1973) Gene assignment by somatic cell genetics. *Journal of Investigative Dermatology* **60**, 399.

SASSA S., SOLISH G., LEVERE R. D. & KAPPAS A. (1975) Studies in porphyria. *Journal of Experimental Medicine* **142**, 722.

SCHLEUTERMANN D. A., BIAS W. B., MURDOCH J. L. & McKUSICK V. A. (1969) Linkage of the loci for the nail-patella syndrome and adenylate kinase. *American Journal of Human Genetics* **21**, 606.

SMITH J. W., TOWNSEND D. E. & SPARKES R. S. (1971) Glucose-6-phosphate dehydrogenase polymorphism: a valuable tool to study tumour origin. *Clinical Genetics* **2**, 160.

STERN C. (1970) Model estimates of the number of gene pairs involved in pigmentation variability of the Negro-American. *Human Heredity* **20**, 165.

STRAUB D. G., LUCAS L. A., McMAHON N. J., PELLETT O. L. & TEPLITZ R. L. (1969) Apparent reversal of X-condensation mechanism in tumours. *Cancer Research* **29**, 1233.

SUTHERLAND B. M. & OLIVER R. (1975) Low levels of photoreactivating enzyme in xeroderma pigmentosum variants. *Nature* **257**, 312.

UHLENDORF B. W. & MUDD S. H. (1968) Cystathionine synthase in tissue culture from human skin; defect in homocystinuria. *Science* **160**, 1007.

VERBOV J. (1970) Hypohidrotic (or anhidrotic) ectodermal dysplasia—an appraisal of diagnostic methods. *British Journal of Dermatology* **83**, 341.

VERBOV J. (1972) Hypohidrotic ectodermal dysplasia: unusual palmprint in a heterozygote. *British Journal of Dermatology* **88**, 92.

WAARDENBURG P. J. (1963) *Genetics and Ophthalmology.* Vol. II. Royal Van Gorcum, Amsterdam.

9

Design and conduct of dermatological trials

R. MARKS

It is often said now, somewhat cynically, that it was not necessary to construct a clinical trial to convince people of the usefulness of penicillin. However, it should be noted that with the advent of the 'Medicines Commission', it is certain that if penicillin were discovered now, clinical trials would be required before it could become registered. (Some in the pharmaceutical industry seriously doubt whether penicillin would ever have become registered had the Medicines Commission existed at that time!)

It is not generally appreciated how much information can be obtained from a well designed and executed trial. It is not only questions concerning the efficacy of particular compounds or total preparations that may be answered but also questions concerning the pathogenesis or aetiology of particular disorders. In addition, subsidiary enquiries can be made such as the incidence of side-effects or level of general acceptability of the preparation to patients. Most of the points to be made concerning clinical trials are plain common sense, but it is surprising just how many people involved in clinical trials forget them. The most important part of any study is in the planning and design stage. It must be firmly kept in mind that the object of the exercise is to obtain an answer to the question posed. The only way in which this end can be accomplished is by sticking to the 'rules' imposed by the design. The clinical trial is as much an experiment as any laboratory procedure. If during the course of an experiment a laboratory worker decided to add a little zest to his day by including gerbils, goats and geese in an experiment in which all the tests were designed for guinea pigs and in which all previous results had been obtained in guinea pigs, then clearly the overall result would be meaningless. The same principles apply to clinical trials. Before entering further into discussion about clinical trials some other general points should be made.

GENERAL POINTS

Questions asked

The first concerns the number of questions to be asked in a clinical trial. It is worthwhile trying to limit these as stringently as possible. It is very easy to

117

become obsessed by the desire to answer all possible enquiries. It is not difficult to be manoeuvred into asking whether 'the wonder drug' in question will also be effective in different concentrations (or doses) or whether it will be effective for other diseases beside the complaint for which it was designed or whether it is more or less effective than yesterday's (and the day before yesterday's) wonder drug(s). It is possible to obtain all this kind of information from a single clinical trial but the more questions that are posed the more the design becomes impossibly complicated. In these circumstances the study often founders because of the difficulties. It is better to conduct a series of studies rather than become bogged down trying to accomplish too much in one study.

Numbers of patients

The second general point is in the nature of another caution—this time concerning numbers of patients. Most clinicians seem to have a rather hazy view of the actual number of patients that they see with a particular disease over say a period of 1 month. The tendency is to be grossly over optimistic and to suggest that three times as many patients with disease 'X' are seen than actually are. Consequently if the trial is designed specifically to treat patients with disease 'X' the trial will take three times longer than originally estimated! Experienced clinical investigators and clinical trials officers in pharmaceutical houses are only too aware of this curious 'disappearing patient syndrome'.

Controls and placebos

Many diseases remit spontaneously and unpredictably and unless an identical group of patients to the test group are observed, then it is impossible to know whether any improvement is a result of the therapy or the result of the natural history of the disease process. For many reasons it has become practice to administer placebo preparations to the control group so as to minimize conscious or unconscious bias from both patient and investigator. This may not be quite so easy as it sounds—especially in some trials of topical agents as the placebo material itself may have a pharmacological action (Tree & Marks 1975). Curiously and regardless of any 'pharmacological' effect that a placebo might have, placebo preparations do appear to possess quite appreciable therapeutic qualities. This has been a notable feature of trials of tetracycline in the treatment of acne (Lane & Williamson 1969) and may be one reason why tetracycline itself has often appeared to produce a relatively small improvement in clinical trials in acne. When a placebo is built into the study then of course it has to be as near a perfect replica of the active drug in appearance, smell and taste as possible. This ideal may not always be attained because of special properties of the active ingredient. For example, if an assessment of the effectiveness of topically applied tetracycline were to be made then difficulties would be experienced in the preparation of a placebo that had the same distinctive colour of tetracycline. Similarly, if two tablet preparations containing active compounds are to be contrasted and their effective dosage is considerably different, then difficulty may be experienced in ensuring that these two drugs are matched in size and appearance both with each other and a placebo.

Assessments

A particular difficulty with dermatological trials is the assessment of change in the patient's disease. Treating psoriasis is not like treating anaemia where a measure of haemoglobin concentration can be used as an indicator of improvement, or like treating peptic ulceration in which there is a good correlation between pain and gastric acid output—which can be measured. There is as yet no adequate way of accurately measuring many of the clinical features of common dermatoses—the extent of the involvement of the skin surface, their redness, scaliness, swelling, ooziness and so on. Inevitably the investigator is driven to constructing some kind of arbitrary scale for the particular features that he most wants to evaluate. This is quite acceptable providing that the arbitrary nature of the scale does not vary from patient to patient or from day to day in the same patient.

If possible, one investigator should be responsible for allotting scores on the arbitrary scale or if it is unavoidable that more than one assessor is involved, then care has to be taken that they are using the identical scales and arbitrary criteria for scoring. One other precaution must be taken when employing arbitrary scales and that is in the statistical handling of the results. The distribution of scores for a particular feature may well be skewed, given 'the population of lesions' in question and, therefore, not suitable for simple statistics. Special 'non-parametric' statistical tests must be employed in this situation.

Whenever possible, advantage should be taken of techniques that avoid possible observer error. More and more methods are becoming available for the accurate evaluation of skin function and the quantitation of abnormalities. The measurement of sebum secretion, sweat secretion, sensitivity to ultraviolet light or itch threshold are now quite well established procedures and should be used whenever possible.

Techniques are also becoming available for the measurement of erythema and for the assessment of scaliness. Although this is not the place for a detailed discussion concerning these techniques a few words should be said concerning them. The assessment of erythema has always bedevilled dermatologists and it should not be imagined that many of the problems have now been solved. Several instruments have been developed for this function and basically they all depend on either comparison with a colour produced by a combination of filters or on reflection spectrophotometry. The most useful instrument at the time of writing appears to be the 'Tintometer' which in our hands is capable of yielding reproducible results and discriminating quite small changes in colour. It is often said that the human eye is the most sensitive instrument for colour comparison. This may be true, but because 'colour memory' is not good then it only applies to comparison between coloured objects seen at one point in time.

Furthermore because it is a qualitative and not a quantitative assessment it is difficult to assess degrees of alteration and to usefully record the observations. As far as 'scaliness' is concerned we have attempted to measure this by using surface contour analysis of skin surface replicas (Nicholls *et al* 1977).

Finally, a cautionary note must be sounded concerning the photographic evaluation of clinical conditions. Unless the possible variables are strictly controlled, photographic assessment can be very misleading. Variables include, camera aperture, patient camera distance, lighting, film, background, development chemicals, development time, enlargement factors and printing paper.

ETHICS OF CLINICAL TRIALS

The only real safeguard for the ethical conduct of clinical studies of any kind is the responsible, compassionate and thoughtful behaviour of the clinical investigator. To obtain 'informed consent' from the participants is not enough. Patients have a child-like belief that their 'doctor' would under no circumstances do anything harmful or withhold treatment known to be effective for their complaint. They will agree only too readily to 'help' in a 'little study' that is being done. There really is no answer to the problem of the recruitment of patients for clinical trials other than the good sense of the investigator. Luckily in most dermatological trials serious ethical problems rarely arise. Clearly the acquisition of knowledge for the 'greater good' can only partially solve the investigator's conscience and the ethical quality of the study. The important consideration is whether the individual patient suffers appreciable harm (of any kind) from the study proposed. The operative word here is 'harm'. Virtually all clinical trials involve the patient in attending the clinic more often than absolutely necessary (which may involve the expense of fares and loss of work). Many require observations and procedures that would otherwise not be required. Furthermore, in the majority of trials these days all or a group of the patients will receive an inactive placebo at some stage in their complaint. Incidentally, some regard it as wrong not to include the most potent preparation available for the particular condition as the control preparation. It is clear from the foregoing that patients who cooperate will at the least suffer a certain amount of inconvenience and this must be kept to a minimum.

It is the practice of most hospitals to insist that all studies involving human subjects (normal volunteers as well as patients) are scrutinized and approved by an 'ethics committee' before being allowed to proceed. Many regulatory bodies insist on the written permission of all participants and some require that the document is witnessed by an independent and disinterested third person. The 'third person' or 'patient's friend' is quite a good way of ensuring that no undue pressure is put on the patient to secure his recruitment. Incidentally, it is reasonable to refund out of pocket expenses but financial inducements for patients ought not to be offered as they constitute 'undue pressure'.

In general clinicals trials on young children, the very old, the mentally sick and the severely subnormal should only be undertaken after the most stringent consideration of the dangers, difficulties and possible benefits. Even if the 'equation' comes down on the side of 'proceed' it is mandatory to seek advice concerning the question of 'consent'. All who want to start a clinical trial are strongly advised to read the Declaration of Helsinki which is contained in an excellent article in the WHO chronicle (1976). Another article worthy of consideration is one by Dollery (1977).

TRIALS OF TOPICAL AGENTS

There are a number of special considerations which apply to trials of topical agents. In particular, it is possible to compare the active and placebo preparation simultaneously in the same patient by treating some lesions with one and some with the other preparation. This has been particularly applied to conditions which symmetrically affect the arms and legs or hands and feet and is, for example, suitable for testing patients with psoriasis or 'chronic hand eczema'. However, this type of trial does have drawbacks. Firstly there is the question of patient compliance—the more complicated the instructions the less likely are they to be followed. Consequently, even the most helpful patient may occasionally become confused and put ointment A where ointment B should be and vice versa (some just do not seem to be able to distinguish left from right).

Secondly, there is the problem of 'ointment crossover'. It has been shown that it is virtually impossible to 'isolate' one ointment treated area from another. Some degree of contamination is almost invariable, so that the ointment A site may unintentionally receive a little of ointment B and vice versa—no matter the precautions taken. Then there is the problem of 'non-homogeneity of lesions'. Theoretically, the fact that the condition may not be entirely symmetrical should even itself out if the treatments are properly randomized and spread over a sufficiently large sized group so that eventually ointments A and B are both tested on a similar population of lesions. However, this may not always be the case and at the end of the trial it is mandatory to check that, for example, all the placebo somehow did not end up on all the worst lesions so that it appears that the 'active' preparation is more active than it actually is.

Lastly, there is the question of absorption of the active ingredient. It is certainly true that active ingredients are absorbed and may reach the placebo treated area, but unless the areas under consideration are quite large (a whole limb for example) it is unlikely that sufficient will be absorbed to have this kind of effect. For all these reasons and despite the halving of numbers of patients and the apparent benefit of using 'each patient as his own control', many experienced trialists do not like this kind of 'laterality study'.

Amount of ointment used

The question of the amount of ointment to be applied frequently crops up. As will be appreciated, the actual dose of the active material delivered to the lesion treated is very difficult to ascertain and in general terms this is a 'bad thing'. Usually the actual amount applied to the lesion is far in excess of that required for the desired effect as it is only that drug held in contact with the lesion at the ointment–lesion interface that is capable of producing any therapeutic effect. Nonetheless, because some ointment may become spread, allowing the ingredient to be absorbed from areas around the lesion, it is wise to indicate just how much ointment should be applied in semiquantitative terms. Often the instructions merely state 'spread thinly to cover the affected areas' and this is probably sufficient. To esure that the materials have been used according to instructions it has become practice to ask the participants in a trial to return the unused ointments at the end, so that the tubes may be weighed and an assessment made as to whether approximately the correct amount was applied or not.

Drop outs

Inevitably in the course of the clinical trial a certain number of patients decide that they prefer the treatment they had previously or just get fed up with the idea of 'being treated as guinea pigs' and decide not to attend the outpatient clinic again. This response is both understandable and invariable in a certain proportion of patients. The actual proportion of 'drops outs' depends on a whole set of factors, many of them intangible. The length of the trial, the number of visits required, the type of assessment at each visit, the degree of improvement achieved and the aesthetic acceptability of the treatment as well as the personality of the investigator are some of the factors that account for the population of patients that do not attend when required. Certainly an analysis of the 'drop outs' is an important check to make, as important and unexpected information can emerge. If 'drop outs' account for an unacceptably large proportion (for example more than 30%) then doubt as to the validity of the findings from the trial must be expected.

Concurrent therapy

It is plainly incorrect to allow the participants in a particular trial to continue to use the treatment that they were previously using or to use some other fresh treatment as well as the trial treatment. The non-uniformity that this freedom would engender in the study would make analysis of the results almost impossible. It may be permissible to allow some other kind of treatment for the patients concurrently, if all individuals in the study receive it. This supplementary treatment must not be anything very potent or anything likely to induce side-effects that confuse the situation with regard to the drug under trial. A bland emollient cleansing preparation may be acceptable as an additional 'treatment' in many dermatological trials as it was in one study of rosacea (Marks & Ellis 1971). It would be totally unacceptable, however, for all individuals in a trial of a new treatment for urticaria to be given one of the antihistamines, as any activity that the new preparation might possess may be swamped.

POINTS ABOUT DESIGN OF CLINICAL TRIALS

Open clinical study

In some circumstances accurate and unbiased documentation of a series of patients treated with the drug under test can give valuable information. Of course, much will depend on the condition treated and the standing of the investigator. This kind of trial is often employed to give preliminary information about the potential usefulness of a preparation.

Controlled clinical trial

In this kind of trial the effect of the test preparation is compared with the effect of another substance the effect of which is well recognized. This control substance can either have a zero activity (ie placebo) or an active material whose potency and other characteristics are well understood and accepted.

Single and double 'blind' controlled trials

We are all biased (consciously or unconsciously). The whole purpose of a clinical trial is to attempt to reach the 'truth' about a drug without bias entering into the judgement, and 'blind' controlled trials are a particular mechanism for this end. In a single blind study the patient does not know whether he is receiving the test or the control material and in a double blind study neither the patient nor investigator knows the identity of the drug that the individual patient is receiving. This type of design has a number of implications. Firstly, there are serious ethical issues which cannot be ducked. The participating patients must give their consent after a full explanation of the nature and the purpose of the study and no pressure of any kind must be used in order to recruit their help (see previously). Secondly, quite a few other individuals are inevitably drawn into the planning and the arranging of the study. Because of the blind nature of the study, the test and the control material should be identical in appearance, taste and smell, and the key as to which patient receives which drug must be held by the pharmacist or by some other permanent stalwart.

Randomization

This ensures that bias does not creep into the selection of patients and that approximately similar types of patients are selected for each treatment group.

There are special randomization tables available to make the selection truly methematically 'random', but for many purposes spinning a coin is an adequate way of ensuring a random distribution.

A 'crossover study'

In this type of trial each patient receives in sequence the test and the control preparation—the actual sequence being determined in most instances by random selection. Thus each patient serves as his own control. This is, of course, not suitable for disorders which will be completely cured on treatment with the active preparation or rapidly fluctuating diseases.

Latin square design

When there is a new treatment (A) that may be superior to a standard therapy (B) either alone or in combination with (B) it is sometimes convenient to arrange the therapy sequentially for each patient, (A, B, AB and O) the actual sequence of therapies being determined by random selection. The number of patients in the study must be divisible by 4. The analysis of this type of result requires special statistical handling but its advantage is that rather fewer patients are required than if there were four separate groups, one per treatment regimen.

Sequential analysis

In this type of trial patients are paired at random and the two therapies (X and Y) under test are allocated at random. The two treatments are assessed as 'X is better', 'Y is better' or 'X and Y are the same'. The result is then entered on to a sequential analysis chart which is modified for the particular study in question, so that when the required degree of significance has been reached the trial

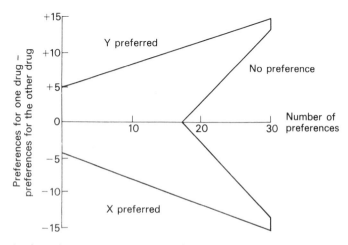

Fig. 9.1 Armitage chart constructed to 5% significant level with 30 paired results.

is stopped. This is obviously 'economic on patients'. Two such types of chart are available and are known as the Bross and Armitage sequential analysis charts (Bross 1952; Armitage 1975). An 'Armitage chart' is shown in Fig. 9.1.

Documentation and recording

It may sound trite to advise the exact reasons for the study should be written down even before attempting to design the trial, but it is essential to have on record the rationale and the specific questions asked. So often a study drags on longer than was planned and the medical personnel change. In these circumstances some kind of written 'protocol' on record is extremely useful. It may also sound somewhat redundant to suggest that it is also mandatory to design 'forms' (proformata) for the recording of the data. There can be few things more annoying than having to analyse the results from a series of scrappy bits of paper and from memory. It is usually convenient to have all the personal data concerning the patient, their 'trial number' and the serial observations all on the same sheet or folder.

ANALYSIS OF RESULTS

This can be quite simple or immensely complex. It is simplest when the results are so clear-cut that statistical handling of the results is completely unnecessary! It is much more difficult (a) when the parameters that have been chosen do not have a simple Gaussian distribution and have to be analysed by non-parametric statistics; (b) when there is only a small difference between the test and control group for the parameters chosen; (c) when there is only a small number of patients; (d) when there are a large number of 'drop outs'; (e) when there are several 'groups', ie several treatments were used as well as the placebo group.

More often than not the clinicians involved in the trial have but the most primitive understanding of statistics and this fact makes itself all too evident in the publications that result. For this reason it should be emphasized that expert help with the statistical analysis is mandatory. In fact, a great deal of time would be saved and far more value could be obtained if statistical advice were taken during the planning stage of the study. The reader is referred to Altman (1977) who gives a useful commentary on the situation.

It should be remembered that an important aspect of the trial record is the number, type and severity of unwanted side-effects. These must be recorded in detail.

STATISTICAL QUAE CLINICAL SIGNIFICANCE

If analysis of the results reveals that the erythema (or scaliness or some other clinical feature) was decreased by a factor of '1' on the arbitrary score it should be obvious that no matter the degree of statistical significance reached the 'improvement' may be of little moment for the patient. This difference between statistical and clinical significance is regrettably not always appreciated. The converse is also true. The remission of a complaint in say 6 out of 12 patients in a test group as opposed to 4 out of 12 in the placebo treated individuals may not reach statistical significance but is highly significant for the two additional patients and may be 'real' in the sense that it did not occur by chance.

REFERENCES

ARMITAGE P. (1975) Sequential Experimentation. In *Sequential Medical Trials*, ed. Armitage P., 2nd edn. Blackwell, Oxford.

ALTMAN D. G. (1977) Statistics in medical papers. *Journal of the Royal College of Physicians* **11**, 274.

BROSS I. (1952) Sequential Medical Plan. *Biometrics* **8**, 188.

Declaration of Helsinki (1976) *WHO Chronicle* **30**, 360.

DOLLERY C. T. (1977) Clinical trials of new drugs. *Journal of the Royal College of Physicians* **11**, 226.

LANE P. & WILLIAMSON D. M. (1969) Treatment of acne vulgaris with tetracycline hydrochloride: a double blind trial with 51 patients. *British Medical Journal* **2**, 76.

MARKS R. & ELLIS J. (1971) Comparative effectiveness of tetracycline and ampicillin in rosacea. *Lancet* ii, 1049.

NICHOLLS S., KING C. S. & MARKS R. (1977) Quantitative and Morphological Evaluation of the Effects of Bath Oil and Emollient on the Stratum Corneum. *Journal of Investigative Dermatology* **68**, 252 (abstract).

TREE S. & MARKS R. (1975) An explanation for the 'Placebo' effect of bland ointment bases. *British Journal of Dermatology* **92**, 195.

FURTHER READING

Aide-memoire for preparing clinical trial protocols. (1977) *British Medical Journal* **2**, 1323.

GOOD, C. S. (1976) *Principles and Practice of Clinical Trials*. Churchill Livingstone, Edinburgh.

HARRIS E. L. & FITZGERALD J. D. (1970) The Principles and Practice of Clinical Trials. E & S Livingstone, Edinburgh.

SWINSCOW T. D. V. (1977) *Statistics at Square One*. British Medical Association, London.

VON FRAUNHOFER J. A. & MURRAY J. J. (1976) *Statistics in Medical, Dental and Biological Studies*. Tri-Med Books Ltd.

10

Measurement of epidermal growth activity

R. MARKS

INTRODUCTION

The epidermis is a constantly self-renewing tissue whose function is the production of a protective but complex outer structure—the stratum corneum. It ought really be thought of as an organ rather than a tissue as it does not consist of just one cell type. However, it is convenient to think of the epidermis as consisting purely of keratinocytes and where this concept conflicts with practical considerations it will be pointed out.

Keratinocytes are generated in the basal layer of the epidermis and to some extent in the immediately suprabasal layer. The anatomical zone of a tissue that is functionally capable of, and responsible for, cell division is known as the *generative compartment*. The proportion of cells in that compartment that are within the time course of one mitotic cycle at any one time is known as the *growth fraction*. As cells are produced either one or both cells move through the epidermis towards the stratum corneum and eventually desquamate at the skin surface as mature corneocytes. For kinetic reasons it is obviously important to know whether both daughter cells stay behind in the basal layer, both ascend or one remains and one ascends. The determining factor for this appears to be the plane of cleavage, ie whether vertical or horizontal to the epidermis (Bullough & Mitrani 1976). This movement towards the surface can be measured by techniques that will be described below. In most situations the more rapid the movement towards the surface the more rapidly cells are being produced in the generative compartment. Thus the shorter the *transit time* the more rapidly keratinocytes are dividing. The process of cell division is known as mitosis and the whole complex but orderly process that the cell undergoes is called the mitotic cycle (see Fig. 10.1). The first part of the mitotic cycle to be considered is the G1 phase (sometimes called interphase). It is the most 'elastic' phase of the cell cycle in that it is capable of considerable variability in length. Very little seems to be taking place in G1 although specific metabolic events certainly take place in the latter part of this section of the mitotic cycle. The next phase is the period when new genetic material (deoxyribonucleic acid—DNA) is synthesized within the nucleus—the synthetic or 'S' phase. During 'S' phase the nucleotide thymidine is incorporated into the DNA and as thymidine does not appear to be utilized in other metabolic pathways this

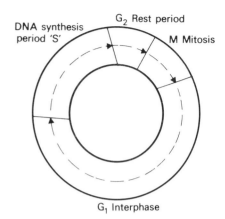

Fig. 10.1 The mitotic cycle.

process can be used as an 'S' phase marker (see below). After the exertions of the synthetic phase the cell 'pauses for breath' for a short time in the phase known as G2. There are some authors who claim that epidermal cells can be 'suspended' indefinitely in the G2 phase (Gelfant 1976) and one must proceed with caution when trying to pinpoint the lengths of individual 'phases' from the autoradiographic labelling index (see below). Immediately following the G2 comes the actual cell cleavage—known as *mitosis* (M phase). During this process there is a rearrangement of nuclear structure and finally the chromosomal DNA divides so that two identical nuclei are produced. Mitosis is conventionally divided into four phases—prophase, anaphase, metaphase and telephase. During prophase the nuclear chromatin network condenses and during anaphase and metaphase it becomes arranged in regular clumps and eventually aligned on the mitotic spindle. In telephase the nucleus is dividing in two. These phases are recognizable in good histological preparations of skin although they may be quite difficult to identify.

The G2 and M phases seem relatively constant in length but the length of 'S' may change within small limits. Some studies have attempted to characterize the individual phase lengths of the mitotic cycle for human epidermis *in vivo* (Weinstein & Frost 1969; Duffil *et al* 1976; Born & Kalkoff 1969). However, disappointingly, these studies have yielded quite different results. It seems quite likely to the writer that the biological variations in these values are quite large in normal epidermis and may be enormous in diseased tissue. In any event the techniques used are actually quite difficult. Nonetheless, a short description of the available methods for phase length determination is included below. Before embarking on a description of the various techniques used in epidermal cell kinetics a few more terms must be defined.

Turnover time is a much used and abused term. It should be accompanied by some constraining description as to whether the term 'turnover' refers to renewal of the whole epidermis or just the generative compartment. The *generation time* refers to the total length of the mitotic cycle.

Sometimes the expression 'G°' is used. This is a theoretical concept to denote cells in the germinative compartment that have opted out (at least temporarily) of the generative process.

Epidermopoiesis is a term used to denote the process of keratinocyte production. Some purists object to this neologism, but as long as all who use it know what it means it seems a convenient portmanteau word without any fundamental objection to its use. It should be appreciated that in life the epidermis is not just simply 'sitting there' as one might get the impression from a study of histological sections but is consistently responding to minor changes in the environment by actively moving and its cells changing in shape. The process of active epidermal cell movement is an essential first step in wound healing (Winter 1972; Rovee *et al* 1972) and is a 'kinetic' process in the true meaning of the word. Active epidermal cell movement (AECM) and mitotic activity seem mutually exclusive but despite the close relationship between these two complementary activities most literary contributions to the consideration of epidermal homeostasis (the processes regulating the constancy of epidermal cell population) or epidermal reactivity appear to ignore AECM. It is true that some writers have considered AECM to be essential in the upward ascent of keratinocytes after mitosis (Etoh *et al* 1975) but it seems likely that 'mitotic pressure' can account for this movement by itself. It is fair to say that the contribution of AECM to everyday epidermal behaviour in the face of the usual minor traumata is unknown. However, it seems likely that it has a significant role which is complementary to mitotic activity.

TECHNIQUES

Estimation of the rate of epidermal cell division

Mitotic counting

The estimation of the numbers of basal epidermal cells in the process of mitosis as a proportion of the total numbers of basal cells (*mitotic index*) is difficult, time-consuming and yields relatively little information. It really takes considerable experience to distinguish a melanocyte from a cell in mitosis and both from a degenerate vacuolated basal epidermal cell. Because mitosis only takes 2–4 hours in man, the number of mitoses seen is extremely small and indeed figures of 0.1–0.2% are to be expected. This signifies that between 1000 and 2000 basal epidermal cells have to be counted before a cell in mitosis can be identified. Thus to obtain consistent results *at least* 5000 basal epidermal cells must be counted. This makes the whole exercise extremely difficult, both because of the time involved and because in the average skin biopsy taken for research purposes in man, there are only about 500 cells per section. Clearly at least ten separate sections have to be evaluated. In addition, care must be taken to see that the same cells are not counted twice so that at least *every other* section should be counted or preferably *every third* section. If this latter course is adopted at least thirty sections must be prepared in order to count ten. To find thirty suitable sections free from artefact can be a tall order and this consideration alone can make the technique impractical.

It must be remembered that it is only interfollicular epidermis that is being evaluated and therefore follicular epidermis must be carefully avoided.

Some workers prefer to express the number of mitoses as a function of the length of the basal layer rather than as a proportion of the total number of basal cells. This is certainly less time-consuming, but does not take into account the presence of non-epidermal cells (or degenerate cells) in the basal compartment, the non-linearity of the basal compartment and the possible variation of epidermal cell size both within a section and between different skin specimens.

As stated above, the recognition of mitoses is not the easiest of tasks. In order for this to be done adequately, the sections should be sectioned as thinly as is consistent with obtaining an entire section and lightly stained with haematoxylin and eosin or Feulgen stain. As mentioned above, care should be taken not to include melanocytes or vacuolated and degenerate basal cells in the mitotic count.

One way of increasing the number of cells to be counted in the mitotic phase and at the same time estimating the numbers of cells entering mitosis per unit time, is by arresting cells in the metaphase stage of the process of mitosis (stathmokinetic technique). A 'mitotic rate' is obtained in this way, as the number of arrested metaphase mitotic 'figures' that are seen, can be regarded as having been 'collected' from the moment of injection of the metaphase arrest agent. Thus, if the stathmokinetic agent is injected 4 hours before the time of biopsy then the metaphase figures have been collected for a 4-hour period and the number of figures that are observed (N) when divided by 4 gives the mitotic rate, i.e. $N/4$ = number of mitoses per hour. The agent most commonly used is colchicine which is an alkaloid containing plant extract. A purified derivative—'colcemid'—was extensively used, but it does not appear to be generally available at the time of writing and such work that is being done with this material relies on the stock on the laboratory shelf. A real disadvantage of the use of colchicine (or its derivatives) is the fact that it is quite toxic and may damage cells non-specifically. If this action is prominent for some reason or other then a false picture may be obtained of the mitotic potential of the tissue. The reason that a 4- or 5-hour period is often chosen between the time of injection and the time of biopsy is that linearity between the numbers of metaphase figures with time is maintained for this period and that 4 or 5 hours allows a reasonable number of mitoses to be collected. However, this has recently been questioned because of its non-specific toxic effects and it seems that we have to be cautious when interpreting results obtained by the colcemid (or colchicine) induced metaphase arrest technique.

Another cytostatic agent has been gaining popularity for the stathmokinetic technique in recent years—vincristine. This material is one of the vinca alkaloids and has substantially the same kind of action on mitosis as has the colchicine alkaloids. It must be said that these stathmokinetic techniques have their main application for work with animal tissues *in vivo*, but are also used for *in vitro* studies. They are in general not suitable for use *in vivo* in man. However, it is worth mentioning two exceptions. The first is a modification of the colchicine technique and was employed by Fisher and Wells (1968). They used a 0.5% colcemid cream to arrest epidermal mitoses in man and obtained very interesting results with this method. The other technique suitable for man is the intracutaneous injection of 1 µg of vincristine—this has recently been utilized by Duffil *et al* (1976) and it seems to be capable of yielding sensible results.

The number of cells in DNA synthesis

As mentioned above the nucleotide thymidine is specifically incorporated into nuclear DNA during the 'S' phase of the generative cycle. Thus, if radioactively-labelled thymidine is employed, the nuclear DNA of the dividing cell becomes radioactive. This radioactive DNA can be traced by the technique of autoradiography or can be directly measured by the scintillation counting method. Either tritium (^{3}H) labelled or carbon 14 (^{14}C) labelled thymidine is used and the general availability of these compounds has transformed the world of cell kinetics and made it available to those with little experience in the laboratory. This is especially true of autoradiographic labelling after exposure of the tissue to tritiated thymidine. The specific activity of the compounds used varies according to the experience and particular technique of the worker concerned, but generally speaking an activity of between 2 and 23 Ci/mmol is used. The tritiated thymidine may be injected into the tissues to be examined *in vivo* (0.1 ml containing 10 µCi of the preparation is usually injected). In animals the substance can also be injected by some other systemic route (0.5–1 µCi/g body weight). Either animal or human tissues may also be exposed *in vitro* to the tritiated thymidine mixed in a nutritive medium.

The length of exposure to tritiated thymidine depends on the particular 'system' used but it is an arbitary time chosen to ensure that all the cells in DNA synthesis at that point in time are adequately exposed to the radioactive precursor. In practice, after injection *in vivo* a period of 45–60 minutes is usually allowed to elapse, while the period of exposure *in vitro* is more variable and may be as short as 30 minutes or as long as 4 hours. There is little published data on the optimal time of exposure *in vitro* but in my and others' experience, it seems that the incorporation 'plateaus' relatively quickly (perhaps after 30 minutes). A longer time is often used to ensure adequate diffusion of the thymidine throughout the tissue as this compound seems to experience difficulties in this respect. Certainly tissue incubated for shorter periods seem to label primarily at the ends of the sections. At the end of the exposure to the radioactive thymidine, the tissues are either removed by biopsy or taken out of culture and treated histologically. The histological section on a glass microscope slide is then 'deparaffinized' (if embedded in paraffin) and then overlaid in the dark with either a layer of photographic emulsion (stripping film technique) or dipped in a photographic emulsion (dipping film technique). The details of these techniques are of importance as without attention to detail poor results are obtained. The success of the technique depends on (a) accurate apposition of a thin layer of sensitive photographic material to the tissue section, (b) exclusion of light from the process.

After the slide bearing the sections has been treated with the photographic material ('nuclear emulsion'), the slides are stored in the dark in 'dark boxes' at 4°C to allow time for the beta particles from the radioactive DNA to fire off the photographic emulsion. As the beta particles only travel a short distance (about 1 μm) only those organelles (almost exclusively the nuclei) in contact with the emulsion which contain radioactive DNA, will produce an accumulation of photographic silver grains above them. The usual period of exposure in the dark is between 1 and 3 weeks. After exposure in the dark box the autoradiographs are developed and fixed—as in conventional photography.

After developing and fixing, the slides are stained through the emulsion. Different workers use different staining regimes but our group found no disadvantage in sticking to straightforward haematoxylin and eosin. The details of the autoradiographic technique used by my own group in Cardiff are appended at the end of this chapter (see p.141). Examination of the autoradiograph under a '×20' objective is usually sufficient although if there is 'light labelling' a higher magnification may be necessary (see Fig. 10.2). A nucleus is counted as labelled if it possesses more than six grains over the number of grains that might be expected in the same area due to 'background' (every autoradiograph has scattered 'background' grains over the section—some are due to cosmic rays and are quite unavoidable). The number of cells in the basal and suprabasal layers that are labelled, expressed as a percentage of the total number of basal cells is usually known as the *labelling index* and is a measure of the number of cells in DNA synthesis at the time of taking the tissue into fixation. The labelled cells in the suprabasal layer may actually be in the suprabasal layer or may appear to be so because of a vagary of sectioning and actually be in the basal layer. Penneys *et al* (1970) estimated that a third of the normal generative compartment was actually in the true suprabasal layer. Sometimes high level cells within the epidermis become labelled—these are probably Langerhans' cells (Schellander & Marks 1972) and should not be included in the estimation of an epidermal labelling index. Another occasional cause of confusion is the presence of dense aggregates of melanin in the epidermis—especially in heavily pigmented individuals. Distinction between melanin and autoradiographic grains is always possible by racking the microscope up and down—the melanin granules are always at a deeper level in the section than the grains.

As thymidine is only incorporated into DNA during the 'S' phase of the mitotic cycle it is also possible to use radioactively-labelled thymidine as a biochemical measure of the rate of DNA synthesis. Both tritiated thymidine and carbon 14-labelled thymidine are widely used for this purpose and the radioactivity incorporated in this way is measured in a 'scintillation-counter'. It is sometimes a problem to know how to express the degree of radioactivity observed. Clearly if one expresses the activity as a specific activity of DNA, ie

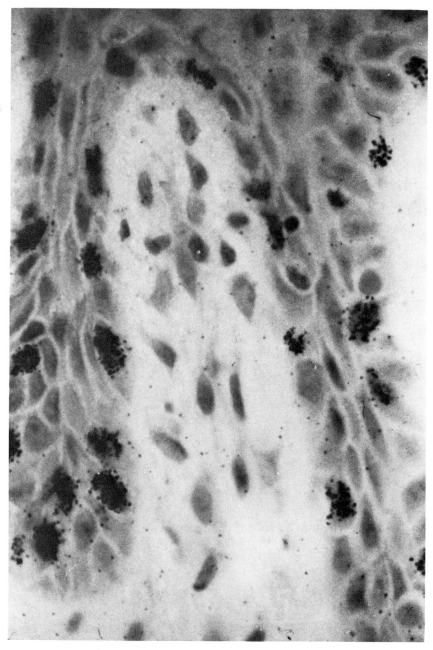

Fig. 10.2 Autoradiograph showing labelled basal cells in hypertrophic epidermis associated with lichenification. (H & E, × 400).

labelled DNA/total tissue DNA, then the figure will represent the rate of DNA production by the whole tissue compartment of DNA, ie from DNA in both the generative and non-generative compartments. This could lead to gross inaccuracies when dealing with the epidermis of higher mammals such as man, as a substantial proportion of the nuclei are no longer 'generative'. The DNA specific activity will be 'diluted' by this non-replicative DNA giving a falsely low estimate of the synthetic capacity. Other possibilities are to express the radioactivity as a function of tissue dry weight (which function still will contain all the non-replicative DNA) or to express the radioactivity per unit surface which may be biologically more relevant. The technique currently employed by our own group in Cardiff to estimate the rate of thymidine incorporation by human epidermis is appended at the end of the chapter (see p.142). A great advantage of this kind of biochemical estimate is the speed with which it can be accomplished. If cell kinetic measurements are ever going to be of use in the management of patients with skin disease a rapid determination of the rate of cell production is obviously of great importance.

Estimation of the rate of epidermal cell transit

Clearly the rate of movement of epidermal cells through the epidermis is to a major extent determined by the rate of epidermal cell production. If tritiated thymidine is injected intracutaneously and the biopsy is performed at a time from 1 to 14 days, subsequently the resulting autoradiograph will demonstrate labelled epidermal cells at various points in the body of the epidermis (see Fig. 10.3). The highest point reached in the epidermis by labelled epidermal cells

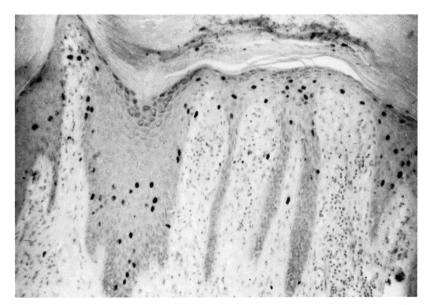

Fig. 10.3 Autoradiograph demonstrating tritium-labelled epidermal cells in a biopsy specimen removed several days after injection of tritiated thymidine. (H & E, ×115).

(h^T) in the test tissue over the height reached by labelled cells in the normal epidermis at that time (h^N) will provide an index of the rate of cell production (P) (r = normal rate of epidermal cell production) ie $h^T/h^N \times r = P$. In some investigations of a particular malady, biopsies have been taken (either from the same or similar individuals) in order to build up a profile of the travel of epidermal cells to the surface. Another technique employed by some groups has been to label epidermal cells with variously labelled radioactive amino acids (glycine, methionine, leucine, histidine, proline etc) as these appear to be incorporated into structural protein of the epidermis. The time taken for the radioactivity to appear in the surface stratum corneum (removed by removing one adhesive tape strip daily after injection of radioactive selenomethionine and estimated by scintillation counting—Porter & Shuster 1967) is a measure of the rate of travel through the stratum corneum. The rate of transit can also be estimated using tritiated amino acids and an autoradiographic technique. Some amino acids are especially incorporated within the granular cell layer of the epidermis (especially histidine) and consequently if the transit through the epidermis and stratum corneum is traced after injection then a very different pattern is seen than when an amino acid is used that is incorporated evenly through the epidermis (Fukuyama & Epstein 1966).

Ethical considerations

Plainly it is undesirable to expose patients to any source of radioactivity, no matter how small. There is a 'special' problem with radioactive thymidine in that because it is specifically taken up by nuclei there is an increased likelihood of a radiation-induced change in the nuclear DNA, with the attendant risks of neoplasia and hereditable genetic damage (if the individual is still in the reproductive period). For these reasons, unless there are very clear-cut and pressing clinical reasons for doing so, the intracutaneous injections of radioactive precursors are best avoided. Of course there may be exceptions to this general rule and the individual investigator must bear the responsibility when he decides not to be constrained by it. For a research project, I consider that the following are essential prerequisites before injection of radioactive precursors *in vivo*.

1   Useful *clinical* information is likely to result.
2   Permission has been obtained from the appropriate ethical bodies.
3   Informed consent has been obtained from the patient.

Estimation of the rate of stratum corneum renewal

Stratum corneum renewal (or turnover) must, of course, be intimately linked to epidermal cell renewal unless one is dealing with an unstable situation, eg at the initiation or healing phase of some of the scaling dermatoses. Kligman and his associates have described two similar techniques for use in human subjects to determine the renewal time of the horny layer. The first (Baker & Kligman 1967) employed tetrachlorsalicylanilide (TCSA) a fluorescent compound in a

1.5% solution. The material was applied for 1–2 hours to the skin surface at the site of the determination and it was examined daily for fluorescence using the long wave ultraviolet emission from a Wood's lamp. As the material penetrated cell layers of the stratum corneum and bound strongly and specifically to it fluorescence persisted until all the horn present at the site and time of application had been shed. This is the stratum corneum renewal time or transit time. Regrettably TCSA is a potent sensitizer and is in addition irritant to many individuals thus increasing mitotic activity at the site of application. The same group from Philadelphia (Jansen *et al* 1974) have, however, improved this technique by substituting the fluorescent dye Dansyl chloride (5-dimethyl amino—1 naphthalene sulphonyl chloride). A 5% ointment (in white soft paraffin) is used with occlusion to the site under investigation. The great disadvantages are of course the necessity for daily observation and the uncertain validity of the method for abnormal skin with disordered keratinization. Another technique employed determines the rate of disappearance of silver stained stratum corneum using a reduced solution of silver nitrate (Ascheim 1968). The amount of silver stain left on the skin surface per day is a function of the rate of desquamation. The degree of silver staining can be determined using a photoelectric reflectance meter. Thus, it is possible to determine the rate of removal of the surface layer by plotting the percentage reflectance against time.

Two other 'manoeuvres' are worth mentioning as far as the stratum corneum is concerned as the writer has been involved with them. Neither are quantitative, they merely give a semiquantitative and indirect estimate of the rate of transit of corneocytes. They both depend on the degree of maturation attained by the ascending horn cell, ie in hyperproliferative disorders the corneocytes will be less mature at any given point within the stratum corneum than in the normally proliferating epidermis. Both techniques employ 'skin surface biopsy' using a cyanoacrylate adhesive (Marks & Dawber 1971). The first depends on the scanning electron microscope appearance of the surface of individual corneocytes (see Fig. 10.4). In hyperproliferative disorders the surface is marked by numerous microvilli (Griffiths & Marks 1973). The second is an enzyme histochemical test which depends on the demonstration of mitochondrial dehydrogenase enzyme activities in the partially mature corneocytes of the hyperproliferative disorders (Marks 1972).

Determination of the phase lengths of the mitotic cycle

This topic will not be dealt with at length because the techniques are quite difficult—if not in execution then certainly in interpretation of the results and a full description would be out of place here. Furthermore, the individual techniques are controversial and seem to yield widely differing results in the hands of different groups of workers. Yet another reason for not becoming too 'fussed' about them is the genuine doubt in the mind of the author concerning the potential usefulness of this type of measurement in the investigation of skin disorders.

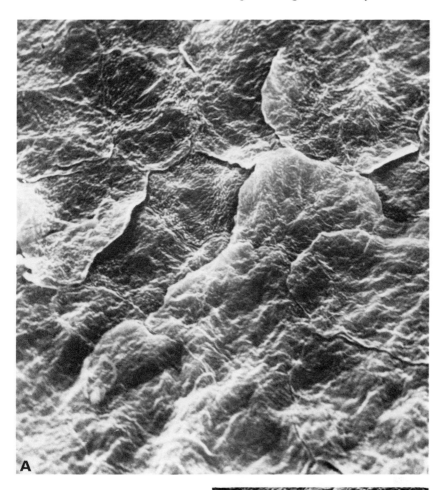

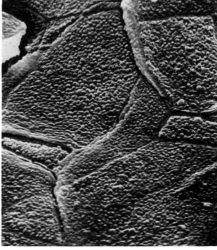

Fig. 10.4 Scanning electron micrograph of skin surface biopsy from (A) normal and (B) psoriatic skin to show the numerous microvilli on the surface of individual corneocytes associated with hyperproliferation in psoriasis.

Labelled mitoses method

For a more detailed description of the technique the reader is referred to
Quastler and Sherman (1959). Essentially tissue is removed at increasing time
intervals after administration of tritiated thymidine and the proportion of
autoradiographically-labelled mitoses of the total number of mitoses, is plotted
as a function of time. An idealized result is portrayed in Fig. 10.5. The time

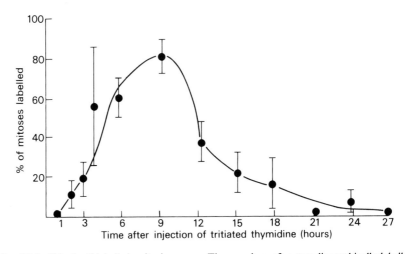

Fig. 10.5 'Idealized'-labelled mitosis curve. The number of autoradiographically-labelled
mitoses is plotted as a function of time after injection of tritiated thymidine.

from the origin to the appearance of the first labelled mitosis is the G2 interval
while the distance between the $37\frac{1}{2}\%$ points on both the ascending and
descending limbs of the curve is the length of 'S' phase. The distance between
the peak of the first and second curves represents the total generation time. Not
only does this method require multiple injections of tritiated thymidine into an
individual but it also necessitates multiple biopsies of the injected sites. Apart
from these ethical problems the assumption has to be made that all the sites
sampled consist of similar cell populations with the same cell kinetics—and
this assumption may not always be justified.

Double labelling method

This can be accomplished using ^{14}C thymidine and tritiated thymidine together
and a double layer of autoradiographic emulsion (so that the stronger beta
emission from the ^{14}C penetrates to the top layer and the tritium-labelled
material only fires off the bottom layer) or tritiated thymidine with two quite
different specific activities (so that the two populations can be characterized by
the quite different degree of nuclear labelling). The experiment is accomplished
by placing the tissue *in vitro* and separately exposing it (with a 1-hour interval
between) to a short pulse of each of the two radioactively-labelled precursor

compounds. The numbers of cells labelled with the first dose of thymidine (Nx) and the numbers labelled with the second dose (Ny) are separately determined in the autoradiograph. The length of 'S' phase is obtained by the term $Ny/Nx = S/t$ where S = 'length of "S" phase in hours' and t = the time interval separating the pulses (1 hour). The labelling index (LI) is also separately determined and the term S/LI will give the whole cell cycle time. This technique has been described for human skin by Heenen and Garland (1971).

Estimation of epidermal cell population size

The estimation of the population size of the epidermis is also a technique worthy of mentioning at this time. As the epidermis is irregular in outline and composed of variably sized keratinocytes this is an intrinsically difficult exercise. The ratio between the length of the basal cell layer and the length of the granular cell layer (B/G ratio) gives a quantitative index of the degree of rete peg hypertrophy and is usually increased in epidermal hyperplasia. The mean epidermal thickness is expressed in cell numbers and is simply measured by counting the numbers of viable nuclei at twelve or twenty vertical random points. It is sometimes useful to measure the actual epidermal thickness. This is not a difficult exercise and merely involves inserting a measuring graticule in the eyepiece of the microscope and ensuring that a representative area of the section has been evaluated and that the section has been cut vertically. Epidermal cell size is another value that may be useful but is for obvious reasons very difficult to obtain. An index of cell size that has been used is the 'mean keratinocyte height' (MKH) in formalin-fixed paraffin sections (Holt *et al* 1976; Holt & Marks 1976). This is simply obtained by dividing the mean epidermal thickness in cell numbers (MECN) into the actual thickness in micrometres (μm) i.e. $MKH = \mu m/MECN$.

The evaluation of potential for active epidermal cell movement (AECM)

There is unfortunately no established way for the investigation of AECM *in vivo* in man. However, numerous investigations of the role that AECM plays in wound healing have been made in experimental animals. The interested reader is referred to Maibach and Rovee (1971).

Attempts have been made to produce standardized wounds that injure the epidermis alone in order to measure the rate of reepithelialization. One such technique employed the 'suction blister' method of producing wounds in hairless hamsters and subsequently measured the rate of reepithelialization both macroscopically and histologically using a computerized image analysing system (Picton *et al* 1976). These techniques are unfortunately time-consuming and costly and thus outside the scope of most smaller laboratories. However, a simple *in vitro* method can provide some information on epidermal cell movement.

A small piece of skin (say 1 cm long by 0.5 cm wide by 0.25 cm deep) is removed and placed immediately in a sterile culture medium (Eagle's minimal essential medium, for example, supplemented with 10% fetal calf serum or autologous serum) in a sterile Petri dish. The dish is then incubated in an atmosphere of 95% oxygen and 5% CO_2 (to maintain a constant pH with the bicarbonate buffer system of the medium) at 37°C for 24–72 hours. At the end of that time the skin is removed, fixed and examined histologically. The epidermis will be found to have migrated from the edges of the skin fragment around the cut edge of the dermis—a process known as epiboly (see Fig. 10.6). The degree of cover of the free dermal aspect can be regarded as a measure of AECM. However, the technique requires serial sectioning as the process of migration is not uniform over the section and quantitation is far from simple (Coombs *et al* 1973, 1974).

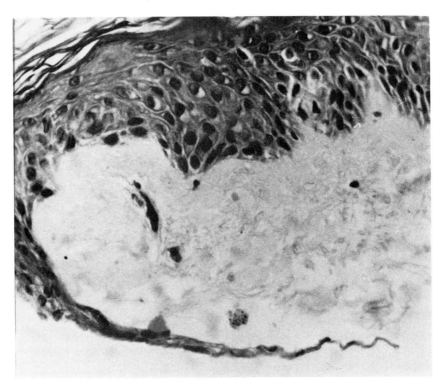

Fig. 10.6 Photomicrograph showing migration of epidermal cells from the edges of a skin fragment maintained in culture—epiboly formation. (H & E, ×250).

SOME FINDINGS USING THE ABOVE TECHNIQUE

The rate of cell production in normal skin at various sites, ages and sexes is not accurately known. However, most laboratories including our own find a thymidine autoradiographic labelling index in the healthy adult of between 4 and 5%.

Table 10.1 sets out some of the findings using some of the techniques discussed. This is meant to give the reader only a 'feel' for the 'order of magnitude' of some of the parameters of epidermal cell kinetics. Many of the figures are disputed and of course many other conditions have been investigated and other parameters documented.

Table 10.1   Some epidermal cell kinetic findings [adapted from Weinstein and Frost (1969)]

Condition	LI%	Labelled cells per cm/basal line	Mitoses per cm/basal line	Cell transit time through epidermis (days)	Phase lengths (h) S	G1	G2	M
Normal	5.2	68.9	7.7	12–14	16	284	6–8	1
Psoriasis	22.7	—	—	4	8.5	24	4	0.3
Basal cell epithelioma	9.2	—	—	—	20	188	7	1.5
Ichthyosis vulgaris	—	49.3	2.5	10–14	—	—	—	—
Epidermolytic hyperkeratosis	—	25.1	40.7	4	—	—	—	—

APPENDIX 1

AUTORADIOGRAPHIC TECHNIQUE

1   Cut 5 μm paraffin sections.

2   Dewax sections and air dry.

3   Melt Ilford Nuclear Emulsion (K2) in a water bath set at 50°C and dilute 1:2 with distilled water.

4   Place emulsion at one end of the slide using a pasteur pipette and spread thinly and evenly over the sections. Hold the slide vertically allowing the excess emulsion to run to one edge from where it can be removed using the pasteur pipette.

5   Place slides in a 'dark box' with silica gel sachets, seal and leave for 2–3 weeks in a refrigerator at 4°C.

6   After exposure remove the slides from the dark box and develop for about 15 minutes in Kodak 'D-19' developer diluted 1:1 with distilled water.

7   Wash the slides briefly in a 1% acetic acid stop bath.

8   Fix the emulsion for 10 minutes in a Kodak 'Kodafix' solution diluted 1:3 with distilled water.

9   After fixing, wash the slides for 15 minutes in running tap water, stain through the emulsion with an appropriate stain (haematoxylin and eosin combination is the one routinely used in our department) and mount as usual.

APPENDIX 2

TECHNIQUE FOR ESTIMATION OF RATE OF INCORPORATION OF THYMIDINE BY HUMAN SKIN

1 Remove skin from the lateral aspect of the thigh with a Castroviejo keratotome set at 0.4 mm. Cut skin into 50 mm² rectangles keeping skin moist at all times with Eagle's minimal essential medium (MEM).

2 Place 3 pieces of skin in a petri dish containing 5 ml of Eagle's MEM. Add 5 µCi of tritiated thymidine (specific activity 2 Ci/mmol) at a concentration of 1 µCi/ml.

3 Place dish in an 'anaerobic' jar containing a small amount of distilled water to maintain a high humidity and 'gas' the jars with 95% oxygen plus 5% carbon dioxide.

4 Incubate at 37°C for 4 hours.

5 After incubation wash each explant with sterile saline and measure areas using graph paper.

6 Store samples at −20°C until processed for scintillation counting.

Procedure for processing tissue for scintillation counting

1 Homogenize in a glass homogenizer with 3 ml distilled water.

2 Transfer homogenate to centrifuge tubes and add 1.5 ml of 10% perchloric acid.

3 Centrifuge for 15 minutes at 800 *g*.

4 Remove supernatant with a pasteur pipette.

5 Wash precipitate twice with 2 ml 2% perchloric acid.

6 Wash precipitate with 2 ml distilled water.

7 Remove supernatant and add 2 ml Soluene (Packard).

8 Agitate until precipitate is dissolved and then transfer 1 ml to a scintillation vial.

9 Add 15 ml toluene based scintillation fluid (12.5 g PPO plus 0.75 g POPOP—2.5 l toluene) and estimate radioactivity in a scintillation-counter.

REFERENCES

ASCHEIM E. (1968) Experimental approach to the renewal of the skin surface. *Nature* **2201,** 1242.

BAKER H. & KLIGMAN A. M. (1967) Technique for estimating turnover time of human stratum corneum. *Archives of Dermatology* **95,** 408.

BORN W. & KALKOFF K. W. (1969) Zur DNS-Synthese der psoriatischen epidermiszelle. *Archives for Dermatological Research* **236,** 43.

BULLOUGH W. S. & MITRANI E. (1976) An analysis of the epidermal chalone control mechanism. In *Chalones,* ed., Houck J. C. North Holland, Elsevier, Amsterdam.

COOMBS V. A., NISSEN B. K., MARKS R. & MORRIS A. (1973) The influence of temperature in epidermal cell migration *in vitro. British Journal of Experimental Pathology* **54**, 673.

COOMBS V. A., NISSEN B. K. & MARKS R. (1974) The epidermal cell migration promoting activity of serum in guinea-pig skin *in vitro. Archives fuer Dermatologische Forschung* **249**, 367.

DUFFIL M., WRIGHT N. & SHUSTER S. (1976) The cell proliferation kinetics of psoriasis examined by three *in vivo* techniques. *British Journal of Dermatology* **94**, 355.

ETOH H., TAGUCHI Y. H. & TABACHNICK J. (1975) Movement of beta-irradiated epidermal basal cells to the spinous-granular layer in the absence of cell division. *Journal of Investigative Dermatology* **64**, 431.

FISHER L. B. & WELLS G. C. (1968) The mitotic rate and deviation in lesions of psoriasis and ichthyosis. *British Journal of Dermatology* **80**, 235.

FUKUYAMA K. & EPSTEIN W. L. (1966) Epidermal keratinization: Localization of isotopically labelled amino acids. *Journal of Investigative Dermatology* **47**, 551.

GELFANT S. (1976) The cell cycle in psoriasis a reappraisal. *British Journal of Dermatology* **95**, 577.

GRIFFITHS W. A. D. & MARKS R. (1973) The significance of surface changes in parakeratotic horn. *Journal of Investigative Dermatology* **61**, 251.

HEENEN M. & GARLAND P. (1971) Cell population kinetics in human epidermis. *In vitro* autoradiographic study by double-labelling method. *Journal of Investigative Dermatology* **56**, 425.

HOLT P. J. A., LAZARUS J. & MARKS R. (1976) The epidermis in thyroid disease. *British Journal of Dermatology* **95**, 513.

HOLT P. J. A. & MARKS R. (1976) Epidermal architecture, growth and metabolism in acromegaly. *British Medical Journal* **1**, 496.

JANSEN L. H., HOJYO-TOMOKO M. T. & KLIGMAN A. M. (1974) Improved fluorescence staining technique for estimating turnover of the human stratum corneum. *British Journal of Dermatology* **90**, 9.

MARKS R. (1972) Histochemical applications of skin surface biopsy. *British Journal of Dermatology* **86**, 20.

MARKS R. & DAWBER R. P. R. (1971) Skin surface biopsy: An improved technique for the examination of the horny layer. *British Journal of Dermatology* **84**, 117.

MAIBACH H. I. & ROVEE D. T. (1972) *Epidermal wound healing.* Chicago Year Book, Medical Publishers, Chicago.

PENNEYS N. S., FULTON J. E., WEINSTEIN G. D. & FROST P. (1970) Location of proliferating cells in human epidermis. *Archives of Dermatology* **101**, 323.

PICTON W., SIM A. W. & MARKS R. (1976) *Methods for evaluating the effects of drugs on reepithelialization.* International Symposium on Wound Healing, Rotterdam. Foundation for International Cooperation in Medical Sciences.

PORTER D. & SHUSTER S. (1967) A new method for measuring replacement of epidermis and stratum corneum in human skin. *Journal of Investigative Dermatology* **49**, 251.

QUASTLER H. & SHERMAN F. G. (1959) Cell population kinetics in the intestinal epithelium of the mouse. *Experimental Cell Research* **17**, 420.

ROVEE D. T., KUROWSKY C. A. & LABUN J. (1972) Local wound healing environment and epidermal healing. *Archives of Dermatology* **106**, 330.

SCHELLANDER F. & MARKS R. (1973) Uptake of tritiated thymidine by high level epidermal cells. *Acta Dermato-Venereologica* **53**, 31.

WEINSTEIN G. D. & FROST P. (1969) Cell proliferation kinetics in benign and malignant skin diseases in humans. *National Cancer Institute Monograph* **30**, 225.

WINTER G. D. (1972) Epidermal regeneration in the domestic pig. In *Epidermal Wound Healing* eds. Maibach H. I. & Rovee D. T. pp. 71–112. Chicago Year Book, Medical Publishers, Chicago.

11

Investigation of fibrinolytic activity

W. J. CUNLIFFE

INTRODUCTION

The quantitative measurement of areas within a tissue section is often a difficult and tedious procedure and the degree of accuracy uncertain. Garner and
Ball (1966) used a point counting technique to measure the proportion of
mineralized and unmineralized bone in samples taken from the iliac crest. They
used a 16 point graticule and moved this over a measured square of bone to
give a total of a hundred fields. The graticule was then rotated through 90° and
the procedure repeated. The statistical basis of this method is given by Hennig
and Meyer-Arendt (1963). The method provides accurate results at the cost of
a large amount of tedious work. We have been interested for several years in
assessing the area of fibrinolysis within tissue sections and have set out to find
a method in which areas of lysis can be easily, quickly and reproducibly
measured. A statistical method devised to give any required degree of accuracy
was used.

MATERIALS AND METHODS

Skin biopsies were taken, usually from standard sites, these being the midpoint
of the palmar aspect of the forearm, medially or the midpoint of the lateral
aspect of the calf. Since blood fibrinolytic activity is affected by exercise, emo-
tion, food and time of day, it is possible that these variables may affect tissue
fibrinolysis. We therefore took the samples between 9 and 10 a.m., the patients
fasting and resting. The biopsies were taken using 2% lignocaine as local
anaesthetic, immediately snap frozen in liquid nitrogen and stored at −20°C.
Samples were never stored for longer than 2 weeks before fibrinolytic
autographs were prepared using Turner and Ryan's (1969) modification of
Todd's technique (1959). In this technique a Perspex frame is placed on a
levelled glass plate to form a trough. The trough is lined with cellophane (400P,
British Cellophane Limited) which has been soaked in Michaelis veronal buffer
(pH 7.4) for 2 hours; the cellophane is smoothed on to the glass with a bent
glass rod. A solution of fibrinogen (Sigma) is made up in Michaelis veronal
buffer (pH 7.4). Originally we used a 2% solution but subsequent batches of

fibrinogen vary in their content of protein and in the proportion of this protein which is clottable. Solutions using new batches are therefore made up to give an equal weight of clottable material to that contained in the original. We realize that different batches of fibrinogen also contain varying amounts of plasminogen activators, for which we make no allowance since in practice it does not affect the reproducibility of the technique. Fibrinogen solution (3.5 ml) is added to 0.1 ml of a solution of bovine thrombin (Parke Davis), 10 units/ml in Michaelis veronal buffer and the mixture immediately poured into the cellophane-lined trough. A fibrin film forms and is left covered by a Perspex lid for 45 minutes. During the 2–3 hours preceding the preparation of the film, cryostat sections (8 μm) are prepared. When the clot has stabilized, the fibrin film and cellophane are cut into strips and placed over the sections. The slides are placed in a humid chamber (a closed Perspex container with a sponge soaked in distilled water, the slides being supported on glass rods) and stored at 4°C for 22 hours. The slides are then transferred to a similar container, previously warmed to 37°C and placed in an incubator at 37°C for 5 minutes; after which the sections are immediately fixed in 10% formalin for 1 hour, the cellophane peeled away, washed in running water for 20 minutes and stained with Loeffler's methylene blue. When dry, the slides are mounted in DPX. The appearance of a section is shown in Fig. 11.1.

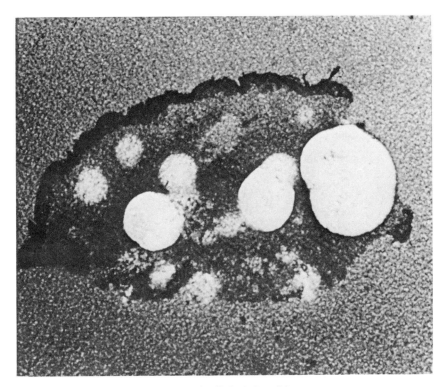

Fig. 11.1   A section of normal skin showing fibrinolytic activity.

Statistical analysis

Consider a section with areas of two types, light (lysis) and dark (no lysis), of which a proportion P is light. If *n* points are chosen at random within the section a proportion p will fall on the light areas. Repeating the process with a different *n* points would provide another value for p, and so on.

These values of p will vary according to a normal distribution with mean P and variance

$$\frac{P(1-P)}{n}$$

(Snedecon & Cochran 1967) (see Fig. 11.2).

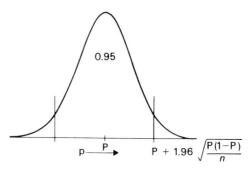

Fig. 11.2   The distribution of p.

We know that 95% of all possible values of p will be within 1.96

$$\frac{P(1-P)}{n}$$

of P. If we require the difference between the p observed in an experiment involving *n* observations and the true proportion of light areas, P, to be at the most 0.05, we use the equation:

$$0.05 = 1.96 \, \frac{P(1-P)}{n}$$

We can then substitute various values for P, and calculate approximate values for *n*. For example, if P is approximately 0.5 then p will be within 0.05 of the true value, P, when n = 400.

Thus by arranging 400 points at random on the section and counting the number falling on light areas we can say, at a 95% confidence level, that P is between p −0.05 and p +0.05. However, *n* can be substantially reduced if P is markedly different from 0.5. If P is approximately 0.20, for example, *n* need only be about 250, whereas if P is 0.10 approximately, *n* need only be about 150. To obtain a greater accuracy than 5%, a larger *n* would be required, and similarly if a higher level of confidence than 95% were required then *n* would have to be increased.

Table 1 Number of points required for a 5% accuracy in the estimation of P.

Approximate percentage of light areas ($P \times 100$)	Required number of points. n
5	75
10	150
20	250
30	330
40	380
50	400
60	380
70	330
80	250
90	150
95	75

Table 11.1 shows the number of random points required to estimate the proportion of light areas to within 0.05 for various values of P. For a 5% accuracy the maximum number of points required to estimate P will never exceed 400.

Practical details

From the above it can be seen that 400 points within a section need to be examined and the incidence of points coinciding with an area of lysis counted. This will give an accuracy of 5% for any percentage estimate of lysis. However, if the percentage is not equal to 50% it is possible to get the same degree of accuracy with fewer readings. Most of our results were around or below 30% and therefore 300 readings were sufficient. To reduce the number of movements of the section and therefore the time taken for each reading, instead of a single crosswire within the eyepiece a 16 point grid graticule (Patterson graticule, type G1, diameter 16 mm) was used. Sixteen points were therefore read at each movement of the slide reducing the number to twenty movements for each skin section. This does impose a certain structure upon the random selection method. However, repeated measurements have shown this to be negligible in affecting the accuracy of the results at the 5% level. Three hundred and twenty points are examined for each section of skin and the number of points on the graticule which coincided with an area of lysis counted and expressed as a percentage of the total number of possible hits, ie 320. The twenty positions of the graticule to make the method statistically significant needed to be determined randomly. The following adjustments were made to a monocular light microscope with a movable stage to enable this procedure to be carried out. Movements of the stage were calibrated using two protractors. The protractors were permanently fixed to the spindle of the controlling knobs. The position of the microscope stage was assessed by pointers (thick fuse wire)

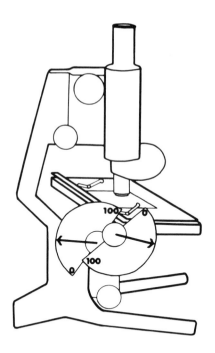

Fig. 11.3 A schematic representation of the microscope.

attached to the movable knobs. When the control knobs were moved the pointers also moved indicating the position of the stage. Thus the stage could be moved from points 0 to 100 on the protractor scale in both directions which represent the x and y axes (see Fig. 11.3). Each section was examined under low power magnification ($\times$ 100). The field at the bottom left hand corner of each section to be examined was located; this was the origin of the graph to be used (see Fig. 11.4, position a). The pointers were then attached to the centre of each controlling knob with the ends at 0 on each protractor. The knob controlling the y axis was then turned to move the field of vision to the limit of the section (see Fig. 11.4, position b) and the reading of each protractor scale noted (in this case 80). The same procedure was carried out on the x axis (see Fig. 11.4, position c with reading 60). The two readings give the limits of the section.

Tables of random numbers in the ranges 0–10, 0–20, etc up to 0–100 have been generated by computer (Tocher 1963). From these, tables with values in the ranges given by the protractor readings are selected (in our example for the y value the 0–80 table, and for the x value the 0–60 table). Pairs of numbers are now read, one from each list and the corresponding knob moved so that the pointer is at the appropriate protractor reading. The field is now examined. For example, if the first numbers generated by computer were 57 on the y axis and 30 on the x axis the graticule would be set to position d (see Fig. 11.4) and the number of hits be 5 out of a possible 16. This is repeated for a further nineteen pairs of numbers read from the table. If the graticule overlaps the edge of the section, the number of intersections coinciding with the sections as well as

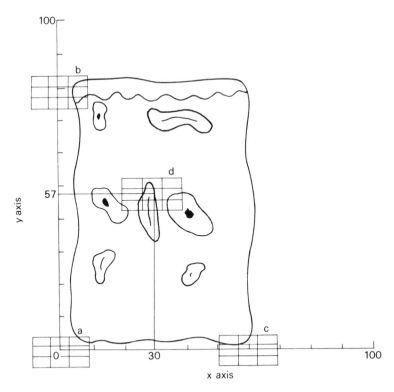

Fig. 11.4   The movements of the graticule over a skin section.

those coinciding with an area of lysis are counted and in this case the total number of possible hits will be less than 320 and additional readings should be taken.

COMMENT

This statistical technique is currently being applied to assess areas of lysis in tissue fibrinolytic and proteolytic autographs. Repeated measurements have demonstrated the reproducibility of the technique. By standardizing the technique significant differences have been found between fibrinolytic activity in different sites of the body (Dodman *et al* 1972) and a reduced tissue fibrinolytic activity in vasculitic lesions (Cunliffe *et al* 1971).

The method described in this paper is simple in operation, the measurement of one section taking less than 10 minutes. It may be adjusted to yield any degree of accuracy required, and involves only minor modifications to any monocular microscope with a movable stage.

We, therefore, feel that this statistical method could be applied not only to areas of lysis but in the measurement of any well defined areas such as blood vessels or glands, occurring within a histological section.

REFERENCES

CUNLIFFE W. J., DODMAN B., HOLMES R. L. & FORSTER R. A. (1971) Local fibrinolytic activity in patients with cutaneous vasculitis. *British Journal of Dermatology* **84,** 420.

DODMAN B., CUNLIFFE W. J. & ROBERTS B. E. (1973) Observations on tissue fibrinolytic activity in patients with cutaneous vasculitis. *British Journal of Dermatology* **88,** 231.

GARNER A. & BALL J. (1966) Quantitative observations on mineralised and unmineralised bone in chronic renal azotaemia and intestinal malabsorption syndrome. *Journal of Pathology and Bacteriology* **91,** 545.

HENNIG A. & MEYER-ARENDT J. R. (1963) Microscopic volume determination and probability. *Laboratory Investigations* **12,** 460.

SNEDECON G. W. & COCHRAN W. H. (1967) Sampling from the binomial distribution. In *Statistical Methods,* 6th Edn., pp. 199–227. Iowa State University Press, Ames, Iowa.

TOCHER K. D. (1963) Pseudo-random numbers. In *The Art of Simulation,* pp. 72–84. English Universities Press, Sevenoaks, Kent.

TODD A. S. (1959) The histological localization of fibrinolysin activator. *Journal of Pathology and Bacteriology* **78,** 281.

TURNER R. H. & RYAN T. J. (1969) Fibrinolytic activity in human skin. *The Transactions of St. John's Hospital Dermatological Society* **55,** 2, 212.

12

Transmission electron microscopy

J. A. A. HUNTER

INTRODUCTION

In this Chapter it is intended to present a practical, though personal, view on the role of transmission electron microscopy in investigative dermatology. No attempt will be made to give a comprehensive account of various techniques as there are already plenty of good books describing them (see Further Reading p.173). However, those special problems posed by skin, which have received little attention in most books, will be emphasized and discussed.

Although most references here will concern work on human skin, the comments should be pertinent to animal studies.

The techniques involved in transmission electron microscopy require skill, patience and experience, and are often finicky and time-consuming. Unfortunately, this Chapter will not be the passport to rapid success though, with luck, it may help to lessen the inevitable number of apparently wasted hours which can be anticipated when embarking on any new technique. The research worker, who asks another laboratory to process his material for electron microscopy, might also find out, in a relatively painless way, what is involved.

The importance of good technique in electron microscopy cannot be overemphasized, but it ought not to be forgotten that in most studies electron microscopy should be used to answer a question rather than to provide beautiful pictures. There is the person who is mesmerized and obsessed by new fixation procedures, osmolalities and different embedding media. The variables in electron microscopic processing are so legion that he could spend a lifetime pottering around with different combinations. He forgets that electron microscopy is a means to an end, avoids asking questions that it can help to answer, and ambles along in an unproductive way deceiving himself that his authoritative publication is just around the corner. On the other hand, there is the person who is apparently brimful and overflowing with ideas, many of which can be solved by a 'quick look' at fine structure. To him the techniques of electron microscopy are little different to those of light microscopy, histochemistry and immunofluorescence—admittedly tricky, but ones which can be mastered by following simple recipes. A technician in his laboratory can sort them out in a few weeks, and a month or so should see the final photographs on his desk. Unfortunately that is just what happens: ghastly photographs appear, and he either makes assumptions from inadequate material or posts them off to a colleague who knows something about electron microscopy. Not surprisingly, the reply can be hurtful. Somewhere between these rather exaggerated extremes is the situation where practical electron microscopy can help to solve well thought out problems.

Although this view has been rather laboured, it is important and leads on to the next point. If there is a problem involving electron microscopy, who should do the work and where?

THE ELECTRON MICROSCOPIC LABORATORY

There are still surprisingly few dermatological laboratories with their own complete electron microscopy units. As the purchase and running costs of an electron microscope are becoming more and more prohibitive there is a lot to be said for having just the preparative (including thin sectioning) and photographic facilities in a skin department and arranging time on a central electron microscope. An advantage of this system is that there is no financial responsibility for the costly maintenance of the machine though a fee for its use should be expected. Personal experience has shown this set-up to be satisfactory. It has the great advantage that all technical procedures can be carried out within the department and under personal supervision. Liaison between workers on a project can also be close and, with practice, there should be no difficulty in dealing with skin, a tissue which presents considerable sectioning problems in most general electron microscopic laboratories.

If many electron microscopic projects are anticipated in a skin department there can be little doubt that the establishment of an electron microscopic unit within that department is the only satisfactory way of facing the problem. A science graduate with an interest in electron microscopy, a technician who enjoys precise work and is good with his hands, and perhaps a technical assistant would be an ideal start. Two small rooms (sectioning room—as draught-free and vibration-free as possible, and a photographic darkroom) and a general processing laboratory are all that is required. The initial major non-recurrent capital expenditure would include the purchase of an ultramicrotome, a knife maker, incubator, light microscope, fridge, photographic enlarger and a print glazer.

If there is no electron microscopic unit in the skin department what is the next best course if fine structural investigations are needed? A local general unit might help out, or fixed specimens can easily be posted to a dermatological electron microscopic unit. A poor knowledge of the problems presented by skin has to be weighed against those problems posed by long distance communications. In any case either alternative is preferable to going it alone in a laboratory devoid of the necessary equipment and expertise.

WHEN TO USE THE ELECTRON MICROSCOPE?

It is really impossible to answer this question properly. There are bound to be exceptions to any rigid view, so perhaps the answer is more a matter of commonsense; that is, if time is made to stop and think! However, there may be some justification in describing the type of situation in which electron microscopy can contribute. These are summarized in Fig. 12.1.

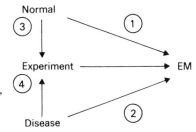

Fig. 12.1 When to use the electron microscope, 1, normal skin; 2, pathological conditions; 3, experiments on normal skin; 4, experiments on pathological skin.

Electron microscopy of normal skin

The necessity for a thorough knowledge of the ultrastructure of normal skin cannot be overemphasized. Normal skin is the ideal material on which to practise preparative schedules and sectioning, and no opportunity should be lost to view it. Abnormality, by definition, is something which does not occur in normal skin, so a comprehensive experience of this tissue is essential. An embarrassing number of abnormal observations have been reported in pathological tissue which experience should have revealed were abnormal due to an error in technique rather than the pathological state.

Electron microscopy of pathological conditions

Electron microscopy may provide two types of information in pathological conditions. Some pointers to the pathogenesis of the disorder may emerge or it may provide clues concerning the function of a particular cell or organelle.

The first category would include the demonstration of viruses. It was only after brick-shaped virus particles were noted electron microscopically that the nature of the recent London smallpox epidemic became apparent (HMSO 1974). Thankfully, dramatic situations like this are rare, but virology departments use electron microscopy as a diagnostic tool in numerous other viral conditions, ranging from the detection of herpes virus to the demonstration of Australian antigen. It is worth mentioning that the electron microscopic detection of virus particles in animal and human malignant melanomas, supported by other techniques, has led a group of workers in Munich to suggest an oncornal virus cause for malignant melanoma (Birkmayer *et al* 1974).

In the second category would be the finding of numerous cells containing Langerhans' cell granules in the lesions of histiocytosis X (Basset *et al* 1965).

Until 1965 most opinion favoured some relationship between melanocytes and Langerhans' cells, but Madame Basset's discovery changed the whole direction of research, and investigations into a macrophage function for the Langerhans' cell were pursued.

A satisfying and possibly more rewarding approach is to single out pathological conditions in which electron microscopy can help to answer a question. Knutson's studies (1974) on the ultrastructure of the wall of the pilosebaceous canal in acne were prompted by the work of others which suggested that follicular hyperkeratosis was important in the pathogenesis of acne. He demonstrated that the cells of the wall of the pilosebaceous canal underwent a metaplastic change in comedones, and caused infundibular obstruction by forming an abnormal keratin layer which did not desquamate and which contained numerous lipid droplets.

Does the Langerhans' cell originate in the thymus, or is it functionally dependent on the thymus? The answer to this question seemed simple when normal Langerhans' cells were found in the epidermis of congenitally athymic nude mice (Hunter *et al* 1976).

Unfortunately, the literature is overflowing with apparently useless and non-contributory electron microscopic observations of various skin diseases. Most seem to be the result of the thoughtless extension of light microscopy, in the vain hope that a higher magnification of structure will reveal hidden clues on the pathogenesis of a disease. For instance, how much has the electron microscope contributed towards the understanding of pityriasis rosea, vasculitis, parapsoriasis and so on? Nevertheless, time has already shown that it is dangerous to scorn the 'lucky dip' approach too much. Did preconceived notions on the ultrastructure of histiocytosis X and contact dermatitis anticipate how the findings would influence thought on the function of the Langerhans' cell?

Electron microscopic experiments on normal skin

This is perhaps the most attractive experimental situation. Normal skin is subjected to some experimental procedure and changes in the ultrastructure noted. If control (preexperimental) and experimental specimens are processed in the same way, and at the same time, minor technical problems should affect both equally, and comparison becomes easier. For instance, suction applied to normal epidermis has been shown to produce paranuclear vacuolization in keratinocytes but not in dendritic cells (Hunter *et al* 1974).

A more elegant experiment in the same category was that of Wolff and Konrad (1972). They produced suction blisters in normal guinea pig skin and injected latex beads of varying sizes into the blister cavities. They showed that lysosomal complexing of the beads within the keratinocytes was a size-dependent phenomenon. Beads with a diameter of 0.1 μm were complexed in groups within lysosomes whilst larger ones (diameter 0.8 μm) were not, and appeared singly in the cytoplasm. Technically, the study is superb, and this naturally instills confidence in the conclusions reached.

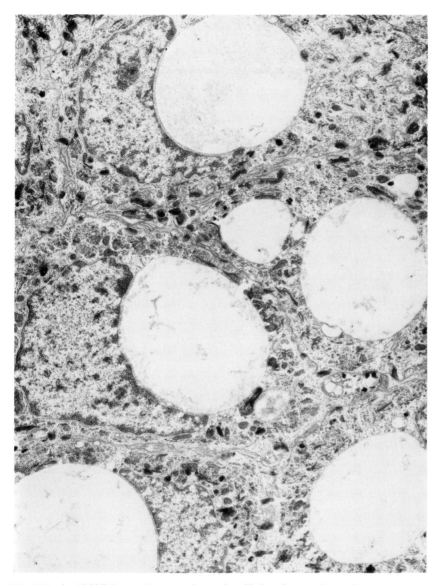

Fig. 12.2   (× 10 000) Paranuclear vacuoles produced in keratinocytes by suction.

Electron microscopic experiments on pathological skin

These are again attractive because a direct comparison of tissue can be made before and after the experimental insult. For example, Schnait *et al* (1975) investigated the immediate response of the skin of erythropoietic protoporphyric patients to ultraviolet irradiation. They concluded that long wave ultraviolet damaged the endothelial cells of the superficial dermal vessels and caused pronounced leakage of vascular contents. This resulted in the accumulation of the perivascular fibrillar material so characteristic of erythropoietic protoporphyric lesions. The multilayered vascular basement membranes were interpreted as consecutive reparative processes following endothelial damage.

It is well worth looking at the studies of Maul and his colleagues (Maul 1969; Maul & Romsdahl 1970) on cultured human malignant melanoma cells. Technically the work is near perfect and the beautiful cellular preservation enabled Maul to spot fine points which had been previously unnoticed. Not surprisingly, his conclusions on the sites of premelanosomal formation differ from those of others, but his views are well supported by the micrographs.

In summary, there can be no fixed rules about when to use the electron microscope. Providing the material is good and the research worker both knowledgeable and observant, a 'lucky dip' approach, particularly in rare conditions, can still provide significant findings. However, the planned project, aimed at answering a simple question, is much more rewarding and, needless to say, there are still unending pathological conditions and experimental situations awaiting investigation.

A word of warning for any electron microscopic enthusiast. Once a reasonable unit is established, requests will come pouring in to look at this and that. A firm grip on the number of projects proceeding at one time is necessary. Halfbaked electron microscopy is not only very unsatisfying, but also dangerous to publish!

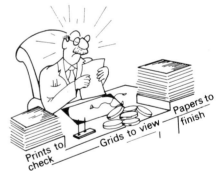

Fig. 12.3 'I am writing to ask you to look at membrane coating granules in ichthyosis.'

ELECTRON MICROSCOPIC CYTOCHEMISTRY

Electron microscopic cytochemistry still remains in its infancy. Its limitations are similar to those of light microscopic histochemistry, but the techniques are often more capricious. There are two main divisions. In the first a chemical is added which reacts with a cellular constituent and the second is concerned with the detection of subcellular enzymatic activity.

Substances which react with or digest cellular constituents

Commonly used fixatives like glutaraldehyde or osmium tetroxide should be included in this category. Although many of their reactions are still obscure, they seem to act as crosslinking agents and produce a stable network by forming chemical bonds between molecules of the cell. Other cellular constituents are caught up and fixed in this network. Although it is a gross oversimplification, glutaraldehyde can be considered to fix mainly proteins and osmium tetroxide mainly lipids. The two fixatives used sequentially are therefore a most satisfactory combination. Routine staining should also be considered in this section. Most of the atoms in animal and plant tissue have a low atomic weight and consequently a poor ability to scatter electrons. Heavy metal salts such as uranyl acetate and lead citrate increase the differential electron scattering power of various cellular components, and are popular stains.

There are, however, more specific dermatological applications in this category. For instance, osmium iodide to stain membrane coating granules (Breathnach & Wyllie 1966) osmium zinc iodide to render parts of Langerhans' cells and granules preferentially visible (Niebauer *et al* 1969) ruthenium red to stain the cell surface coats of keratinocytes in pemphigus vulgaris (Hashimoto & Lever 1970) lanthanum nitrate to outline the Langerhans' cells and granules preferentially visible (Niebauer *et al* 1969) (see Fig. 12.4) and differential enzymatic digestion to determine the nature of

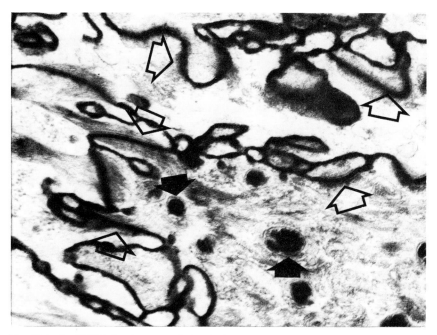

Fig. 12.4 (× 15 200) Lanthanum outlining the intercellular space just below the granular cell layer. Note permeation of desmosomes (open arrows) by tracer. Arrows point to melanosomes within a keratinocyte.

cytoplasmic components of keratinocytes (Wolff & Schreiner 1971). Specific antibody can be bound covalently to ferritin (Singer 1959) or enzymes such as horseradish peroxidase (Nakane & Pierce 1967) and used to detect the site of antigen at a subcellular level.

Tracer substances such as thorotrast, horseradish peroxidase and ferritin have also been used to mark phagosomes and lysosomes. For example, Wolff and Schreiner (1970) using horseradish peroxidase and Sagebiel (1972) using ferritin, have shown that keratinocytes are more phagocytic than Langerhans' cells, and Wolff and Hönigsmann (1971) used thorotrast to investigate the phagocytic nature of keratinocytes and demonstrated acid phosphatase activity in the phagosomes.

The subcellular detection of enzymatic activity

This technical problem became much easier when Sabatini *et al* (1963) recorded that certain dialdehydes (including glutaraldehyde) not only fixed cellular structures but also stabilized proteins in such a form that enzyme activity was preserved. A compromise is made between prolonged fixation with loss of enzyme activity but good cellular preservation, and incomplete fixation with good enzyme activity but poor cellular detail. After partial fixation, the tissue is incubated in a specific substrate which is broken down by enzymatic

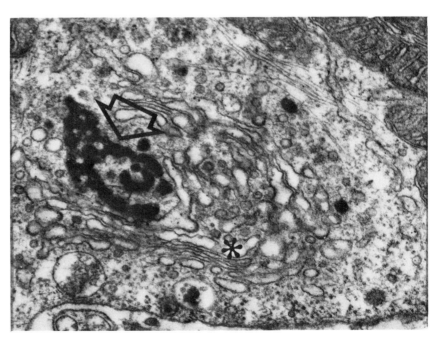

Fig. 12.5 (× 43 000) Ultrastructural dopa reaction, malignant melanoma. Reaction product (open arrow) is present in tumour cell in endoplasmic reticulum adjacent to the Golgi apparatus (*).

activity in the tissue. If the reaction product so formed is not already electron dense it is 'captured' by the addition of a further substance in the incubating medium so that an electron dense product is finally formed. In Barka and Anderson's (1962) modification of Gomori's (1952) lead sulphide method for the detection of acid phosphatase, sodium β-glycerophosphate is used as a substrate, and the phosphate released is captured by the addition of lead nitrate to the medium. If all goes well, insoluble electron dense lead phosphate is precipitated at the site of enzyme activity. This technique is becoming more frequently used, as membrane-bound acid phosphatase activity is now accepted as a marker of lysosomes (Novikoff 1963).

Tyrosinase (or dopa oxidase) in melanocytes and melanoma cells can be most conveniently detected as the reaction product produced by its action on the colourless tyrosine or dopa (in the medium) is the electron dense melanin. Of course relevant control experiments are necessary to establish the more precise nature of the enzyme involved (Hunter *et al* 1970; Okun *et al* 1970; Brumbaugh *et al* 1973).

ELECTRON MICROSCOPIC AUTORADIOGRAPHY

Electron microscopic autoradiography has extended the possibilities for experimentation and further levels of analysis. It has proved invaluable in the study of tissue and cell dynamics. Living material, which cannot be viewed under an electron microscope, is used and the synthesis, turnover and migration of substances can be followed. The resolution is about ten times better than with light microscopic autoradiography (Jacob 1971). The techniques involved in electron microscopic autoradiography are tricky, time-consuming and, initially, often frustrating. Anyone contemplating this sort of work would be well advised to attend a course on the subject, or liaise with a laboratory with experience of the technique. Reviews of the subject have been written by Salpeter and Bachman (1965) and Jacob (1971). Nakai and Shubik (1964), Blois and Kallman (1964), Zelickson *et al* (1965) and Toda and Fitzpatrick (1971) have, for example, already revealed the scope of the technique when using labelled DOPA to investigate the intracellular site of melanin synthesis.

ANALYTICAL ELECTRON MICROSCOPY

If electron microscopy cytochemistry is in its infancy, then the use of the electronprobe microanalyser in combination with high resolution transmission electron microscopy (analytical electron microscopy) is at an embryonic stage. In this instrument a thin beam of electrons (probe) is directed on to an area of specimen which can be monitored by transmission or scanning electron microscopy. X-rays are emitted and their spectrometric analysis allows identification of elements bombarded by the probe. Care has to be taken in choosing the type of stains and grids as lead, uranium and copper will all be recorded. Diffusable ions also present obvious problems and the mastery of special fixation regimes and cryoultramicrotomy will be important. However the prospects are exciting. Already machines with this capability are commercially available.

TECHNIQUES AND PROBLEMS IN ROUTINE TRANSMISSION ELECTRON MICROSCOPY

Some golden rules:

1 Establish a satisfactory preparation schedule and stick to it. Good fixation is all important and, if wrong, time spent afterwards is wasted.
2 Good records are essential. Faults cannot be traced without them.
3 Avoid short cuts, but if they are unavoidable then record details.
4 Changes in the routine schedule should be for a good reason; not because the pubs are open.
5 Plan tomorrow's experiments today. Start punctually.
6 Arrange for 'cold' experiments to start on Monday morning.
7 Scrupulous cleanliness. Dust becomes rocks when looked at with the electron microscope. Water can be as big an enemy.
8 Treat toxic chemicals with respect. Osmic acid can damage eyes. Cacodylate buffer is poisonous. Institute adequate precautions if specimens are taken home to finish processing as children will explore and interfere.
9 Don't fiddle with knobs on an electron microscope if their function is unknown. Preferably ask a technician to help.
10 Patience, endless patience.

As mentioned in the opening paragraph this Chapter is not meant to be a list of recipes; neither can it be a comprehensive review.

If a burning desire to take up electron microscopy is felt then one immediate and sensible course is obvious—a visit for a substantial period to an electron microscopic unit, not necessarily dermatological. The individual must at some stage gain a working knowledge of *every* process involved. This does not mean just a chatty morning of abortive thin sectioning; it will entail hours of patient effort aimed at mastering each technique in the laboratory. It is appreciated that, eventually, it will neither be necessary nor expedient to do everything oneself. However, the whole point of a good training period is to become so thoroughly acquainted with the techniques that help can be given when work is piling up or, perhaps more important, that the origins of faults can be quickly detected and corrections made. It is also helpful to be able to walk into the laboratory and appreciate exactly what is, or is not, happening at a given moment. Short cuts and sloppiness in technique should be spotted rapidly with the result that high standards are more easily maintained.

A routine schedule is outlined in Table 12.1 though different laboratories have their own preferences. Details of more rapid processing schedules have also been published.

Table 12.1 Timetable of a routine processing schedule

Day 1	Biopsy and fixation. Hold overnight in buffer.
Day 2	Post fixation, block staining, dehydration and infiltration with plastic. Overnight in plastic-propylene oxide mixture.
Day 3	Impregnation in polythene troughs.
Day 4	Blocks transferred to capsules containing fresh plastic mixture. Orientate blocks. Capsules placed in incubator.
Days 5–7	Polymerization in incubator.

If specimens are received on a Monday then processing can be completed by the end of that week and the material studied any time afterwards.

Collection of material

It is mandatory that biopsy or other specimens are fixed immediately after removal. Delays of over 30 seconds may be costly in terms of tissue preservation. For skin, a shave biopsy is particularly satisfactory providing that the study only concerns a level above mid dermis. On a number of occasions personal experience has confirmed that, if the operator is skilled, this procedure can be easily tolerated even without local anaesthetic. Usually only a small sliver of skin is needed (eg 3 mm^2) to provide 8–10 blocks.

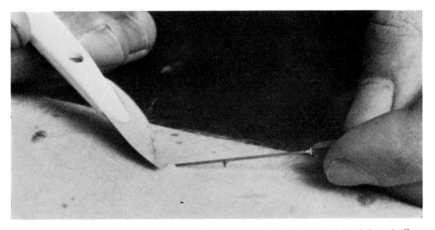

Fig. 12.6 Shave biopsy. Under sterile conditions, skin is raised with a needle and shaved off.

Fixation

The specimen is immersed immediately into a labelled bottle. If glutaraldehyde is in the primary fixative the specimen should be removed after about 1 minute, when the consistency is crisper and more suitable for trimming. This is carried out under a drop of the fixative on dental wax. The traumatized edges are trimmed with a new razor blade (edge cleaned) and discarded; the rest of the tissue is then diced into small cubes of not larger than 1 mm³, but often much smaller. Perfusion fixation may be preferable in animals.

Most popular regimes depend on double fixation, i.e. fixation initially in glutaraldehyde and postfixation in osmium tetroxide. Although is has a high osmolality a paraformaldehyde (2%)-glutaraldehyde (2.5%) mixture (Karnovsky 1965) has been found to be the most suitable all purpose fixative for skin in our laboratory. It does, however, have to be made-up carefully and therefore the recipe (a modification employed by Wolff's group in Austria) is worth detailing:

Stock Solutions:

1 Sodium cacodylate buffer 0.2 M pH 7.4.
2 Sodium cacodylate buffer 0.1 M pH 7.4.

Method

Paraformaldehyde (2 g EM grade) + 20 ml fresh glass distilled water in 125 ml cork stoppered conical flask. Heat at 60°C on stir plate for 45 minutes. Don't boil. When moisture forms on sides of flask add four drops of 1N NaOH and stir (magnet) until solution clears (eg after 15 minutes). Cool under tap to room temperature. Add 10 ml of 25% glutaraldehyde + 20 ml sodium cacodylate buffer 0.2 M pH 7.4. Add 25 mg CaCl₂ (fused granular). Take pH which should fall in range of pH 7.2–7.4. There is now a total of 50 ml. Add 50 ml of sodium cacodylate buffer 0.1 M pH 7.4 for a 1:1 dilution. Check pH is exactly 7.4.

This concentration may be changed by adding/subtracting the sodium cacodylate 0.1 M. With a 1:1 dilution the concentration of glutaraldehyde is 2.5% and the paraformaldehyde is 2%.

In a busy laboratory it should be made up fresh twice weekly, but for special experiments it is best to make it up on the same day as fixation.

NB: Glutaraldehyde deteriorates on standing—even in the fridge. If more than four drops of NaOH have to be added it has probably become too acidic. A check of the pH of glutaraldehyde should therefore be carried out occasionally if the turnover is slow.

After fixation the blocks should be thoroughly rinsed in buffer; 0.1 M cacodylate is our preference as this is used in the fixative. The specimens can be stored overnight at 4°C in the buffer with or without added sucrose to increase the molality.

Postfixation and dehydration

Different regimes can be found in all technical books (see Further Reading p.173). We have found Professor Wolff's routine very satisfactory. Each step is ticked off on a sheet after completion (see Table 12.2). The sheets are kept in

Table 12.2

EM No: Name: Procedure:	Diagnosis:	Date: Histology No:
	Time	Temperature
Karnovsky 1:1	5 h	Room

0.1 M cacodylate buffer
  pH 7.4
	20 min + 20 min + 20 min
	            overnight
		Fridge

Cytochemistry	See below	
OsO_4. 3% in dH_2O	1 h 30 min	Icebath
0.1 M cacodylate buffer pH 7.4	5 min + 5 min	Fridge
Uranyl acetate 0.5% in VA buffer pH 7.2	45 min	Fridge
Alcohol 50%	5 min	Fridge
Alcohol 70%	5 min + 5 min	Fridge
Alcohol 95%	5 min + 5 min	Fridge
Alcohol absolute	20 min 20 min 20 min	Fridge Cold Room
Propylene oxide: plastic (2:1)	1 h	Room
Propylene oxide: plastic (1:1)	3 h	Room
Propylene oxide: plastic (1:2)	Overnight	Room
Plastic impregnation	24 h	Room
Polymerization Plastic formula:	3 days	60°C
Cytochemistry:		

a book which does not leave the processing laboratory. Block staining with uranyl acetate after postfixation produces sections of greater contrast. Membrane damage is probably lessened by omitting the use of 100% propylene oxide.

Embedding media

Today epoxy resins are the routine embedding media in most laboratories. Available supplies may dictate whether this is Epon 812 or Araldite and mixtures of the two are becoming popular. Epon is easier to work with even though it is more hygroscopic that Araldite. Stock solutions of Epon have to be covered and precautions taken to prevent the uptake of water vapour in the air. Dermal preservation in particular seems superior when Epon is used, but Epon is probably more tricky to section than Araldite.

Orientation

Proper orientation of the block in the tip of the capsule or side of the mould can save much frustration later on when cutting sections. After postfixation in osmium tetroxide there should be little difficulty, especially if a dissecting microscope is used, in establishing which is epidermis (homogeneous dark brown to black) and dermis (uneven gingery brown).

Bubbles within the resin in the capsule are removed with a needle—again under a dissecting microscope. The small cubes are allowed to float to the bottom of the capsules of their own accord and then aligned with a needle so that both epidermis and dermis lie on the flat bottom surface of the capsule. Before the capsules are put into the incubator each one should contain a label identifying the specimen, within the resin.

Sectioning

It is always worthwhile cutting thick (1–2μm) sections of the whole face of the block. These are stained rapidly with toluidine blue (see Fig. 12.7).

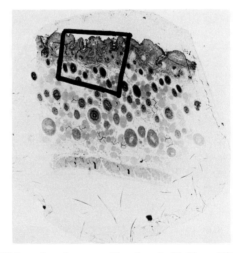

Fig. 12.7   (× 36) Thick section of mouse epidermis embedded in araldite stained with toluidine blue. A suitable area can be chosen for making a pyramid (eg as outlined) and then for cutting thin sections.

An area in the thick skin is then chosen for thin sectioning. The pyramid is trimmed so that its flat top coincides with this area. It is preferable to cut in a direction along the dermoepidermal junction (see Fig. 12.8).

Ultramicrotomy principles relevant to other tissues apply (see Further Reading p.173). Using Araldite of medium hardness, satisfactory 50–60 nm sections can be obtained using glass knives with an edge angle of 45° and a clearance angle of 4°. A cutting speed of 2 mm/s seems appropriate for most skin specimens.

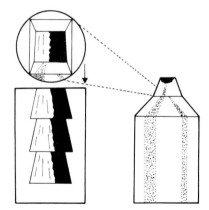

Fig. 12.8 Epoxy resin block on right with tissue embedded in tip. On left is a diagrammatic representation pyramid fact (top) with epidermis illustrated in black. Bottom left shows sections coming off knife edge into trough. Note pyramid is made so that final direction of cut is along dermoepidermal junction.

Staining of sections

No special problems are presented by skin, and the reader is referred to the books mentioned at the end of this Chapter (see Fig. 12.9).

Use of electron microscope

Again, there are no problems particularly relevant to skin. it is imperative to receive good technical coaching on the use of any machine. Although each machine has its own idiosyncrasies, the basic rules are the same for all. Much time and frustration will be saved if a few sessions are spent with someone who is familiar with the ultrastructure of skin, and normal skin should be viewed and photographed time and again until the individual is familiar with the tissue. The best pictures are those which are taken quickly though carefully, as too long spent focusing will result in specimen contamination causing loss of detail in the pictures. Astigmatism should be corrected at each session, if photographs of magnification greater than × 20 000 are anticipated.

Careful records should be kept. A good habit is to summarize the findings of each session in a personal laboratory book—particularly as it is not necessary to photograph absolutely everything. If something of real interest is noticed then care should be taken to record the whereabouts on the grid for future referral.

Photography

Some general points are worth mentioning. An enlarger with a point source is recommended as this yields high contrast prints of fine detail. An automatic print processing machine will save an enormous amount of time though occasionally hand developing is preferable for tricky prints. A working knowledge of photographic procedures is a great help and even acceptable pictures can be obtained from poor negatives by juggling with enlarger exposure

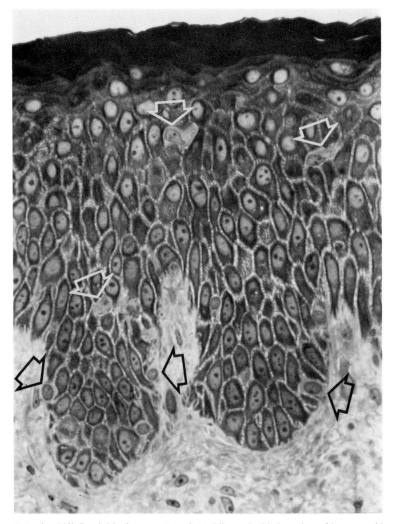

Fig. 12.9 (× 540) Semi-thin (approx. 1 μm) Araldite embedded section of human epidermis stained with toluidine blue. Note that Langerhans' cells (white arrows) and melanocytes (black arrows) are clearly distinguishable from keratinocytes.

times, paper grades and developing methods. It is an incomplete electron microscopist who has not spent hours in a photographic darkroom.

All photographs should be enlarged to a reasonable size (eg 20 × 15 cm) for routine inspection. If this is deemed unnecessary then it is unlikely that the photo should ever have been taken in the first place. Routine enlargements should be permanently fixed and the negative number, specimen number and magnification recorded on the back.

Inspection of prints

All photographs should be studied with the help of a magnifying glass. Peace and quiet are essential as this requires real concentration. As it is tiring, only a few should be inspected at one time, but it is always worth looking at prints again or showing them to different people. Interesting ones can be marked with an indelible felt tip pen and remarks recorded in the margin. Special ones can be enlarged further if necessary. Rectangles and squares can be drawn to outline areas for publication prints or slides. When a mass of prints has accumulated, a good filing system is essential to avoid chaos.

Measurement

The measurement of size does not pose too many problems. The magnification recorded on the machine cannot be depended on for accuracy. It alters according to servicing and variations in lens current and high voltage. For moderate resolution work it is always worth inserting a calibration grid into the machine at the end of a session, particularly if important material has been looked at. Calibration-grids are replicas of a diffraction grating in which the distance between the parallel lines is accurately known. An accurate magnification of the negative can easily be worked out using a simple formula. For high

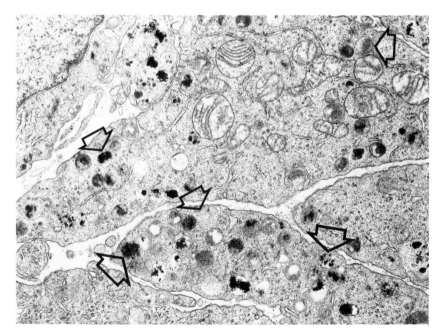

Fig. 12.10 (× 12 400) Tumour cells in malignant melanoma. As the cellular preservation is good, details of the abnormal melanosomes (arrows) can be easily studied.

resolution work polystyrene spheres of known diameter may be sprayed on to specimens mounted on grids, and direct measurements made.

Quantitative measurements are a real problem in standard transmission electron microscopy. The 'linear scanning' technique is useful for determining volume ratios of cells or organelles within a tissue, providing an adequate number of photographs are sampled. The application and details of the method have been outlined by Carpenter and Lazarow (1962) and Zelickson and Mottaz (1968) have shown how it can be used to quantitate epidermal cell populations in various pathological and experimental situations. Computerized methods of quantitation are also now available. A computer can be trained to recognize certain shapes and sizes and will scan negatives and record them.

SIGNIFICANCE AND INTERPRETATION OF RESULTS

Although photographs never tell lies, their interpretation can often lead to a conclusion far from the truth. How do we know which and what to believe? The technical quality of micrographs is not difficult to appreciate. The ideal picture should show good cellular preservation and demonstrate clearly the point which is under discussion, so that the reader with only scant electron microscopic knowledge is convinced by the evidence (see Fig. 12.10).

The more discerning reader should be able to spot poor technique. Even conclusions based on good technique may be open to doubt, but those based on artefact should never reach a debateable stage. If the best pictures in a paper show artefact, are out of focus (providing that the journal is not responsible), or demonstrate some other failure in technique, then who can blame anyone for wondering what the material left out of the publications was like? An argument cannot be persuasive if the evidence is suspicious (see Figs. 12.11 and 12.12).

It has already been stressed that there is no substitute for personal experience in all stages of preparative procedures in electron microscopy. This makes interpretation of micrographs so much more simple and the cause of faults, if they exist, easier to detect. Terms like 'swollen mitochondria' and 'increased number of desmosomes' are accepted as being all but meaningless, because they are most likely due to fixation faults or subjective hunches.

This train of thought leads on to another related theme—the subjective element of electron microscopy. It is human nature to notice things which are being looked for and to miss those which are not expected. For instance, different groups of workers have reported different findings on tape stripping of the epidermis. Mishima and Pinkus (1968) were impressed by the dissolution of the tonofilament-desmosomal connections, keratinocyte phagocytosis of retracted desmosomes and the presence of melanosomes within phagocytic vacuoles of Langerhans' cells (Mishima 1966). Mottaz and Zelickson (1970) and Mottaz *et al* (1971) were struck initially by the phagocytic nature of the keratinocytes which contained phagocytosed parts of Langerhans' cells, and later by the fact that many melanocytes contained melanosomes within

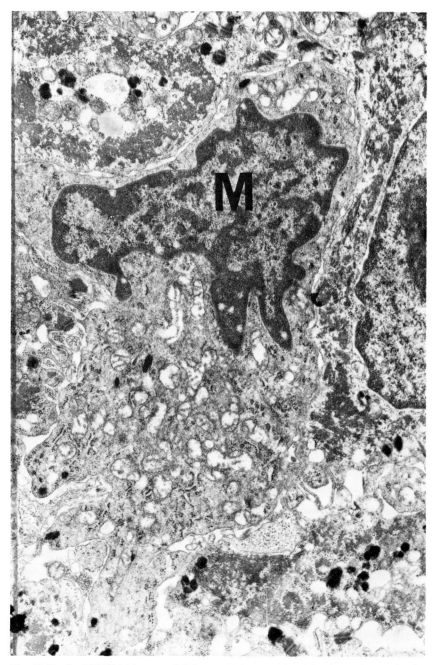

Fig. 12.11 (× 15 000) Melanocyte (M) in normal human skin epidermis. Inadequate fixation has resulted in poor membrane preservation. The mitochondrial cristae have ruptured and these organelles are also bloated.

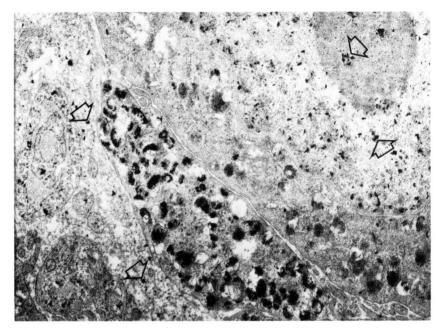

Fig. 12.12 (× 12 000) Malignant melanoma. Ultrastructural acid phosphatase reaction. There is random artefactual deposition of reaction product (open arrows) throughout the section.

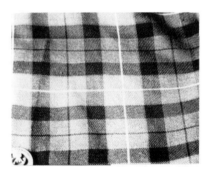

Fig. 12.13   Hunter tartan.

autophagic vacuoles, showed increased tyrosinase activity and phagocytosis of parts of Langerhans' cells. The micrographs presented in all the papers are convincing, but serve as a reminder that what one person sees is not necessarily the same as another.

Fig. 12.13 is a picture of the Hunter tartan. A snip taken from one area could be white, from another red and from a third green. Each could represent a block of tissue processed for electron microscopy. If the overall pattern was not appreciated then one worker would conclude that the material was white, whilst others would consider it red or green.

Sampling can be a huge problem in electron microscopy. Numerous pictures of an interesting appearance may be obtained, but they could all come from the same cell, or from a tiny area in the tissue. It is most important to check that any findings are representative of the whole tissue, rather than freak occurrences in a single cell. Natural enthusiasm must be kept firmly in check by an honest and scientific approach.

ACKNOWLEDGEMENT

It is a pleasure to acknowledge the technical help of D. J. Fairley.

REFERENCES

BARKA T. & ANDERSON P. J. (1962) Histochemical methods for acid phosphatase using hexazonium pararosanilin as coupler. *Journal Histochemistry and Cytochemistry* **10**, 741.
BASSET F., NEZELOF C., MALLET R. & TURIAF J. (1965) Nouvelle mise en Évidence, par la Microscopie Électronique, de particules d'allure Virale dans une seconde forme Clinique de l'Histiocytose X, le Granulome Éosinophile de l'os. *C.r. hebd. Séanc. Acad. Sci., Paris* **261**, 5719.
BIRKMAYER G. D., BALDA B. R. & MILLER F. (1974) Oncorna-viral information in human melanoma. *European Journal of Cancer* **10**, 419.
BLOIS M. S. & KALLMAN R. F. (1964) The incorporation of C^{14} from 3.4. Dihydroxyphenyl-alanine. 2'. C^{14} into the melanin of mouse melanomas. *Cancer Research* **24**, 863.
BREATHNACH A. S. & WYLLIE L. M. (1966) Osmium iodide positive granules in spinous and granular layers of guinea pig epidermis. *Journal of Investigative Dermatology* **47**, 58.
BRUMBAUCH L. J., BOWERS R. & LEE K. (1973) Histochemical evidence that peroxidase does not affect melanin formation in feather melanocytes. *Yale Journal of Biology and Medicine* **46**, 523.
CARPENTER A. M. & LAZAROW A. (1962) Component quantitation of tissue sections. *Journal of Histochemistry and Cytochemistry* **10**, 329.
GOMORI G. (1952) *Microscopic Histochemistry*. University Press, Chicago. P. 189.
HASHIMOTO K. (1970) Lanthanum staining of Langerhans' cell. *Archives of Dermatology* **102**, 280.
HASHIMOTO K. & LEVER W. F. (1970) An ultrastructural study of cell junctions in pemphigus vulgaris. *Archives of Dermatology* **101**, 287.
HER MAJESTY'S STATIONERY OFFICE (1974) *Report of the Committee of Inquiry into the Smallpox Outbreak in London in March and April 1973*. HMSO, London.
HUNTER J. A. A., FAIRLEY D. J., PRIESTLEY G. C. & CUBIE H. A. (1976) Langerhans' cells in the epidermis of athymic mice. *British Journal of Dermatology* **94**, 119.
HUNTER J. A. A., McVITTIE E. & COMAISH J. S. (1974) Light and/electron microscopic studies of physical injury to the skin. I. Suction. *British Journal of Dermatology* **90**, 481.
HUNTER J. A. A., MOTTAZ J. H. & ZELICKSON A. S. (1970) Melanogenesis: ultrastructural histochemical observations on ultraviolet irradiated human melanocytes. *Journal of Investigative Dermatology* **54**, 213.
JACOB J. (1971) The practice and application of electron microscope autoradiography. *International Review of Cytology* **30**, 91.
KARNOVSKY M. J. (1965) Vesicular transport of exogenous peroxidase across capillary endothelium into the T system of muscle. *Journal of Cell Biology* **27**, 49A.
KNUTSON D. D. (1974) Ultrastructural observations in acne vulgaris: The normal sebaceous follicle and acne lesions. *Journal of Investigative Dermatology* **62**, 288.
MAUL G. G. (1969) Golgi-melanosome relationship in human melanoma *in vitro*. *Journal of Ultrastructural Research* **26**, 163.

MAUL G. G. & ROMSDAHL M. M. (1970) Ultrastructural comparison of two human malignant melanoma cell lines. *Cancer Research* **30,** 2782.

MISHIMA Y. (1966) Melansomes in phagocytic vacuoles in Langerhans' cells. Electron microscopy of keratin-stripped human epidermis. *Journal of Cell Biology* **30,** 417.

MISHIMA Y. & PINKHUS H. (1968) Electron microscopy of keratin layer stripped human epidermis. *Journal of Investigative Dermatology* **50,** 89.

MOTTAZ J. H., THORNE E. G. & ZELICKSON A. S. (1971) Response of the epidermal melanocyte to minor trauma. *Archives of Dermatology* **104,** 611.

MOTTAZ J. H. & ZELICKSON A. S. (1970) The phagocytic nature of the keratinocyte in human epidermis after tape strapping. *Journal of Investigative Dermatology* **54,** 272.

NAKAI T. & SHUBIK P. (1964) Electron microscopic radioautography. The melanosome as a site of melanogenesis in neoplastic melanocytes. *Journal of Investigative Dermatology* **43,** 267.

NAKANE P. K. & PIERCE G. B. (1967) Enzyme-labelled antibodies for the light and electron microscopic localization of tissue antigens. *Journal of Cell Biology* **33,** 307.

NIEBAUER G., KRAWCZYK W. S., KIDD R. L. & WILGRAM G. F. (1969) Osmium zinc iodide reactive sites in the epidermal Langerhans' cell. *Journal of Cell Biology* **43,** 80.

NOVIKOFF A. B. (1963) Lysosomes in Physiology and Pathology of Cells: Contribution of Staining Methods. In *Ciba Foundation Symposium on Lysosomes,* eds., de Reuk A. V. S. & Cameron M. P. Little Brown, Boston.

OKUN M. R., DONNELLAN B., PATEL R. P., LEON M. & EDELSTEIN M. D. (1973) Subcellular demonstration of peroxidatic oxidation of tyrosine to melanin using dihydroxyfumarate as co-factor in mouse melanoma cells. *Journal of Investigative Dermatology* **61,** 60.

SABATINI D. D., BENSCH K. & BARRNETT R. J. (1963) Cytochemistry and electron microscopy. The preservation of cellular ultrastructure and enzymic activity by Aldehyde fixation. *Journal of Cell Biology* **17,** 19.

SAGEBIEL R. W. (1972) *In vivo* and *in vitro* uptake of ferritin by Langerhans' cells of the epidermis. *Journal of Investigative Dermatology* **58,** 47.

SALPETER M. M. & BACHMANN (1965) In *The Use of Autoradiography in the Investigation of Protein Synthesis,* ed. Harris R. J. C. Academic Press, New York.

SCHNAIT F. G., WOLFF K. & KONRAD K. (1975) Erythropoietic protoporphyria—submicroscopic events during the acute photosensitive flare. *British Journal of Dermatology* **92,** 545.

SINGER S. J. (1959) Preparation of an electron dense antibody conjugate. *Nature* **183,** 1523.

TODA K. & FITZPATRICK T. B. (1971) The Origins of Melanosomes. In *Biology of Normal and Abnormal Melanocytes,* eds., Kawamura T., Fitzpatrick T. B. & Seiji M. p. 265. University Park Press, Baltimore.

WOLFF K. & HÖNIGSMANN H. (1971) Permeability of the epidermis and phagocytic activity of keratinocytes. *Journal of Ultrastructural Research* **36,** 176.

WOLFF K. & KONRAD K. (1972) Phagocytosis of latex beads by epidermal keratinocytes *in vivo. Journal of Ultrastructural Research* **39,** 262.

WOLFF K. & SCHREINER E. (1970) Uptake intracellular transport and degradation of exogenous protein by Langerhans' cells. An electron microscopic-cytochemical study using peroxidase as tracer substance. *Journal of Investigative Dermatology* **54,** 37.

WOLFF K. & SCHREINER E. (1971) Differential enzymatic digestion of cytoplasmic components of keratinocytes: electron microscopic observations. *Journal of Ultrastructural Research* **36,** 437.

ZELICKSON A. S., HIRSCH H. M. & HARTMANN J. F. (1965) Localization of melanin synthesis. *Journal of Investigative Dermatology* **45,** 458.

ZELICKSON A. S. & MOTTAZ J. H. (1968) Epidermal dendritic cells. A quantitative survey. *Archives of Dermatology* **98,** 652.

FURTHER READING

GLAURT A. M. (1973–1977) *Practical Methods in Electron Microscopy,* Vols 1–5. North Holland Publishing Co., Amsterdam.

GRIFFIN R. L. (1972) *Ultramicrotomy.* Baillere Tindall, London.

KAY D. H. (1965) *Techniques for Electron Microscopy.* Blackwell, Oxford.

LANGFORD M. J. (1973) *Basic Photography.* 3rd edn. The Focal Press, London.

MEEK G. A. (1970) *Practical Electron Microscopy for Biologists.* Wiley Interscience, London.

MERCER E. H. & BIRBECK M. S. C. (1972) *Electron Microscopy: A Handbook for Biologists.* 3rd edn. Blackwell, Oxford.

*WEAKLEY B. S. (1972) *A Beginners Handbook in Biological Electron Microscopy.* Churchill Livingstone, Edinburgh.

*Highly recommended for the beginner.

13

Application of scanning electron microscopy to dermatology

N. MOORE AND R. MARKS

INTRODUCTION

The scanning electron microscope (SEM) first became commercially available in the mid 1960s. Since that time the instrument has amply illustrated that it has the capability of inspecting the surface of all types of structure at high resolution and great depth of focus. The micrographs that can be obtained with the instrument have a 'natural' appearance and a pleasing 'solid' quality. For this reason the micrographs are more easily interpreted than by conventional microscopy.

A modern SEM has a resolution of between 5 and 10 nm in the emissive mode compared with about 200 nm for a light microscope and less than 0.5 nm for a transmission electron microscope. Although resolution is an important feature of SEM, perhaps the feature that recommends itself to most users is the great depth of focus it allows. Experience has shown that for many purposes the SEM is used at magnifications well within the resolving power of a light microscope. However, at these magnifications the depths of focus of a light microscope is of the order of 1μm. Therefore, an 'in focus image' cannot be obtained of any surface having features larger than 1μm. The SEM in contrast has a depth of focus of about 1mm at these magnifications and can give a clear image of comparatively uneven surfaces. It is this ability of the SEM to show the detail of uneven surfaces that is of particular interest. Paradoxically, it is this same ability to provide an unusually sharp vision of surfaces which previously were too uneven to be seen entirely in focus at one and the same time which has resulted in confusion and abuse. Confusion because it is sometimes difficult to interpret the nature of the surface projections, pits or other contoured features of membranes and correlate them with data obtained by transmission electron microscopy. Abuse, because this unusual and aesthetically pleasing image has a surrealistic aura about it, which permits the belief that novel and useful data is being generated. The 'lunar surface look' to many scanning electron micrographs and the difficulty in fusing the image of the particular structure examined with more conventional ultrastructural views has led to a kind of cynicism by some who do not understand the potential of this type of examination. This cynicism has not been helped by publications which merely record the SEM appearance of this that or the other tissue.

The real usefulness of the SEM is that it is possible to examine cell surface membranes and in particular determine how structures interrelate on cell surfaces and how individual cells or cells and microorganisms interrelate.

The SEM, in common with the transmission electron microscope, needs an evacuated column down which the electrons pass. The electrons in general are obtained by thermionic emission from an electrically heated tungsten filament and are accelerated down the column by a voltage of between 2 to 50 kV. This beam of electrons is progressively reduced in diameter by successive electromagnetic condenser lenses until it has a cross-section at the specimen of 5–10 nm. The fine beam of electrons is scanned across the specimen by electromagnetic coils in a raster (a rectangular array of lines similar to that on a television screen) which typically contains 1000 lines. When the beam of primary electrons strikes the specimen, some of the electrons are reflected, and some cause the production of secondary electrons from the surface. It is these reflected and secondary electrons which are collected and used to form the image in the 'emissive mode' of operation. The collected electrons are amplified and the signal obtained is used to determine the brightness of the spot on a cathode ray tube (c.r.t.), which is scanning a raster moving synchronous to the raster of the primary beam. For this reason there is at any instant a direct relationship between a point on the specimen and a point on the c.r.t. screen; the brightness of the point on the c.r.t. is dependent on the number of electrons collected from the corresponding point on the specimen. The magnification is achieved by making the size of the raster on the specimens small compared with the size of the c.r.t. screen. The linear magnification then is the width of the c.r.t. screen divided by the width of the raster on the specimen. By this method magnifications in excess of 100 000 can be obtained. The image is normally viewed on a c.r.t. having a long persistence phosphor. At low magnifications and large spot sizes, television scan speeds may be used to give a flicker-free image. Higher magnifications require a smaller spot size and a slower scan rate to achieve the required resolution. A photographic record is obtained from a c.r.t. having a short persistence phosphor and the recording time for the photographs is usually between 40 and 100 seconds. This relatively long recording time reduces the amount of 'noise' that is recorded and improves the amount of detail that is photographed. The noise which is generated in the amplifying system depends on the spot size and so tends to be a problem at high magnifications. By careful selections of spot size and recording time the effects of noise can be reduced and the micrographs should always show more detail than is visible on the viewing screen.

So far we have only mentioned the emissive mode of operation, but let us consider the other effects which occur when an electron beam strikes a specimen. If the specimen is suitably thin, some primary electrons will penetrate through the specimen and may be collected under the specimen and used to form an image. This is called the 'transmission mode' of operation and shows up details from within the specimen.

The primary beam can also generate X-rays in the specimen, some of these X-rays are characteristic of the individual elements contained within the specimen. The characteristic X-rays can be used to identify the constituents of the sample, their concentrations and position (a type of electron probe X-ray microanalysis). Light is also generated by the primary beam and this can be used to form the so-called 'cathode luminiscence image'.

Finally, electrons are absorbed within the specimen itself and in conducting samples can be used to form a 'conducting mode image' but in the specimens of interest the absorbed electrons generate heat and often tend to damage the specimen.

PHOTOGRAPHY

Good scanning electron micrographs are essential to be able to draw conclusions from SEM experiments. Considerable experience with a particular SEM is necessary before good photographs can be produced and it is really worthwhile mastering 'the art' before any value can be obtained from 'the science'. Particular attention should be given to 'focus' and it is usual practice to first focus on a particular feature at two magnification settings on the machine higher than is intended for the actual photograph. Careful attention must also be given to the astigmatism and signal strength controls or else distorted or poor contrast pictures will be produced. The photographs should be of sufficient size (half plate is usually sufficient) and it is the authors' preference to print these on high gloss paper. It is not infrequently the case that large numbers of photographs emanate from an 'SEM project' and at this stage professionalism really shows in the ability to file (and later retrieve!) these in a logical and simple way.

PREPARATION OF SPECIMENS FOR SEM

All tissues and biological structures examined by SEM must be dehydrated as they are examined in a vacuum chamber. However, minimum if any fixation is required and this allows a relatively artefact-free view of cell membranes.

Stratum corneum

For examination of the surface of the stratum corneum it is customary to take replicas of the skin surface, although early workers did examine the surface of ordinary skin biopsies. Replicas are taken in two stages. In the first the 'negative' is taken by applying a silicone rubber material such as is used to take dental impressions (Silflo is routinely used in our department) to the area to be examined. After a minute or so the material dries and then is gently lifted off the skin. Some practice is required in mixing the components of the silicone rubber material before applying to the skin to avoid the production and trapping of bubbles. The 'negative' is then placed on a glass microscope slide and coated with a hard drying plastic used for mounting histological specimens on

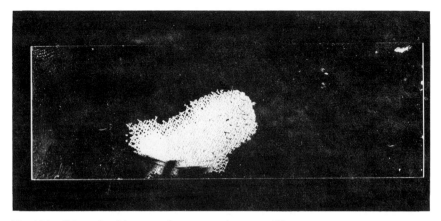

Fig. 13.1   Skin surface biopsy as taken onto a microscope slide.

microscope slides and known as DPX (R. A. Lamb, London)—another stage in which bubbles may be produced. The preparation is then hardened by dehydration in a desiccator for 6–12 hours after which time the negative and DPX positive can be separated without great difficulty.

In order to examine the internal structure of the stratum corneum, microbial invaders of the stratum corneum or detailed surface structure of individual corneocytes it is necessary to take skin surface biopsies (SSBs). This technique described by Marks and Dawber (1971) involves the removal of 3–5 intact cell layers of the stratum corneum with a rapidly bonding cyanoacrylate adhesive. The adhesive (the one used in our department is Permabond—Staident Products Ltd., Staines) is placed on the skin surface and a glass microscope is then placed over the drop and slight pressure applied for about 30 seconds. The glass slide is then removed from the surface of the skin by progressively lifting one of its ends. In this way an intact layer of stratum corneum stuck to the glass slide should be removed (see Fig. 13.1). Because the cyanoacrylate is transparent and has similar optical properties to glass it is also possible to examine these preparations by light microscopy. No specific dehydration or fixation is necessary for the examination of SSBs or replicas by SEM.

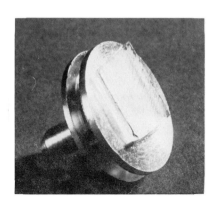

Fig. 13.2   Skin surface biopsy mounted on SEM 'stub'.

In order to examine SSBs and replicas by SEM it is first necessary to mount the preparations on special mushroom shaped holders made of aluminium and known as 'stubs'. This is simply done by cutting the specimen to the required size and sticking them to the stub (see Fig. 13.2). The edges of the specimen are painted with a silver paint known as 'silver dag' in order to make the edges electrically conducting.

Hair

Samples of hair for examination are merely stuck to double-sided adhesive tape so that the hairs may be stuck to one sticky face while the other sticky face is stuck to the stub.

Viable tissue

The examination of viable tissues from the skin is slightly more complex as some type of fixation as well as dehydration is sometimes necessary. As there is no difference in principle (and often in practice) between the preparation of skin tissues and the preparation of other kinds of tissue and there is some disagreement amongst various groups of workers, 'the beginner' in the field is advised to read widely and at the same time develop his own techniques which suit him and his particular object of interest best. At the end of this chapter there is a selected bibliography which covers various preparative techniques. In general, two types of 'tissue sample' may be examined in the SEM. The first is a dispersion of cells (lymphocytes, fibroblasts, malignant cell lines, microorganisms etc), which may originate directly from the organism concerned or from cell or microbial culture. The second is a tissue 'face' of some kind such as the cut margins of a tissue sample or even the surface of a tissue section prepared for either light or transmission electron microscopy.

Clearly the way that the sample is prepared for SEM depends on the size, structure and the stability of the specimen. Viable tissue or cell suspensions can be prepared for SEM by either freeze drying in a Pearse tissue drying apparatus or by treatment in a critical point drying apparatus (Anderson 1951; Boyd *et al* 1972). This latter method in general produces the better results with fragile tissues. It relies on the replacement of the water content of the tissue under conditions of low pressure and its replacement by an inert gas such as carbon dioxide. If preservation of tissue architecture is not vital air drying after dehydration in graded acetone solutions can be used. If freeze drying or critical point drying is employed only 'limited fixation' is required. Cell suspensions are often fixed for periods of 30–60 minutes in a 2.5% buffered glutaraldehyde solution. Microtomized sections, of course, do not need fixation (however paraffin sections have to be deparaffinized in xylene before any other kind of preparative technique).

Specimen coating

The specimens obtained by the methods outlined above are of course non-conducting and if examined in the SEM at normal voltage, the electron beam will cause a build-up of electrostatic charge on the surface. This charge is unstable and can adversely affect the image quality. The charge can deflect and defocus the primary beam causing loss of resolution and gross astigmatism. Increased emission from charged areas give bright bands on the image and no detail can be discerned within the bright areas of 'charge'. Areas adjacent to the charged sites appear much darker than normal leading to a loss of detail. It is possible to examine non-conducting samples at low voltage (about 2 kV), and at magnifications up to about × 1000 without charging becoming apparent (eg hair). The resolution under these conditions is very much reduced. For operations at high resolution it is necessary to coat the sample with a thin layer of conducting material. The most common materials used are gold or gold/palladium alloy. A layer 40–50 nm thick is usually adequate. In addition, to prevent charging the coating has other useful functions. Gold is a good source of secondary electrons, it is relatively opaque to the primary beam and is a good conductor of heat. A good source of secondary electrons is important to give a bright noise-free image. As it is relatively opaque to the primary beam most secondary electrons are generated close to the surface and few secondary electrons generated from within the specimen can escape, be collected and confuse the image. It also follows that if less of the primary beam penetrates into the specimen, less heat will be generated in the specimen as some of that heat will be conducted away by the coating, less specimen damage will result.

There are two main methods which are used to coat samples with the required thickness of metal prior to examination. The most common method until quite recently was by evaporation in a vacuum of less than 10^{-4} mmHg. A small loop of the coating metal is placed on a 'V' shaped tungsten wire. The amount of metal in the loop is calculated by assuming that it is all spread evenly of the required thickness, over the surface of a sphere, with a radius equal to the filament-sample distance. The system is evacuated and a high current up 60 A is passed through the tungsten wire to first melt and then evaporate the coating metal comprising the loop. The process is usually observed through welder's goggles to ensure that all the coating metal is evaporated; this is usually judged to happen when the tungsten filament reaches an even colour. In order to ensure that the coating has reached all parts of the specimen, the samples are rotated. More even coating will be obtained if the samples can be made to follow a planetary path, and there are several commercially available units which can perform this. One disadvantage of this method of coating is that the samples are exposed to the radiant heat from the tungsten evaporation source. To overcome this problem and to avoid the necessity of moving the samples during coating many microscopists have turned to 'sputter coating' with gold. Sputter coating takes place at a much higher pressure (ie less of a vacuum) than filament evaporation, typically at approximately 0.1 mmHg. A rotary vacuum pump is sufficient to achieve this pressure, making the pumping system less sophisticated and easier to operate. In a 'sputter coater' a beam of argon ions is directed at a gold target, gold atoms are knocked from the surface of the target and are deposited on the specimens and other nearby surfaces. As the pressure in the chamber is relatively high, the atoms of gold suffer many collisions with the gas atoms and therefore reach the specimens from all directions. This ensures an even coating of all facets of the sample. The rate of sputter coating for any instrument is known (approximately 20 nm/min) the thickness of coating being determined by the time of sputtering.

Carbon is sometimes used as a coating material, but it is not recommended for organic material as it is so easily penetrated by the primary beam. However, it does have some advantages: it causes less interference when analysis is performed in the SEM, and is considerably less expensive than other coatings. Carbon coating is carried out in a vacuum evaporator at a pressure of approximately 10^{-4} mmHg, and a current of about 30 A is passed through the junctions of two carbon rods. The rate of coating is very fast (of the order of 20 nm/sec) and care must be exercised so as not to overcoat.

OPERATION OF THE SEM

There is a rigid sequence of manoeuvres that must be performed to ensure that a vacuum exists in the column and before the filament can be activated. This varies with each model and must be carefully learnt to save damaging expensive apparatus. Let us assume that the SEM is in fact ready for use. The stub is placed in the appropriate slot in the specimen chamber at the bottom of the vacuum column and then the chamber is sealed and the column evacuated (which takes approximately 2 minutes depending on the machine). When the column is at low vacuum the electron beam is allowed to strike the specimen. The exact site for inspection is chosen after 'scanning' the specimen at very low power. The 'tilt angle' (angle at which the electron beam strikes the specimen) is also selected—this is usually 45° for most biological materials. Details concerning the particular controls and the sequence of operation is different for each SEM and is usually well set out in the handbook accompanying the SEM.

SOME FACTS AND ARTEFACTS IN SEM OF SKIN COMPONENTS

Stratum corneum (SC)

Excellent views of both the internal structure and the actual surface of the SC may be obtained by SEM. Samples for the first may be obtained by skin surface biopsy (SSB—see above) and samples for the second may be obtained by a replica technique (see above). For many purposes the two techniques are interchangeable and give surprisingly similar pictures of the SC in the horizontal plane. At low power ($\times$ 25–100 magnification) and at a tilt angle of 45° the skin surface morphology can be seen as a regular series of valleys and ridges (see Fig. 13.3) interspersed with the pores of the eccrine sweat ducts and the more complex and variably sized hair follicle ostia. The overall pattern differs in different sites and should information about the gross morphology of the skin surface be required the production and inspection of a replica at low magnification in the SEM is ideal. Similarly, considerable information on the eccrine sweat pores and their abnormalities can be obtained using the same technique. Papa (1972) demonstrated the usefulness of this approach in the investigation of anhidrosis. Surprisingly hairs may also be seen in SSBs—despite the fact that it is purely the under surface of the split off portion of the SC that is being inspected. The explanation is that some of the hair are distracted at the time of taking the specimen but remain in the portion of the hair canal in the SSB.

Luckily the SSB splits between individual corneocytes rather than through cells—a tribute to the toughness of the plasma membranes of corneocytes. The cyanoacrylate adhesive appears to penetrate no further than to the second cell layer of the SC and as the SSB is five or more cells thick the adhesive never permeates to the surface of the SSB and should never be seen on SEM. At higher magnifications ($\times$ 500–2000) individual corneocytes can be seen. Tremendous detail can be seen in replicas at this magnification nonetheless when a detailed inspection of corneocytes is necessary it is best to examine SSBs. It is our routine practice to particularly note certain features when examining SSBs at high magnification.

Corneocyte surface pattern

The surface of the normal corneocyte plasma membrane is usually somewhat undulating but otherwise disappointingly featureless (see Fig. 13.4). (A series of low ridges is occasionally seen on some corneocytes interspersed amongst the more numerous corneocytes with a relatively featureless surface). On the palm or the sole, the surface of corneocytes is studied with numerous small projections or microvilli. When there is a high rate of cell production by the epidermis the stratum corneum that is produced is composed of corneocytes that have the same or even more prominent microvillous pattern (Marks & Griffiths 1973) and this feature is best seen in psoriasis (see Fig. 13.5).

Intercorneocyte gaps

Normally the corneocytes overlap each other slightly in an orderly manner but gaps become visible with the disorderly SC production of some inflammatory dermatoses or after treatment with keratolytics (Davies & Marks 1976) or after hydration (Nicholls *et al* 1978).

Corneocyte margins

In some situations the corneocyte margins appear 'ragged' (as after treatment with keratolytics (Davies & Marks 1976) or swollen 'cylinder-like' (as after hydration). At times intercorneocyte connections can be seen in the form of

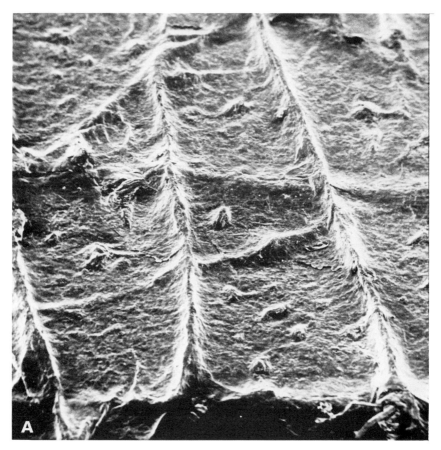

Fig. 13.3 A, SEM micrograph of skin surface biopsy from patients with ichthyosis (machine mag. × 30); B, SEM micrograph of skin replica from leg (machine mag. × 220).

tube-like bridges and presumably these are the remnants of desmosomes. Attention should also be paid to the number of single desquamating corneocytes and desquamating clumps of corneocytes. In the ichthyotic disorders very few solitary desquamating cells are visible compared to normal although partially detached clumps of corneocytes aggregated together may be seen (Nicholls *et al* 1977). Apart from these morphological considerations the diameter of the corneocytes should be estimated—either by use of the 'mu marker' if there is one on the SEM being used or with a special 'magnification ruler' (Polaron Ltd) or by measurement with a ruler and calculation. Of course note must be taken of the presence of other extraneous material—such as microorganisms. Difficulties that may be encountered include 'charging' (see above) due to uneven coating which will produce bright and fuzzy areas on the scanning field 'astigmatism' (see above) the inadvertent burning of holes in the specimen due to the scanning of small areas (at high magnification) with a high

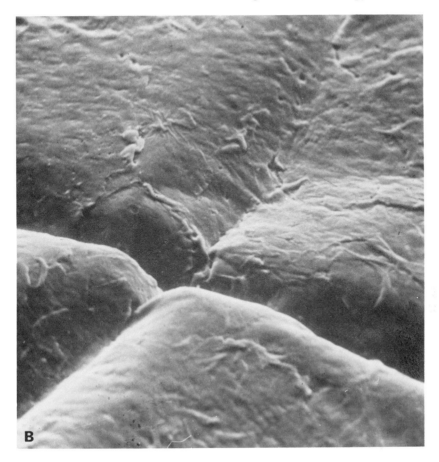

kilo voltage beam (see Fig. 13.6) and too thick a coating of conducting material which will obscure all fine detail.

Hair

Hair can be seen uncoated if the accelerating voltage is low (2 kV) or can be treated as SC specimens and coated, after fixing samples to SEM stubs, and viewed at a higher accelerating voltage. The normal cuticular scale can be clearly seen at magnifications of × 200 or more. The individual cuticle cells closely overlap each other normally and have a featureless surface apart from the occasional pit and or small protuberance. The free edges of the cuticle cells are characteristically somewhat angulated (see Fig. 13.7). Several lengths should be inspected or else intermittent abnormalities such as trichorrhexis

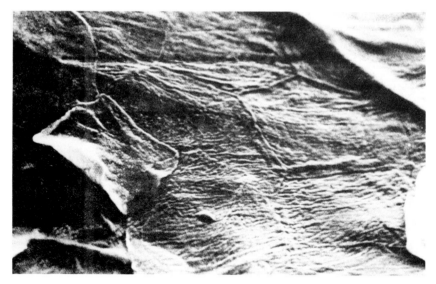

Fig. 13.4 Micrograph to show normal corneocyte surfaces taken from skin surface biopsy of forearm (machine mag. × 3900). A faint ridge pattern can be seen.

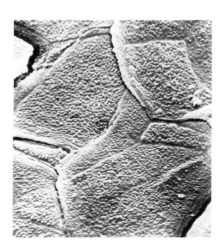

Fig. 13.5 Psoriatic corneocytes from skin surface biopsy (machine mag. × 1150). A microvillous pattern is seen.

nodosa may be missed (see Fig. 13.8). Similarly, disorders of orientation of the shaft may be missed if only short sections are examined (see Fig. 13.9). Areas of loss of scale are often seen towards the tip of the hair shaft from 'weathering and grooming'. During examination of a hair shaft, its width should be measured and recorded. If possible, more than one hair should be examined to avoid missing abnormalities in which every hair is not affected as in some infections.

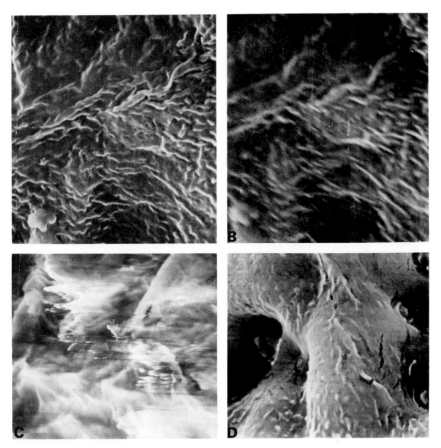

Fig. 13.6 A and B demonstrate the effects of astigmatism. A shows a normal corneovyte. B shows the same field with the effects of astigmatism (machine mag. × 3900). C, the effects of 'charging' (skin surface biopsy machine mag. × 3900); D, the effects of beam overheating or 'burning' (machine mag. × 3900). Numerous fissures are seen as a heating effect.

Dermatophytes

These microorganisms can be examined either *in vivo* (Marks & Dawber 1972; Marks *et al* 1972) in the stratum corneum or directly after culture (De Nollin *et al* 1977). The former technique is more important in learning about host parasite interactions and the latter technique of importance in the understanding of the biology of the infecting microorganism and of the effect of antimicrobial drugs on it. The authors have had more experience of the *in vivo* technique and have been surprised at the relative ease with which microorganisms can be adequately examined by taking skin surface biopsies from infected areas (see Fig. 13.10). The exact relationship of the microbe with the horn should be recorded. For example do the mycelial strands penetrate the

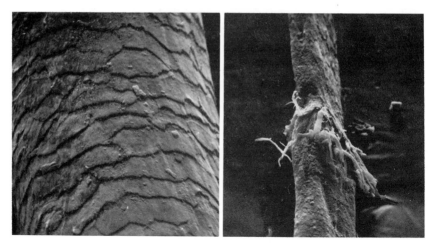

Fig. 13.7 (left)   Normal hair shaft (machine mag. × 1200). (With courtesy of Dr. R. R. P. Dawber)

Fig. 13.8 (right)   Micrograph of hair with trichorrhexis nodosa (machine mag. × 300). (With courtesy of Dr. R. R. P. Dawber)

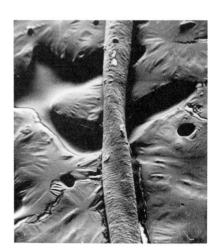

Fig. 13.9   Hair showing pili torti (machine mag. × 120). (With courtesy of Dr. R. R. P. Dawber)

Fig. 13.10   Both 'A' and 'B' are micrographs of the erythrasma microorganism *in vivo* from skin surface biopsies taken from the groin (A—machine mag. × 3500) (B—machine mag. × 1700).

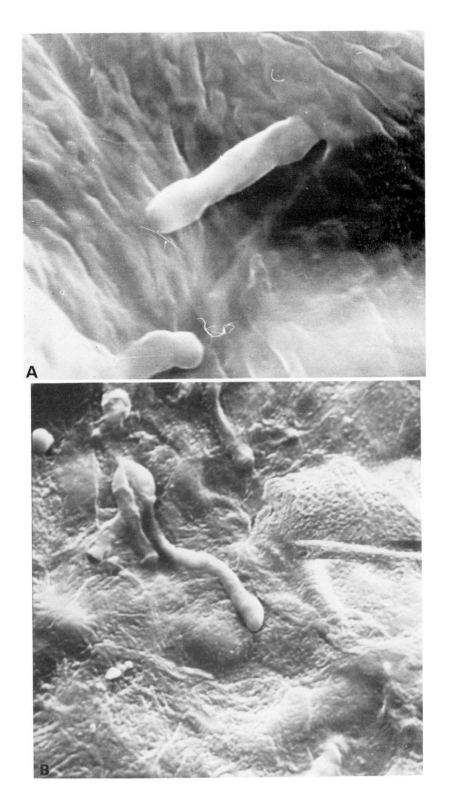

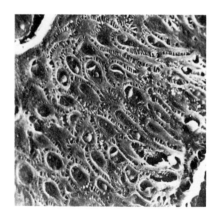

Fig. 13.11 Micrograph of human epidermis (biopsy of patient with lichenized eczema) from paraffin section (machine mag. × 100).

corneocytes or do they travel predominantly between the cells? The types of microbial structure and the relative amounts of each of the host stratum corneum and the presence of 'abnormal forms' of microbial structure should also, of course, be recorded. We believe that this type of study will be of increasing use in the study of the biology of human dermatophyte infections and their treatment.

The epidermis

As yet there have been few SEM studies of the epidermis normal, stimulated or diseased and this could be a fertile field for valuable experimental work. Wong and Vickers (1972) and Marks and Bhogal (1974) describe techniques for examining either fresh skin (either after biopsy or from culture) or of paraffin sections (see Fig. 13.11). Holbrook and Odland (1975) published the results of a beautiful correlative study in which they examined the fine structure of human fetal epidermis by transmission electron and light microscopy as well as by SEM.

The dermis

The same comment can be made for this important component as has for the epidermis. However, mention should be made of the study by Brown (1973) who cleverly designed a technique for studying the orientation of the connective tissue fibres after stressing human skin.

CONCLUSION

In general, the techniques of SEM are less arduous and time-consuming than for transmission electron microscopy. The resulting micrographs are often in addition more aesthetically pleasing. These 'advantages' should be handled carefully as without doubt they are double-edged and have led to needless opprobrium being piled on to a potentially useful technique. As with all 'techniques' SEM is only a means to an end. The 'end' is of course the answer to a scientific question. The value of any investigation (SEM studies included) depends on the interest and validity of the 'question' and on the interpretation of the results obtained as well as being dependent on the proficiency with which the particular technique is used.

REFERENCES

ANDERSON T. F. (1951) Techniques for the preservation of three dimensional structure in preparing specimens for the electron microscope. *Transactions of the New York Academy of Science* **13**, 130.

BOYDE A., WEISS R. A. & VESELY P. (1972) Scanning electron microscopy of cells in culture. *Experimental Cell Research* **71**. 313.

BROWN I. A. (1973) A scanning electron microscope study of the effects of uniaxial tension on human skin. *British Journal of Dermatology* **89**, 383.

DAVIES M. & MARKS R. (1976) Studies on the effect of salicylic acid in normal skin. *British Journal of Dermatology* **95**, 187.

DE NOLLIN S., BORGERS M. & VAN BELLE H. (1977) The effects of miconazole on the ultrastructure of candida albicans. *Proceedings of the Royal Society of Medicine* **70**, Supplement 4. p.19.

HOLBROOK K. A. & ODLAND G. F. (1975) The fine structure of developing human epidermis: light scanning and transmission electron microscopy of the periderm. *Journal of Investigative Dermatology* **65**, 16.

MARKS R. & DAWBER R. R. P. (1971) Skin surface biopsy: An improved technique for the examination of the horny layer. *British Journal of Dermatology* **84**, 117.

MARKS R. & DAWBER R. R. P. (1972) *In situ* microbiology of the stratum corneum. *Archives of Dermatology* **105**, 216.

MARKS R., RAMMARAIN N., BHOGAL B. & MOORE N. (1972) The erythrasma microorganism in situ: Studies using the skin surface biopsy technique. *British Journal of Clinical Pathology* **25**, 799.

MARKS R. & GRIFFITHS W. A. D. (1973) The significance of surface changes in parakeratotic horn. *Journal of Investigative Dermatology* **61**, 251.

MARKS R. & BHOGAL B. (1974) Scanning electron microscopy of the normal epidermis and the epidermis *in vitro*. *British Journal of Dermatology* **89**, 387.

NICHOLLS S., KING S. & MARKS R. (1978) Quantitative and morphological evaluation of the effects of bath oil and an emollient on the stratum corneum. *Journal of the Society of Cosmetic Chemists* **29**, (10).

NICHOLLS S., KING C. S. & MARKS R. (1977) Quantitative assessment of physical changes in the horny layer of patients with ichthyosis. In *The Ichthyoses*, eds., Marks R. & Dykes P. MTP Press.

PAPA C. M. (1972) Mechanisms of eccrine anidrosis. *Journal of Investigative Dermatology* **59**, 295.

WONG C. K. & VICKERS H. R. (1972) A study of vertical sections of normal human skin with the scanning electron microscope. *Dermatologica* **145**, 371.

FURTHER READING

HASHIMOTO K. & TAMOTSU K. (1975) Surface ultrastructure of human skin. *Acta Dermato-Venereologica* **55**, 413.

HOLT D. B., MUIR M. D., GRANT P. R. & BOSNARVA I. M. (1974) *Quantitative Scanning Electron Microscopy*. Academic Press, London.

DAWBER R. & COMAISH S. (1970) Scanning electron microscopy of normal and abnormal hair shafts. *Archives of Dermatology* **101,** 316.

SWIFT J. A. & BROWN A. C. (1972) The critical determination of fine changes in the surface architecture of human hair due to cosmetic treatment. *Journal of the Society of Cosmetic Chemists* **23,** 695.

MENTON D. N. & EISEN A. (1971) Structure and organization of mammalian stratum corneum. *Journal of Ultrastructure Research* **35,** 247.

MAKITA T. & SANDBORN E. B. (1971) Identification of intracellular components. *Experimental Cell Research* **67,** 211.

HAYES T. L. (1968) The scanning electron microscope: principles and applications in biology and medicine. *Advances in Biological and Medical Physics* **12,** 85.

14

Techniques for investigating collagen in pathology

Ch. M. LAPIERE

Collagen pathology at the molecular level is becoming one of the best examples of pathology related to one specific protein. This is due to recent characterization of the multiple steps required to achieve, from the genetic information, an architecturally perfect supporting framework.

Information relating to the clinical symptomatology and the inheritance of most connective tissue diseases can be found in the treatise *Heritable Disorders of the Connective Tissue* (McKusick 1972). A definition of the disorders at the molecular level (Lapiere & Nusgens 1976) is published as a chapter in *Biochemistry of Collagen* (Ramachandran & Reddi 1976).

A basic background of knowledge is required to understand the significance of the various tests usable in human clinical conditions. It can be found in several review articles, most of them being included in the above mentioned treatise (Ramachandran & Reddi 1976). This information can be summarized as follows. Collagen is a large protein forming the main fibrous framework that insures the mechanical strength of the skin. It is associated with elastin, another fibrous protein, forming with acid glycoproteins the elastic fibres. The resistance of these fibres to stress is minimal but their involvement in the ultimate fine mechanical properties of skin and the architectural organization of the polymers is very significant.

The fibroblast, defined as any cell capable of synthesizing at least the fibrous proteins, collagen or elastin, uses under some ill-defined control, part of its genome to produce messenger-RNA coding for specific collagen polypeptides and associated enzymes that are synthesized using the classical machinery for protein synthesis. Five different types of collagen polypeptides can be produced (α_1 I–IV and α_2) whose ultimate helical association into trimers will form the four main types of collagen. Collagen type I$[\alpha_1(I)_2\alpha_2]$ is most common and found in large amounts in the reticular dermis, bone and tendon; collagen type II$[\alpha_1(II)]_3$ is present in cartilage; collagen type III$[\alpha_1(III)_3]$ is most important in embryonic skin, blood vessels, gut and the papillary dermis while collagen type IV$[\alpha_1(IV)_3]$ is a component of basement membranes. A common feature of all these fibrous proteins are posttranscriptional enzyme-mediated covalent modifications of the molecules. Shortly after the formation of a few peptide bonds, the hydroxylation of specific prolyl- and lysyl-residues giving rise to hydroxyproline and hydroxylysine occurs, catalysed by prolyl or

191

lysyl hydroxylase using two cosubstrates (molecular oxygen and α-ketoglutarate) and two cofactors (Fe^{++}, ascorbate). Hydroxyproline is required to stabilize the triple helix at body temperature through hydrogen bonding. In skin, some hydroxylysines are glycosylated through the action of sugar transferases adding first one galactose residue and then a glucose to the galactose. In bone, only the first reaction occurs. The substituted polypeptides, extended at both extremities by additional non-helical sequences containing disulphide bridges, represent the intracellular precursor of collagen.

A partly processed procollagen seems to be secreted by the fibroblast and released in the extracellular space where it undergoes additional changes through the action of two enzymes. The first one is lysyl oxidase catalysing a deaminative oxidation of defined lysyl and hydroxylysyl residues to transform them into the corresponding aldehydes. The second one is procollagen peptidase, an endopeptidase removing all the peptide extensions of the precursor and allowing the collagen molecules to pack into the fibres and form a crystalline lattice that becomes stabilized by reaction of the aldehydes first into labile and ultimately into stable crosslinks.

The architectural organization of the fibres in the tissue is provided by multiple factors among which the relative proportion of type I and type III collagen seems important in defining bundle size (Lapiere *et al* 1977) while mechanical forces intervene to orient them (Lapiere *et al* 1975). All types of collagen polymers require a specific protease to be degraded. Collagenase produced by several strains of cells results, in most instances, from the activation of an inactive enzyme. Additional proteases and cathepsins are responsible for further degradation to smaller peptides and free amino acids. A defined proportion of peptide bound and free hydroxyproline, hydroxylysine and its glycosides is excreted in the urine. Most connective tissues undergo a constant turnover, the rate being higher in bone, lower in skin and probably under the control of endocrine secretions.

Any one of the above mentioned steps required to allow the expression of the specific function of the connective tissue can be tested in human pathology using the skin. They represent most valuable tools for investigating diseases either inherited or acquired since the dermis contains all types of collagen, except type II specific for the cartilage, and expresses many of the pathological defects by alteration of its composition, structure and/or function.

My goal in this chapter is to survey the available techniques that can provide the most complete answer up to the molecular level.

PHYSICAL PARAMETERS

Skin can be defined in terms of its physical properties and many pathological disorders will affect these.

The thickness of the skin

This can be measured using various techniques that provide measurements of the same order of magnitude and are capable of disclosing differences as a function of sex, age and localization.

1 By histology, the direct measurement on sections perpendicular to the skin surface from the epidermis to the hypodermis can give reliable information (Shuster *et al* 1975) provided fixation and dehydration does not modify the initial structure.

2 Experienced investigators measuring the skinfold thickness at identical locations and under constant pressure using either the Harpenden skinfold caliper (Tanner & Whitehouse 1955) or the micrometer screw gauge (Kirby & Munro 1976) can obtain reproducible data.

3 Direct measurements of the thickness of the compressed dermis by tangential X-rays has been described by Sheppard and Meema (1967) by Black (1969) and by Marks *et al* (1975).

The mechanical properties of skin

These can be tested *in vivo* by tonometric measurements relating force to a deformation obtained by pulling, pressing, stretching or twisting. The significance of the results varies as a function of the direction of the force.

1 The suction method has been successfully used by Grahame (1970). It consists in measuring the deflection of the skin surface aspirated in a bell-shaped cup under a known depression. It measures with little accuracy, the extensibility of the whole dermis and its adherence to the underlying fascia.

A more simple technique that we use (Pierard & Lapiere 1976) can provide similar information. It is based upon measuring the deformation, recorded by a micrometer, as a function of traction produced by a force applied perpendicular to a constant skin surface. At high traction, it measures the deformability of the dermis and its adherence to the underlying fascia. It can also be used to estimate the biological elasticity, ie the time dependent recovery of the initial position of the skin surface, in relationship to the tension of the fibrous components. At low force (around 1 N) traction extends more specifically the papillary dermis and measures its mechanical properties. When related to the skinfold thickness, all these parameters provide meaningful and reproducible information allowing one to specify various mechanical properties of the dermis as a function of age, sex, location, disease and the effect of therapy.

2 Two techniques can relate force to pressure. The first (Kirk & Kvorning 1949) uses indentation under determined pressure to measure not only the resistance of the dermis but also the deformability of the underlying tissue. The second method is the ballistometric technique of Tosti *et al* (1976) recording the height of the successive rebounds after a drop impact on the skin surface. It measures the tension and the elasticity of the fibrous components of the dermis and also the tension of the hypodermis.

3 Several methods are suitable for measuring the stress–strain relationship for a force applied parallel to the skin surface, in two axes perpendicular to one another (Kenedi *et al* 1965). Such techniques requiring sophisticated equipment mainly prove useful to record not only breaking strength of healing wounds but also deformability.

4 Mechanical properties of the dermis can also be tested by torsion on the plane of the skin surface. It theoretically minimizes the resistance of the dermo-hypodermal junction (Burton & Shuster 1973).

MORPHOLOGY

Structural examination is an integral part of the investigation of a connective tissue. A high degree of precision can be achieved at the ultrastructural level and by combination with immunohistochemistry.

Standard histological section

When stained with the Masson technique a standard histological section provides some information on the structural architecture of the collagen fibres and the state of tension of its bundles of fibres (Flint *et al* 1975). Silver impregnation will contrast reticulin fibres, probably made of type III collagen. Orcein will stain the elastic fibre framework. The region of the basement membrane can be identified by its PAS reactivity. The relative amount and the spatial relationship between these components is disturbed in many pathological processes.

Transmission electronmicroscopy (TEM)

On thin sections stained with uranyl acetate, phosphotungstic acid or lead citrate TEM will provide information on cell structure and permit the identification of the collagen fibres recognized by their typical repeating 670 Å (640–680) asymmetrical cross striation (Bruns 1976). No obvious difference in this pattern is capable of defining the formation of the different types of collagen fibres. The calibre of the fibre is, however, smaller for type III than for type I. When comparing the fibre structure and arrangement in areas of skin of the same location and at the same depth, some parameters are of potential significance, ie in longitudinal section the direction of the banding pattern and their registration in adjacent fibres, their parallel arrangement and the spatial relationship between collagen, elastin and proteoglycans; in transverse section, fibre diameter, shape, spacing between fibres and bundle size (number of fibres per bundle).

Scanning electronmicroscopy

This provides a three dimensional view of bundles allowing one to better define size, composition and arrangement, resulting in the architectural organization of the fibrous framework. It is also most useful for observing the modifications in organization induced by mechanical force on specimens fixed at the tension they have *in vivo*. Comparison between samples should also be made on parts of the dermis collected from similar locations, since the architecture of the connective tissue varies extensively from place to place and within the depth of the skin, as well as in the proximity of adnexial glands, hair, nerves and vessels.

Immunohistochemistry

Immunohistochemistry has been developed to provide most significant information through the use of antibodies specific for the various types of collagen (Nowack *et al* 1976), associated proteins and some enzymes.

END PRODUCT ANALYSIS

A logical sequence of procedure and chemical analyses allows the determination of a defect in any one of the chemical events involved in the building of a normal fibrous framework.

The sample of tissue from which the hypodermal layer of adipose tissue has been removed is immediately frozen in liquid nitrogen. It is crushed in a mortar and pestle until rendered into a thin powder that can be stored frozen at $-70°C$. Roughly speaking, the dry weight of skin is 30–40% of the wet weight. It is composed of 70–80% collagen polypeptides. Aliquots are collected for the following procedures and analyses.

Extractability

The proportion of collagen extractable in 0.5 M NaCl or 0.1 N acetic acid at $4°C$ is indicative of the rate of metabolic turnover (Legrand *et al* 1969) since insolubilization is a process which slowly progresses with time, irrespective of the amount of molecule synthesized. The proportion of extractable collagen is also increased when crosslinking is impaired as in lathyrism (Levene & Gross 1959), homocystinuria (Kang & Trelstad 1973) or in penicillamine therapy (Harris & Sjoerdsma 1966). Collagen extracted in neutral saline in the presence of a cocktail of protease inhibitors (0.02 M sodium ethylendiamine tetraacetate (EDTA), 0.001 M phenylmethane sulphonyl fluoride (PMSF), 0.1% *N*-ethylmaleimide (NEM), pepsatin, Trasylol, etc) is most suitable for detecting procollagen molecular species in increased proportion as in the Ehlers-Danlos syndrome type VII (Lichtenstein *et al* 1973) or in dermatosparaxis (Lenaers *et al* 1971).

A 20 mg aliquot (wet weight) of frozen skin powder is suspended in 2 ml of cold 0.5 M NaCl, unbuffered containing proteases inhibitors. After shaking in the cold ($4°C$) for 24 hours, the undissolved material is removed by centrifugation at 18 000 rev/min for 20 minutes. A sample of 250 µl collected very carefully in the centre of the supernatant solution is transferred to a small 0.8

cm × 10 cm) pyrex tube. After adding 750 µl of 8 N HCl, the tube is sealed and hydrolysis is performed at 138°C for 3 hours. After removing all the extract, the residue is also hydrolysed in 6 N HCl. Activated charcoal is added to the hydrolysates which are filtered through a glass fibre filter rinsed twice with 1 ml of distilled water. The clear solution is dried under reduced pressure. Hydroxyproline is measured by a scaled-down method derived from the Bergman and Loxley technique (1963). Extractibility is expressed in per cent.

Identification of collagen polypeptides

Although the technique of acrylamide gel electrophoresis used to characterize the collagen polypeptides would allow only these polypeptides to penetrate the gel at acid pH, a large excess of other proteins could reduce the penetration of collagen polypeptides inside of the gel. For this reason, we prefer to perform the analysis on collagen partly purified either by salt precipitation or after limited pepsin digestion.

The rest of the above mentioned extract is made 2.4 M in NaCl by adding cold 5 M NaCl. After resting in the cold for 24 hours, the precipitate is collected by centrifugation at 3000 X g and the supernatant discarded. Five hundred µl of NaCl 0.15 M Tris 0.05 M pH 7.4 are added to the precipitate which is allowed to dissolve by shaking in the cold and after 24 hours the undissolved material is removed by centrifugation at 40 000 X g. Cold absolute ethanol is added to reach a 30% concentration (v/v); the collagen precipitate is collected after 15 minutes by centrifugation at 12 000 X g and the supernatant completely discarded. Two hundred µl of a glycine 0.05 M acetate buffer pH 4 made 6 M in urea are added and the collagen denatured by heating at 60°C for 10 minutes. Half of the sample is collected into another tube into which dithiothreitol (DTT, ±0.5 mg) is added, denaturation being repeated at 60°C for another 10 minutes. Collagen type III is indeed found in the tissue in the form of a trimer linked by disulphide bridges. Up to 100 µl of the solution (optimal amount 30 µg of collagen polypeptides) is laid on the top of an acrylamide gel and electrophoresis (PAGE) performed at 100 volts (± 3 mA per tube 5 mm in diameter and 5 cm long) for 3 hours according to the technique described by Lenaers *et al* (1971) and Lenaers and Lapiere (1975). The technique of interrupted electrophoresis (Sykes *et al* 1976) is even more suitable for analysing collagen polypeptide species in skin. It is performed on a single sample, the first half of the run allowing separation of α_1 and α_2 before reduction and the second half of the run after reduction, permitting α_1 (III) to migrate into the gel.

If the identification of collagen precursors is not required, a better and simpler technique for quantitating α_1(I), α_2 and α_1(III) is extraction under limited proteolysis. Wet tissue (10 mg) is sufficient. The crushed dermis is incubated at 15°C for 48 hours in 2 ml of 0.5 M acetic acid containing 100 µg of pepsin per ml. The supernatant is collected after centrifugation in the cold, 1 ml of 1.0 M Tris (base) added followed by 1.5 ml of cold absolute ethanol. The collagen precipitate collected by centrifugation is processed as previously described for the identification of the polypeptides by PAGE.

Proteolysis by pepsin does not dissolve all the collagen present. The only available technique to determine the total polypeptide composition relies on cyanogen bromide digestion of a fragment of dermis and determination of the peptides pattern by acrylamide gel electrophoresis as already described (pH 5.5–10% gels) (Nusgens & Lapiere in preparation) or in 7.5% gel in the presence of sodium docecyl sulphate (Weber *et al* 1977).

Amino acid analysis

In terms of detection of pathological features in collagen, amino acid analysis is only useful on small biopsies to detect reduced hydroxylation of prolyl and/or lysyl-residues. To perform a correct analysis, the collagen should be adequately purified. Collagen (1 mg) extracted after pepsin digestion, fractionated or not by NaCl to separate type III (1.5 M NaCl) and type I (2.4 M NaCl) is largely sufficient for obtaining reliable results by liquid chromatography of a hydrolysate in an adequate system allowing the separation of hydroxyproline and hydroxylysine.

Crosslinks

The detection of the aldehydes and their reaction products provide direct information on the function of lysyl oxidase and indirect information on the type of collagen involved as well as its rate of turnover. Type III and type I collagen crosslinks are identical in structure but not in proportion (Fuji *et al* 1976) and their reaction products change with increasing maturation of the polymers in the tissues.

Frozen powdered skin (10 mg) are suspended in 1 ml of 0.4 M potassium phosphate buffer and one drop of a 0.1% antifoam C (used in tissue culture procedure) solution is added. Tritiated sodium borohydride (300 µg) (of high specific activity) dissolved in 0.2 ml of 0.01 N NaOH are added in fractions of 50 µl every five min. Five minutes after the last addition, the content of the tube is transferred to a dialysis bag and dialysed against a large volume of distilled water (10 l at least) 4 times for 24 hours. The sample is hydrolysed for 24 hours in 5.6 N distilled HCl in a tube sealed after flushing with dry nitrogen. The hydrolysate is dried under vacuum solubilized in 3 ml of distilled water and dried again to eliminate all the free tritium ions.

The fractionation of the labelled amino acid derivatives, the aldehydes and the crosslink derivatives, is performed by liquid chromatography (Bailey *et al* 1970) and the radioactivity measured by liquid scintillation. This procedure is qualitative and even if completely standardized in terms of reagents, pH, time and temperature of reaction, can hardly be supposed to be quantitative.

ENZYME IDENTIFICATION AND QUANTITATION

All the enzymes involved in the posttranscriptional modelling of the various collagen polypeptides can be identified and measured with some accuracy. For most of them, the procedure is quite complex since it requires the preparation of a suitable substrate and often delicate techniques. The amount of effort necessary to set them up makes it not worthwhile for casual use and collaboration with specialized laboratories is advisable. Only principles of the techniques will be provided here.

Prolylhydroxylase

The substrate is unhydroxylated collagen α chains prepared in tissue or cell cultures in the presence of highly labelled tritiated proline (3.4³H Proline) and in the absence of oxygen or ascorbic acid, or better still, in the presence of a chelating agent as $\alpha-\alpha'$, dipyridil. The assay is based upon the release of tritium by the hydroxylation reaction in the presence of the required cosubstrate (oxygen and α ketoglutarate) and cofactors (Fe^{++} and ascorbate). The released tritiated water is collected by distillation (Prockop & Juva 1965) or by a simpler technique of ion exchange chromatography (Blumenkrantz & Asboe-Hansen 1976).

Lysyl-hydroxylase

The substrate is prepared as above but using tritium-labelled lysine. The assay is similar (Kivirikko & Prockop 1967).

Sugar transferases

The substrate is collagen extracted from skin and denatured in diluted acid and heating (gelatinization). The assay consists of the addition of labelled galactose or glucose to the substrate plus the enzyme preparation in question and adequate cofactors. The products, hydroxylysine-galactose or hydroxylysine-galactose-glucose, are isolated after alkaline hydrolysis either by paper chromatography (Spiro & Spiro 1971a, 1971b) or ion exchange chromatography (Risteli & Kivirikko 1976).

Lysyl oxidase

The substrate (collagen and/or elastin) is prepared in cell or tissue culture incubated in a medium containing (6³H) or (4–5³H) lysine of high specific activity in the presence of βamino-propionitrile (βAPN). The enzyme is extracted in saline containing urea (2 M) to increase the yield and the assay performed by incubation at 37°C both in the absence and in the presence of βAPN. The radioactivity released by the oxidative deamination induced by the enzyme is the difference in counts between the reaction mixture in the absence and the presence of inhibitor (βAPN) (Pinnel & Martin 1968).

Procollagen peptidases

The substrates are collagen precursors, procollagen type I collected from dermatosparactic skin or fibroblast culture or procollagen type III collected from fetal skin or cell culture. The enzyme is collected from skin homogenates. The incubation is performed at 26°C and the collagen collected by adding absolute ethanol (50% of the reaction volume) and centrifugation (Lapiere & Pierard 1974). The proportion of cleaved α-chains versus uncleaved precursor in the absence and in the presence of EDTA (inhibitor) is measured on the recorded pattern of an acid pH acrylamide gel electrophoretic separation of the reaction mixture.

Collagenase

The safest technique for measuring collagenase is the release of radioactivity from a suspension of fibres of ^{14}C-glycine-labelled collagen polymerized *in vitro* according to Nagai *et al* (1966). The blank is either the supernatant after centrifugation of the unreacted substrate, or the reaction mixture inhibited by EDTA.

Only granulocyte collagenase can be extracted in its active form. From all other cells and tissues, incubation *in vitro* is required to release active enzyme.

TURNOVER

Indirect measurement

The metabolic activity of the connective tissues can be estimated by the urinary excretion of specific breakdown products of collagen and related proteins. The measurement of urinary hydroxyproline has been extensively used and most laboratories of medical chemistry can perform it. Although several procedures have been described, the most frequently used is that of Prockop and Udenfriend (1960) which is somewhat tedious to perform but allows the most reliable results. This procedure has to be used for hydroxyproline measurement when the samples (urine or biological products) contain high amounts of metabolites of various origin (urea, catabolites of proteins or nucleic acids, drugs . . .) interfering with oxidation or colour development in the Bergman and Loxley technique (1963).

The quantitation of proline can easily be performed on the same hydrolysate (by the technique of Troll & Lindsley 1955). It may provide additional information on collagen metabolism when compared to the excretion of hydroxyproline. In normal adults, and in the absence of heavy proteinuria, the ratio of proline to hydroxyproline lies around 2.5. In collagen, this ratio is 1.1. When collagen catabolism is increased specifically, the ratio between the two amino acids in the urines tends to reach the 1.1 found in collagen (Nusgens & Lapiere 1973). An increased amount of the urinary hydroxyproline and a lower than 2.5 ratio of proline to hydroxyproline means that catabolism of collagen is increased without specifying the tissue of origin of the stimulated degradation process, bone and skin being the two main sources of these products. Additional information can be obtained by analysing urinary collagen catabolites for hydroxylysine and its glycosides. Hydroxylysine-galactose is found in higher proportion in bone collagen while hydroxylysine-galactose-glucose is predominant in skin collagen. The procedure for this analysis is more complex since it requires ion exchange chromatography as described by Askenasi (1975).

Direct estimation

Several of the enzymes involved in the posttranscriptional modelling of the collagen polypeptides can be used for obtaining an estimate of the metabolic activity of the fibroblasts in a tissue sample. Prolyl hydroxylase, lysyl hydroxylase, sugar transferases (Ristelli & Kivirikko 1976) and procollagen peptidase (Lapiere & Pierard 1974) are known to be related in amount of activity to growth and connective tissue development.

Collagen synthesis can also be measured by isotope incorporation in skin biopsies as described by Uitto (1970) and improved in our procedure (Broux *et al* in preparation).

A rectangular biopsy 16 mm long, 5 mm wide, is sectioned immediately after collection, in 16 equal sections of 1 mm in thickness. The sections are dipped immediately in 5 ml of Eagle basal medium free of proline and glutamine. Tritiated proline (40 µCi per ml) of high specific activity is added. A mixture of 95% oxygen and 5% CO_2 is bubbled for 2 minutes into the flask which is then incubated under constant stirring at 37°C. One piece of tissue is collected at 2, 4, 6 and 8 hours, gassing being repeated after each opening. The samples, dipped in 14% ethanol in NaCl 0.15 M, Tris 0.05 M pH 7.4 can be kept frozen in this medium until processed. A larger sample (8 slices) is collected after 8 hours of incubation.

The isolated slices are crushed to a fine powder in a mortar after being frozen in liquid nitrogen. The powder is collected into a centrifuge tube and incubated in 0.5 ml of a solution of pepsin (100 µg per ml of 0.5 M acetic acid). Proteolysis is allowed to proceed at 15°C for 48 hours and 0.25 ml of 1 M Tris are added to raise the pH 7.5 and collagen is precipitated by adding 400 µl of cold absolute ethanol. The total insoluble material (collagen + residual dermis) is collected by centrifugation (10 000 rev/min for 15 min) and washed at least three times with 0.5 ml, 30% cold ethanol after mixing throughout until no extractable radioactivity remains. The specific radioactivity of hydroxyproline is measured by the technique of Juva and Prockop (1966).

The large sample (8 slices) collected at 8 hours of incubation is used for investigating the differential synthesis of type I and type III collagen, *in vitro,* a representation of the cell activity *in vivo*. It can be obtained by measuring the radioactivity associated with these two molecular species separated by acrylamide gel electrophoresis. The gel is sliced into 1 mm sections that should be combusted for optimal recovery of the radioactivity.

CELL FUNCTION

Fibroblast culture is required to substantiate connective tissue alterations related to premature ageing such as a reduced doubling potential (Martin *et al* 1965) and many of the defective lysosomal functions responsible for storage diseases (Hers & Van Hoff 1973). It can help in identifying a defective enzyme activity in the posttranscriptional modelling of collagen or elastin (see Lapiere & Nusgens 1976 for examples). Fibroblast culture has also proved of interest for investigating the nature of the collagen produced by the connective tissue from which the cells have been collected; allowing, for example, one to substantiate the lack of collagen type III synthesis in Ehlers-Danlos type IV (Pope *et al* 1975). It has, however, to be pointed out that the phenotypic expression of the fibroblasts can be modified by conditions of cell or tissue culture. Primary culture of fibroblasts or secondary culture have also been extensively used for studying the activity of drugs or biological products. One has to keep in mind most certainly that such cells have lost the regulatory mechanisms which control their activity in the tissues. It makes it difficult to extrapolate the resulting information to *in vivo* conditions.

CONCLUSION

Although one of the main goals in using the above described procedures is to pinpoint the basic defects in connective tissue disorders, one has to be aware of a large variety of possible secondary chemical lesions that can be disturbing. Let us consider, for example, the crosslinking process. Defective crosslinking might result from the absence of lysyl oxidase activity due to lack of enzyme, absence of a required cofactor such as copper, or the presence of an inhibitor as in lathyrism. Also the following conditions will express themselves as tissue fragility through defective crosslinking; absence of hydroxylation of lysine; absence of procollagen peptidase or presence of bulky steric inhibitors of the aldehydes (such as penicillamine). This example is provided to demonstrate that one single technique is capable of disclosing one alteration and that only a whole array of procedures will provide the correct answer.

Finally, one has to be aware that collagen alone does not form the connective tissue. Various other specific compounds (proteoglycans, glycoproteins, elastin, etc) are most certainly important in conditioning polymer organization, structure and function. Little, however, is known of their involvement in defining the mechanical properties of the dermis although we know that pathology may result from an abnormal relationship of the fibres within the bundle or of impaired arrangement of the bundles, one in respect to another. Nothing is known of how they hold together to form the kind of network required for insuring the suppleness of the resistant envelope that is the dermis. Besides the known compounds and their complex metabolism, there could exist other substances whose role might be as significant as that of the fibrous proteins.

REFERENCES

ASKENASI R. (1975) Urinary excretion of free hydroxylysine, peptide-bound hydroxylysine and hydroxylysl glycosides in physiological conditions. *Clinica Chimica Acta* **59**, 87.

BAILEY A. J., PEACH C. M. & FOWLER L. J. (1970) Chemistry of the collagen cross-links. Isolation and characterization of two intermediate intermolecular cross-links in collagen. *Biochemical Journal* **117**, 819.

BERGMAN I. & LOXLEY R. (1963) Two improved and simplified methods for the spectrophotometric determination of hydroxyproline. *Analytical Chemistry* **35**, 1961.

BLACK M. M. (1969) A modified radiographic method for measuring skin thickness. *British Journal of Dermatology* **81**, 661.

BLUMENKRANTZ N. & ASBOE-HANSEN G. (1976) Simplified method for determination of protocollagen proline hydroxylase. *Clinical Biochemistry* **79**, 256.

BROUX M., PIERARD G. E., NUSGENS B. V. & LAPIERE Ch.M. Measurement of collagen biosynthesis in human skin *ex vivo*. Manuscript in preparation.

BRUNS R. R. (1976) Supramolecular structure of polymorphic collagen fibrils. *Journal of Cell Biology* **68**, 521.

BURTON J. L. & SHUSTER S. (1973) A rapid increase in skin extensibility due to prednisolone. *British Journal of Dermatology* **89**, 491.

FLINT M. H., LYONS M. F., MEANEY M. F. & WILLIAMS D. E. (1975) The Masson staining of collagen—an explanation of an apparent paradox. *Histochemical Journal* **7**, 529.

FUJII K., TANZER M. L., NUSGENS B. V. & LAPIERE Ch.M. (1976) Aldehyde content and cross-linking of type III collagen. *Biochemical and Biophysical Research communications* **69**, 128.

GRAHAME R. (1970) A method for measuring human skin elasticity in vivo with observations on the effects of age, sex and pregnancy. *Clinical Science* **39**, 223.

HARRIS E. D. & SJOERDSMA A. (1966) Effect of penicillamine on human collagen and its possible application to treatment of scleroderma. *Lancet* **ii**, 996.

HERS H. G. & VAN HOFF F. (1973) *Lysosomes and storage diseases.* Academic Press, New York.

JUVA K. & PROCKOP D. J. (1966) Modified procedure for the assay of ^{3}H-or ^{14}C-labelled hydroxyproline. *Analytical Biochemistry* **15**, 77.

KANG A. H. & TRELSTAD R. L. (1973) A collagen defect in homocystinuria. *Journal of Clinical Investigation* **52**, 2571.

KENEDI R. M., GIBSON R. & DALY C. H. (1965) Bio-engineering studies of the human skin II. In *Biomechanics and Related Bio-Engineering Topics*, ed., Kenedi R. M., p.147. Pergamon Press, Oxford.

KIRBY J. D. & MUNRO D. D. (1976) Steroid induced atrophy in an animal and human model. *British Journal of Dermatology* **94**, suppl 12, 111.

KIRK J. E. & KVORNING S. A. (1949) Quantitative measurements of the eleastic properties of the skin and subcutaneous tissue in young and old individuals. *Journal of Gerontology* **4**, 273.

KIVIRIKKO K. I. & PROCKOP D. J. (1967) Enzymatic hydroxylation of proline and lysine in protocollagen. *Proceedings of the National Academy of Science* **57**, 782.

LAPIERE Ch. M. & NUSGENS B. (1976) Collagen pathology at the molecular level. In *Biochemistry of Collagen*, eds. Ramachandran G. N. & Reddi A. H. Plenum Press, New York.

LAPIERE Ch. M. & PIERARD G. (1974) Skin procollagen peptidase in normal and pathological conditions. *Journal of Investigative Dermatology* **62**, 582.

LAPIERE Ch. M., NUSGENS B. & PIERARD G. E. (1977) Interaction between collagen type I and type III in conditioning bundles organization. *Connective Tissue Research* **5**, 21.

LAPIERE Ch. M., NUSGENS B., PIERARD G. & HERMANNS J. F. (1975) The involvement of procollagen in spatially orientated fibrogenesis. In *Dynamics of Connective Tissues Macromolecules*, eds., Burleigh M. & Poole R. North Holland, Amsterdam.

LEGRAND Y., LAPIERE Ch. M., PIGNAUD G. & CAEN J. (1969) Microméthode d'extraction du collagène à partir de biopsie de peau humaine. Application à l'étude des maladies du saignement. *Pathologie Biologie* **17**, 991.

LENAERS A. & LAPIERE Ch. M. (1975) Type III procollagen and collagen in skin. *Biochimica et Biophysica Acta* **400**, 121.

LENAERS A., ANSAY M., NUSGENS B. & LAPIERE Ch. M. (1971) Collagen made of extended α-chains, procollagen in genetically defective dermatosparaxic calves. *European Journal of Biochemistry* **23**, 533.

LEVENE Ch. I. & GROSS J. (1959) Alteration in state of molecular aggregation of collagen induced in chick embryos by β-amino-propionitrile (Lathyrus factor). *Journal of Experimental Medicine* **100**, 771.

LICHTENSTEIN J. R., MARTIN G. R., KOHN L. D., BYERS P. H. & MCKUSICK V. A. (1973) Defect in conversion of procollagen to collagen in a form of Ehlers-Danlos syndrome. *Science* **182**, 298.

MARKS R., DYKES P. J. & ROBERTS E. (1975) The measurement of corticosteroid induced dermal atrophy by a radiological method. *Archives of Dermatological Research* **253**, 93.

MARTIN G. M., GARTLER S. M., EPSTEIN C. J. & MOTULSKY A. G. (1965) Diminished lifespan of cultured cells in Werner's syndrome. *Federation Proceedings* **24**, 678.

MCKUSICK V. A. (1972) *Heritable Disorders of Connective Tissue*. 4th edn. C. V. Mosby, St. Louis.

NAGAI Y., LAPIERE Ch. M. & GROSS J. (1966) Tadpole collagenase. Preparation and purification. *Biochemistry* **5**, 3123.

NOWACK H., GAY S., WICK G., BECKER O. & TIMPL R. (1976) Preparation and use in immunohistology of antibodies specific for type I and type IV collagen and procollagen. *Journal of Immunological Methods* **12**, 117.

NUSGENS B. & LAPIERE Ch. M. (1973) The relationship between proline and hydroxyproline urinary excretion in human as an index of collagen catabolism. *Clinica Chimica Acta* **48**, 203.

NUSGENS B. V. & LAPIERE Ch. M. Estimation of collagen type I and type III by acrylamide gel electrophoresis at acid pH of cyanogen bromide peptides. Manuscript in preparation.

PIERARD G. E. & LAPIERE Ch. M. (1976) Skin in dermatosparaxis. Dermal microarchitecture and biomechanical properties. *Journal of Investigative Dermatology* **66**, 2.

PINNELL S. R. & MARTIN G. R. (1968) The cross-linking of collagen and elastin: enzymatic conversion of lysine in peptide linkage to α-aminoadipic-δ-semialdehyde (allysine) by an extract from bone. *Proceedings of the National Academy of Science* **61**, 708.

POPE F. M., MARTIN G. R., LICHTENSTEIN J. R., PENTTINEN R., GERSON B., ROWE D. W. & MCKUSICK V. A. (1975) Patients with Ehlers-Danlos syndrome type IV lack type III collagen. *Proceedings of the National Academy of Science* **72**, 1314.

PROCKOP D. J. & JUVA K. (1965) Synthesis of hydroxyproline in vitro by the hydroxylation of proline in a precursor of collagen. *Proceedings of the National Academy of Science* **53**, 661.

PROCKOP D. J. & UDENFRIEND S. (1960) A specific method for the analysis of hydroxyproline is tissues and urine. *Analytical Biochemistry* **1**, 228.

RAMACHANDRAN V. N. & REDDI A. H. (1976) *Biochemistry of Collagen*. Plenum Press, New York.

RISTELLI J. & KIVIRIKKO K. I. (1976) Intracellular enzymes of collagen biosynthesis in rat liver as a function of age and in hepatic injury induced by dimethylnitrosamine. Changes in prolyl hydroxylase, lysyl hydroxylase, collagen galactosyl-transferase and collagen glucosyltransferase activities. *Biochemical Journal* **158**, 361.

SHEPPARD R. H. & MEEMA H. E. (1967) Skin thickness in endocrine disease. *Annals of Internal Medicine* **66,** 531.

SHUSTER S., BLACK M. M. & McVITIE E. (1975) The influence of age and sex on skin thickness, skin collagen and density. *British Journal of Dermatology* **93,** 639.

SPIRO R. G. & SPIRO M. J. (1971a) Studies on the biosynthesis of the hydroxylysine-linked disaccharide unit of basement membrane and collagens. I. Kidney glucosyltransferase. *Journal of Biological Chemistry* **246,** 4899.

SPIRO M. J. & SPIRO R. G. (1971b) Studies on the biosynthesis of the hydroxylysine-linked disaccharide unit of basement membranes. II. Kidney galactosyltransferase. *Journal of Biological Chemistry* **246,** 4910.

SYKES B., PUDDLE B., FRANCIE M. & SMITH R. (1976) The estimation of two collagens from human dermis by interrupted gel electrophoresis. *Biochemical and Biophysical Research Communications* **72,** 1472.

TANNER J. M. & WHITEHOUSE R. H. (1955) The Harpenden skinfold caliper. *American Journal of Physical Anthropology* **13,** 743.

TOSTI A., GOMPAGNO G., VILLARDITA S. & FAZZINI M. L. (1977) A ballistometer for the study of the plasto-elasticity of human skin: measurement of physical properties of skin. *Journal of Investigative Dermatology* **69,** 315.

TROLL W. & LINDSLEY J. (1955) A photometric method for the determination of proline. *Journal of Biological Chemistry* **215,** 655.

UITTO J. (1970) A method for studying collagen biosynthesis in human skin biopsies in vitro. *Biochimica et Biophysica Acta* **201,** 438.

WEBER L., MEIGEL W. N. & RAUTERBERG J. (1977) SDS polyacrylamide gel electrophoretic determination of type I and type III collagen in small skin samples. *Archives of Dermatological Research* **258,** 251.

15

Techniques in cutaneous microbiology

W. C. NOBLE

ROUTINE IDENTIFICATION

To the extent that much clinical microbiology still depends on obtaining a pure primary culture on a nutritious medium, microbiology can be said to have changed little since its inception. Indeed, Pasteur and Koch would find much that was familiar in even the most modern laboratory (provided that disposable plastic were substituted for glass). Once pure primary cultures have been obtained, however, the available techniques are different, and are changing at an increasing rate. Identification of common pathogens has been speeded by the introduction of enzyme assays and standardized substrates. This is most easily seen with certain of the Gram-negative rods, the tiresome group frequently lumped as the 'coliforms' more correctly the Enterobacteriaceae.

Formerly it was necessary to assemble a rack of 'sugars', 5 ml or 25 ml bottles containing sugars such as lactose or other substrates and to incubate these for long periods, a week was commonly used. In Crookshanks *Textbook of Bacteriology*, the fourth edition of which was published by H. K. Lewis in 1896, only a year after Pasteur's death, the following tests are used to identify *Bacillus (= Salmonella) typhosus* and to distinguish it from *Bacillus (= Escherichia) coli communis*; Motility, indole production, gas from glucose, milk coagulation (= lactose fermentation), gelatin liquifaction. In a modern textbook of bacteriology, Cruickshank, Duguid, Marmion and Swain's *Medical Microbiology*, 12th edition published by Churchill Livingstone (1975) the tests include motility, gas from glucose, and acid from lactose, whilst gelatin liquifaction is used in tests to separate the sub-genera of Salmonellae.

However, modern techniques use prepared substrate systems in which essentially only a suspension of the organism in water needs to be added to a series of open ended blisters on a plastic strip, each blister containing a dried substrate and indicator. Overnight incubation only is needed to achieve identification. Such systems have brought repeatability to the laboratory and have reduced the space needed for storage and incubation as well as technician time needed for identification of 'coliforms'. Descriptions of API, one of a number of such systems, can be found in Washington *et al* (1971), Smith *et al* (1972), Robertson *et al* (1976).

A recent development, APIZYM, makes it possible to detect the activity of enzymes on 19 substrates in four hours and Humble *et al* (1977) have applied this to identification of medically important bacteria. There seems no doubt that diagnostic microbiology will become increasingly simpler and less time-consuming.

RESEARCH TECHNIQUES

Research techniques used cover the whole area of microbiology and biochemistry, and it would be tedious to enumerate them all. The most satisfactory way of reporting these may be to discuss very briefly specific areas of research in cutaneous microbiology and to indicate the techniques being used.

Microorganisms as tools

The use of microorganisms to assay antibiotics is probably familiar to all but other antagonistic substances can also be detected and measured by microbial assay. Noble *et al* (1975) reported the assay of therapeutic methotrexate in the body fluids and tissues of patients receiving this drug for treatment of psoriasis, *Lactobacillus* sp. and certain *Streptococcus* sp. require folic acid and this can be quantitatively antagonized by methotrexate. Daniels (1965) described the use of *Candida albicans* to assay phototoxic material, a culture of the yeast is flooded onto a nutrient medium and exposed first to the test substance and subsequently to a specific wavelength of light. Inhibition zones indicate the presence of a phototoxic agent.

Antibiotic production

Two areas need to be considered here; one is the production of well characterized antibiotics by dermatophyte fungi, studied in relation to antibiotic allergy and selection of resistant organisms; the other, the production of unknown antibiotics or antagonists by cocci and diphtheroids is studied for possible therapeutic use.

Dermatophyte fungi have been shown to produce penicillin, 6-amino penicillanic acid, a streptomycin-like antibiotic, a fusidic acid type antibiotic, azalomycin-like and other, as yet uncharacterized, antibiotics *in vitro* (Youssef *et al* 1978); and to produce penicillin and other substances in natural dermatophyte lesions of patients (N. Youssef, personal communication). This has involved growing dermatophytes in fluid culture and on human or porcine stratum corneum adhering to sticky tape such as 'Steridrape', a technique described by Knight (1972). Detection of antibacterial or antifungal agents is accomplished by bringing the test organisms or extracts of growth media in contact with indicator organisms in fluid or in solid media. Inhibition of the indicator cultures shows that an antagonist is present, use of penicillinase (β-lactamase) will demonstrate whether or not the antagonist belongs to the penicillin group of substances. Further identification is made by using a panel of solvents for paper strip chromatography and comparing R_F values with standards (Betina 1964). The position of the antibiotic on the paper strip is detected by laying the strips on plates of agar growth medium seeded with an indicator organism; diffusion of the antibiotic results in a zone of inhibition, the whole process usually being referred to as 'bio-autography' (e.g. Leeming *et al* 1970).

Antibiotic or antagonist production by members of the cutaneous flora has been described by Selwyn (1975) as having a protective value. Patients admitted to hospital with antibiotic producing organisms in lesions of eczema or psoriasis are less frequently infected by *Staph. aureus* than are those lacking producer organisms.

Extraction of an antibiotic from a growth medium can involve precipitation of protein by salting out, drying and separating by column chromatography on Sephadex. Such techniques were used by Marsh (1975) in a study of antibiotic production by cutaneous cocci.

Microbial genetics

In studies of antibiotic resistant staphylococci, genetic variants of *Staphylococcus aureus* were found on differing areas of the human body (Noble 1977, Noble & Naidoo 1978). This is attributable to gain or loss of 'plasmids', non-chromosomal, covalently linked closed circular DNA rings which in staphylococcus are transferable by phage. Acquisition and loss of resistance plasmids can be demonstrated by examination of cultures by conventional sensitivity tests, by plating on agar growth media containing combinations of antibiotics, by manipulations designed to cause loss of non-chromosomal DNA such as culture in sodium dodecyl sulphate or ethidium bromide, by transduction of resistance using phage derived from a resistant organism to lysogenize a previously sensitive one [see Lacey (1975) for a review of Staph. genetics], or by agarose gel electrophoresis of plasmid DNA extracted from cells (Meyers *et al* 1976). Using these techniques, Naidoo and Noble (in preparation) have shown that gentamicin resistance can be transferred between strains of *Staph. aureus* naturally on the skin of patients admitted to hospital and treated with topical antibiotics or experimentally on the skin of human volunteers or of mice in the absence of antibiotic.

A combination of techniques has been used in the studies on staphylococcal epidermolytic toxin conducted by Arbuthnott, Lyell and their colleagues in the UK and by Glasgow, Melish and their coworkers in the USA. Electrophoretic separation of the toxin (Arbuthnott *et al* 1974) demonstration that the genes governing abundant toxin production are located on a plasmid (Rogolsky *et al* 1974) and electron microscopic studies on the plane of splitting will be found summarized in the extensive reviews published by Wuepper *et al* (1975) and Elias *et al* (1977).

Taxonomy

The techniques most associated with taxonomy are computer handling to cope with the volume of data generated. In a study of cutaneous coryneforms (diphtheroids) Pitcher (1977) conducted tests on reference strains and wild strains isolated from human skin. Application of computer programs devised by Sneath and his colleagues (Pitcher & Noble 1978) to banks of data yields a dendrogram in which organisms are arranged in order of similarity or a matrix in which the relation of each organism to every other is printed. Nevertheless, much of our current concept of the taxonomy of cutaneous coryneforms is based on studies of the cell wall composition. This involves identification of the diamino acids, sugars and lipids of cell walls by thin-layer or paper chromatography or the use of gas-liquid chromatography (g.l.c.) for comparative studies, g.l.c. is already an established technique for the identification of the non-sporing anaerobic Gram-negative rods (e.g. Bacteroides) by separation of the volatile end products of glucose metabolism. *Bacteroides fragilis* infection can also be diagnosed by g.l.c. determination of bacterial fatty acids in pus (Nord 1977). Though this has not yet been applied extensively in cutaneous microbiology, examination of head space gas has been used in a study of methane thiol production by skin and cheese organisms (Sharpe *et al* 1977).

Analysis of cell wall fatty acids by g.l.c. and assessment of the degree of similarity of organisms with varying lipid patterns can be facilitated by computer derivation of dendrograms. Identification of cell wall lipids can be made by mass spectroscopy allied to gas chromatography. Sesardic (personal communication) has applied these techniques to a study of human cutaneous coryneforms.

Polyacrylamide gel electrophoresis has been used in a taxonomic study of enzymes produced by *Brevibacterium*, a genus recently discovered to be a member of the normal skin flora (Foissy 1974).

Chemostat studies

Stated simply, a chemostat is a pot of fluid culture medium in which not merely the temperature of incubation can be controlled, but also the pH, Eh, availability of new nutrient material and removal of toxic products. Marsh and Selwyn (1977a, b) have described studies in which strains of cutaneous cocci and coryneforms were allowed to compete in a chemostat. By using a coccus which produced an antibiotic and others which were sensitive or resistant to that antibiotic the authors were able to study interaction. An attempt was made to devise a 'solid medium' chemostat (Milyani & Selwyn 1978) in which microbes growing on a solid surface exchanged nutrient and waste products with a fluid flowing at the underside of the solid support.

Alternatively the growth of one microbe, specifically *Propionibacterium acnes*, can be studied under changing conditions of oxygen tension, pH etc. (Roberts 1975).

Immunology

Since microbiology and immunology might be said to be twin subjects it is not surprising to find that any, perhaps every, immunological technique has been used, even in cutaneous microbiology. Some current examples are the use of immunofluorescence in studies on localization of *P. acnes* in tissue (Imamura *et al* 1969) and in demonstration of C3 in inflammatory acne lesions (Dahl & McGibbon 1976). Immune deposits are being sought in the viscera of patients with acute glomerulonephritis following streptococcal pyoderma (Ossi *et al* 1976; Hallett *et al* 1977). Lymphocyte transformation has been studied in patients with nodulocystic acne (Puhvel *et al* 1977) whilst adult patients with staphylococcal scalded skin syndrome have been studied for abnormal neutrophil chemotaxis and T lymphocyte function (Peterson *et al* 1977). Immunoelectrophoresis has been used by Massey, Mowbray and Noble (1978) to demonstrate that C3 is cleaved by the alternative pathway by *P. acnes*. Finally since the realization that *P. acnes* and *Corynebacterium parvum* represent the same species, attention has been turning to the immunological effect of *P. acnes* for example in relation to potentiation or suppression of immune response (e.g. Nagoya *et al* 1977).

SUMMARY

Cutaneous microbiology covers a vast field of taxonomy, ecological genetics, secondary metabolite production, enzyme synthesis and immunology. The choice of techniques used in these studies is correspondingly wide and a selection only is given in this paper.

REFERENCES

ARBUTHNOTT J. P., BILLCLIFFE, B. & THOMPSON W. D. (1974) Isoelectric focusing studies of staphylococcal epidermolytic toxin. *F.E.B.S. Letters* **46**, 92.

BETINA V. (1964) A systematic analysis of antibiotics using paper chromatography. *Journal of Chromatography* **15**, 379.

DAHL M. C. & McGIBBON D. H. (1976) Complement in inflammatory acne vulgaris. *British Medical Journal* **4**, 1383.

DANIELS F. (1965) A simple microbiological method for demonstrating photo-toxic compounds. *Journal of Investigative Dermatology* **44**, 259.

ELIAS, P. M., FRITSCH P. & EPSTEIN E. H. (1977) Staphylococcal scalded skin syndrome. Clinical features, pathogenesis, and recent microbiological and biochemical developments. *Archives of Dermatology* **113**, 207.

FOISSY H. (1974) Examination of *Brevibacterium linens* by an electrophoretic zymogram technique. *Journal of General Microbiology* **80**, 197.

HALLETT A. F., ADHIKARI M., COOPER R. & COOVADIA H. M. (1977) Post-streptococcal glomerulonephritis in African children. *Transactions of the Royal Society of Tropical Medicine and Hygiene* **71**, 241.

HUMBLE M. W., KING A. & PHILLIPS I. (1977) APIZYM: a simple rapid system for the detection of bacterial enzymes. *Journal of Clinical Pathology* **30**, 275.

IMAMURA S., POCHI P. E., STRAUSS J. S. & McCABES W. R. (1969) The localization and distribution of *Corynebacterium acnes* and its antigens in normal skin and in lesions of acne vulgaris. *Journal of Investigative Dermatology* **53**, 143.

KNIGHT A. G. (1972) Culture of dermatophytes upon stratum corneum. *Journal of Investigative Dermatology* **59**, 427.

LACEY R. W. (1975) Antibiotic resistance plasmids of *Staphylococcus aureus* and their clinical importance. *Bacteriological Reviews* **39**, 1.

LEEMING R. J., PORTMAN-GRAHAM H., SWAN C. H. J. & BLAIR J. A. (1970) The application of tetrazolium bio-autography to the identification of folic acid derivatives. *Journal of Clinical Pathology* **23**, 411.

MARSH P. D. (1975) In vitro studies of antagonism among human skin bacteria. Ph.D. Thesis, University of London.

MARSH P. D. & SELWYN S. (1977a) Studies on antagonism between human skin bacteria. *Journal of Medical Microbiology* **10**, 161.

MARSH P. D. & SELWYN S. (1977b) Continuous culture studies of interactions among human skin commensal bacteria. *Journal of Medical Microbiology* **10**, 261.

MASSEY ANNIE, MOWBRAY J. & NOBLE W. C. (1978) Complement activation by *Corynebacterium acnes*. *British Journal of Dermatology*. **98**, 583.

MEYERS J. A., SANCHEZ D., ELWELL L. P. & FALKOW S. (1976) Simple agarose gel electrophoretic method for the identification and characterization of plasmid deoxyribonucleic acid. *Journal of Bacteriology* **127**, 1529.

MILYANI R. M. & SELWYN S. (1978) Quantitative studies on competitive activities of skin bacteria growing on solid media. *Journal of Medical Microbiology*. In press.

NAGOYA T., KOBAYASHI F. & NOMOTO K. (1977) Immunological properties of *Propionibacterium acnes*. *1* Potentiation and suppression on antibody response to sheep and hamster erythrocytes in mice. *Microbiology and Immunity* **21**, 33.

NOBLE W. C. (1977) Variation in the prevalence of antibiotic resistance of *Staphylococcus aureus* from human skin and nares. *Journal of General Microbiology* **98**, 125.

NOBLE W. C. & NAIDOO J. (1978) Evolution of antibiotic resistance in *Staphylococcus aureus*. The role of the skin. *British Journal of Dermatology*. **98**, 481.

NOBLE W. C., WHITE P. M. & BAKER H. (1975) Assay of therapeutic doses of methotrexate in body fluids of patients with psoriasis. *Journal of Investigative Dermatology* **64**, 69.

NORD C. E. (1977) Diagnosis of anaerobic infections by gas-liquid chromatography. *Acta pathologica et microbiologica Scandinavia* B. Suppl. **259**, 55.

OSSI E., PREZYNA A., SEPULVEDA M., ELWOOD C. & ANDRES G. (1976) Immune deposits in the spleen of a patient with acute post-streptococcal glomerulonephritis (APSGN). *Clinical Immunology and Immunopathology* **6**, 306.

PETERSON P. K., LAVERDIERE M., QUIE P. G. & SABATH L. D. (1977) Abnormal neutrophil chemotaxis and T lymphocyte function in staphylococcal scalded skin syndrome in an adult patient. *Infection* **5**, 128.

PITCHER D. G. (1977) Rapid identification of cell wall components as a guide to the classification of aerobic coryneform bacteria from human skin. *Journal of Medical Microbiology* **10**, 439.

PITCHER D. G. & NOBLE W. C. (1978) Aerobic diphtheroids of human skin. In *Coryneform Bacteria*, eds. I. J. Bousfield & A. G. Callely, p. 265. Academic Press, London.

PUHVEL S. M., AMIRIAN D., WEINTRAUB J. & REISNER R. M. (1977) Lymphocyte transformation in subjects with nodulocystic acne. *British Journal of Dermatology* **97**, 205.

ROBERTS C. D. (1975) The role of bacteria in acne vulgaris. Ph.D. Thesis. University of Leeds.

ROBERTSON E. A., MACKS G. C. & MacLOWNY J. D. (1976) Analysis of cost and accuracy of alternative strategies for *Enterobacteriaceae*. *Journal of Clinical Microbiology* **3**, 421.

ROGOLSKY M., WARREN R., WILEY B. B., NAKAMURA H. T. & GLASGOW L. A. (1974) Nature of the genetic determinant controlling exfoliative toxin production in *Staphylococcus aureus*. *Journal of Bacteriology* **117**, 157.

SELWYN S. (1975) Natural antibiosis among skin bacteria as a primary defence against infection. *British Journal of Dermatology* **93**, 487.

SHARPE M. E., LAW B. A., PHILLIPS B. A. & PITCHER D. G. (1977) Methane thiol production by coryneform bacteria: strains from dairy and human skin sources and *Brevibacterium linens. Journal of General Microbiology* **101,** 345.

SMITH P. B., TOMFOHRDE K. M., RHODEN D. L. & BALOWS A. (1972) API system: a multitude method for identification of *Enterobacteriaceae. Applied Microbiology* **24,** 449.

WASHINGTON J. A. II, YU P. K. W. & MARTIN W. J. (1971) Evaluation of accuracy of multitest micromethod system for the identification of *Enterobacteriaceae. Applied Microbiology* **22,** 267.

WUEPPER K. D., DIMOND R. L. & KNUTSON D. D. (1975) Studies on the mechanisms of epidermal injury by a staphylococcal epidermolytic toxin. *Journal of Investigative Dermatology* **65,** 191.

YOUSSEF N., WYBORN C. H. E., HOLT G., NOBLE W. C. & CLAYTON Y. M. (1978) Antibiotic production by dermatophyte fungi. *Journal of General Microbiology.* **105,** 105.

16

Laboratory investigation of the porphyrias

G. H. ELDER

The porphyrias are a group of disorders of haem biosynthesis in which characteristic clinical features are accompanied by over-production of haem precursors. The main types are listed in Table 16.1 where they are subdivided according to the site of accumulation of haem precursors within the body. Primary enzyme defects (Fig. 16.1) which, in most types, are inherited have now been identified and patterns of haem precursor accumulation and excretion defined for the porphyrias. These patterns reflect increases in the concentrations of the substrates of the defective enzymes, brought about in order to maintain the rate of haem synthesis in the presence of the enzyme defects.

The clinical features of the porphyrias are of two types: skin lesions and acute attacks of severe abdominal pain, peripheral neuropathy and mental disturbance, and which are often precipitated by drugs, such as the barbiturates. The skin lesions are due to photosensitization caused by porphyrins and therefore occur in all porphyrias in which there is porphyrin over-production, that is in all except acute intermittent porphyria (AIP) (Table 16.1). Acute attacks of porphyria are always accompanied by markedly increased excretion of the porphyrin precursors, porphobilinogen (PBG) and

Table 16.1 Classification of the porphyrias

Site of haem precursor over-production	Type of porphyria	Inheritance	Major clinical features	
			Acute attacks	Skin lesions
Erythropoietic	Congenital erythropoietic porphyria (CEP)	Recessive	0	+
Erythrohepatic	Protoporphyria (PP)	Dominant	0	+
Hepatic	Acute intermittent porphyria (AIP)	Dominant	+	0
	Hereditary coproporphyria (HC)	Dominant	+	+
	Variegate porphyria (VP)	Dominant	+	+
	Porphyria cutanea tarda (PCT)	Less than 10% of cases are familial	0	+

212

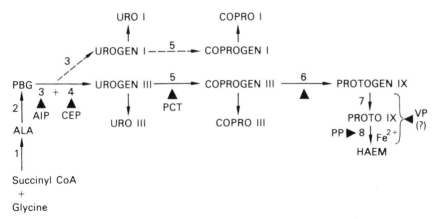

Fig. 16.1 The sites of primary enzyme defects in the porphyrias. Porphyrinogens with 7, 6, 5 and 3 carboxyl groups which are formed as intermediates during the conversion of UROGEN to COPROGEN and COPROGEN to PROTOGEN are not shown. The porphyrias are abbreviated as in Table 16.1. (1) 5-Aminolaevulinate (ALA) synthase. (2) Porphobilinogen (PBG) synthase. (3) Uroporphyrinogen (UROGEN)-I-synthase. (4) UROGEN-III cosynthase. (5) UROGEN-decarboxylase. (6) Coproporphyrinogen (COPROGEN)-oxidase. (7) Protoporphyrinogen (PROTOGEN)-oxidase. (8) Ferrochelatase.

Table 16.2   Haem precursors: reference values

Erythrocytes	Coproporphyrin	0– 4 µg/dl packed RBC
	Protoporphyrin	4– 52 µg/dl packed RBC
Urine	PBG	0– 2 mg/24 h
	Coproporphyrin	0–160 µg/24 h
	Uroporphyrin	0– 30 µg/24 h
Faeces	Coproporphyrin	0– 27 µg/g dry wt
	Protoporphyrin	0– 75 µg/g dry wt
	Ether-insol. porphyrin	0– 21 µg/g dry wt

5-aminolaevulinate (ALA), and are restricted to AIP, hereditary coproporphyria (HC) and variegate porphyria (VP). In AIP they are the only clinical manifestation. Patients with HC or VP may present either with skin lesions alone or with acute attacks, alone or accompanied by skin lesions. Since identical clinical features occur in more than one type or porphyria, precise diagnosis depends on accurate laboratory investigation of the pattern of over-production of haem precursors. In recent years, methods have been introduced for the measurement of the activity of some of the defective enzymes and have been shown to be of particular usefulness for the diagnosis of latent porphyria in family studies.

This chapter describes the laboratory investigation of patients presenting with skin lesions suggesting a diagnosis of porphyria. The porphyrins have recently been reviewed in detail by Meyer and Schmid (1978).

CHEMISTRY

The structure of uroporphyrin III is shown in Fig. 16.2. Replacement of the four acetate substituents by methyl groups gives coproporphyrin III. Protoporphyrin IX differs from coproporphyrin III in that the 2- and 4-propionate groups are replaced by vinyl (—CH=CH$_2$) groups. There are four position isomers of uroporphyrin according to the order in which the substituents are arranged around the macrocycle. All natural porphyrins belong to, or are derived from, position isomers belonging to the I or III series. Apart from protoporphyrin IX, the intermediates of haem biosynthesis are not porphyrins but porphyrinogens (Fig. 16.1). These are colourless hexahydro-derivatives of porphyrins which become oxidized to porphyrins when they accumulate in tissues and during excretion.

Porphyrin carboxylic acids are soluble in dilute aqueous acids and alkalis. Minimum solubility in aqueous solutions is reached at the isoelectric point which is around pH 3.5. At this pH they can be completely extracted into ether, ethyl acetate or butan-1-ol, a process which is facilitated if some acetic acid is present. Solubility in ether is inversely proportional to the number of carboxylic acid substituents, the octacarboxylic uroporphyrin being ether-insoluble. Porphyrins can be extracted from ether with dilute mineral acids. The strength of hydrochloric acid (in g/dl) required to extract two-thirds of the porphyrin from an equal volume of ether is known as the 'HCl number', and is 0.09 for coproporphyrin and 2.5 for protoporphyrin. The methyl ester derivatives of porphyrin carboxylic acids are soluble in organic solvents such as chloroform, carbon tetrachloride and benzene, as well as in the more polar organic solvents in which the free acids are soluble.

Porphyrins in solution have characteristic visible and ultraviolet absorption spectra (Falk 1964; Smith 1975a; Fuhrhop & Smith 1975) with an intense absorption band, the Soret band, around 400 nm. The high molar absorption coefficient ($1.5-5.5 \times 10^5$ litre mol^{-1} cm^{-1}) of this band makes it very useful

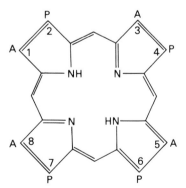

Fig. 16.2   Uroporphyrin III. A = acetate (—CH$_2$.CO$_2^-$); P = propionate (—CH$_2$.CH$_2$.CO$_2^-$). In uroporphyrin I the sequence of the substituents at positions 7 and 8 is reversed.

for the spectrophotometric determination of porphyrin concentrations. Absorption coefficients for natural porphyrins, with a formula and factors for correcting for interference from other substances absorbing in the Soret region, are given by Fuhrhop and Smith (1975). The wavelengths of the absorption maximum of the absorption bands in the Soret and visible regions, with their relative intensities, are important physicochemical characteristics for the identification of the different porphyrins.

Porphyrins also show bright orange or red fluorescent when irradiated with light around 400 nm (Wood's filter). This property is widely used for their detection on chromatograms and in solution and provides an alternative method of quantification, which is more sensitive, but more susceptible to interference, than spectrophotometry (Schwartz *et al* 1960).

THE EXTRACTION, SEPARATION AND CHARACTERIZATION OF PORPHYRINS

Fresh urine and faeces may contain both porphyrinogens and porphyrins. Although methods have been devised for the determination of these compounds separately in urine, in most techniques for porphyrin estimation porphyrinogens are oxidized to porphyrins and thus contribute to the measured porphyrin concentration. Oxidation may be accomplished by treatment with dilute aqueous iodine or benzoquinone derivatives (2,3-dichloro-5,6-dicyanobenzoquine; 2,3,5,6,-tetrachloro-4-benzoquinone) (Fuhrhop & Smith 1975; Schwartz *et al* 1960) or by exposure to air and light under mildly acidic conditions.

Extraction of porphyrins

Porphyrins with five or less carboxylic acid substituents can be extracted quantitatively from erythrocytes, urine or faeces by grinding or shaking with ether or ethyl acetate containing acetic acid (10–25%, v/v) (Rimington 1971). The acetic acid is then removed by washing with excess dilute aqueous sodium acetate or alkali to prevent loss of porphyrins with low HCl numbers. Uroporphyrin is insoluble, and porphyrins with seven and six carboxyl groups only sparingly soluble, in ether. Uroporphyrin is extracted from aqueous solutions at pH 1.5 by cyclohexanone, at pH 3.2 by ethyl acetate or at pH 3.5 by butan-1-ol, which at this pH conveniently extracts all natural porphyrins. Complete extraction of ether-insoluble porphyrins from the solid residues left after solvent extraction of erythrocytes or faeces may be difficult. Aqueous ammonia (10%) has been used but the most efficient extractant appears to be 45% (w/v) urea, containing 4% (v/v) Triton X-100, which was introduced by Rimington *et al* (1967) for the determination of hydrophilic porphyrin conjugates ('X-porphyrin').

Preparation of porphyrin methyl esters

Porphyrin carboxymethyl esters are more easily separated by chromatography and characterized than the corresponding carboxylic acids. Fuhrhop and Smith (1975) list a number of esterification techniques; that using methanol–H_2SO_4 is the most convenient for hospital laboratories. Ideally samples for esterification should be dry, which can be achieved either by evaporating organic solvents such as ether or ethylacetate in a stream of N_2 at temperatures of 50°C or less, or by adsorbing porphyrins from aqueous solutions at pH 3.5 on to talc, which is collected by centrifugation or filtration and dried (Doss 1974). The porphyrins are then dissolved in methanol–H_2SO_4 (19:1 v/v). Uroporphyrin will be esterified after 24 h at room temperature in the dark and shorter times suffice for porphyrins with fewer carboxyl groups. With (1973) has shown that the presence of small amounts of water retards, but does not prevent, esterification. Even uroporphyrin is completely esterified in 24 hours by 10% (v/v) H_2SO_4–methanol containing 10% water. Porphyrin methyl esters may be recovered from the esterification mixture by adding chloroform or ether, followed by excess water, with subsequent washing of the organic phase with 10% NH_4OH (Fuhrhop & Smith 1975).

Separation techniques

A large number of methods have been described for the separation of porphyrins with or without prior conversion to methyl ester derivatives (Doss 1974; Fuhrhop & Smith 1975; Jackson 1977). In general, separation of porphyrins with different numbers of carboxyl groups or other hydrophilic substituents presents few problems, while separation of position isomers is much more difficult.

(a) *Separation by solvent partition*

In the most widely used methods for their determination, porphyrins are fractionated according to their solubility properties. Urinary porphyrins can be divided into an ether-soluble coproporphyrin fraction and an ether-insoluble uroporphyrin fraction by extracting the urine at pH 3–4 with ether (Rimington 1971). The ether-soluble porphyrin fraction from faeces frequently contains pigments derived from dietary chlorophyll, which show red-fluorescence in ultraviolet light. These pigments have high HCl numbers and remain in the ether phase after porphyrins related to haem synthesis have been extracted, and divided into coproporphyrin and protoporphyrin fractions, by shaking with 0.1 M HCl, followed by 5% (w/v) HCl (Rimington 1971). Similarly, erythrocyte coproporphyrin and protoporphyrin can be separated from haem, which is soluble in ether and ethyl acetate, but has too high an HCl number to be extracted by 5% (w/v) HCl. Solvent partition techniques have the disadvantage that the components of the fractions, which often contain mixtures of porphyrins, are not positively identified. In most instances, it is correct to assume that uroporphyrin, coproporphyrin and protoporphyrin are the main components of the fractions named after them, but occasionally other porphyrins of similar HCl number may predominate. For example, on occasion, the coproporphyrin fraction from faeces may contain largely bacterial metabolites of protoporphyrin or, in PCT, isocoproporphyrin (Elder 1975).

(b) *Separation by chromatography*

(i) *Thin layer chromatography*. Paper chromatography has now been largely superseded by thin-layer chromatography (t.l.c.) for the separation of porphyrins. A number of solvent systems have been described for the separation of porphyrin methyl esters on silica gel plates (Doss 1974; Elder 1972; Smith 1975b; Jackson 1977). Benzene ethyl acetate–methanol (85 : 13.5 : 1.5, by vol.) (Doss 1974) is a widely used solvent system that gives excellent separations but benzene, in addition to its toxicity, has the disadvantage of promoting the photo-oxidation of protoporphyrin and other porphyrins with unsaturated substituents. The benzene may be replaced by toluene (Smith 1975b) and similar separations are also obtained with kerosene–chloroform–methanol mixtures (Elder 1972). In these systems porphyrin esters are separated according to the number of methoxycarbonyl groups they contain, the rate of migration being inversely proportional to the number of such groups. Separation of the more polar porphyrins can be improved by increasing the proportion of ethanol or methanol in these systems. Free hydroxyl groups and unesterified carboxyl groups retard migration; an effect which, in the case of hydroxyl groups, can be abolished either by conversion to acetyl or trimethylsilyl derivatives. Complex mixtures of methyl esters can be resolved by two-dimensional t.l.c. (Elder 1971).

Porphyrins are located on chromatograms by their colour and by their red fluorescence in ultraviolet light (Wood's filter). Spots invisible in ordinary light are readily revealed by their fluorescence, which is intensified if kerosene is present in the solvent system or sprayed onto the plate. Some green chlorophyll derivatives and purple biliviolins, which may be present in faeces, also show red-fluorescence in ultraviolet light but can be distinguished by their characteristic colours and chromatographic mobilities. After separation, porphyrin esters may be quantified by spectrophotometry after elution from the plates with chloroform–methanol (4 : 1, v/v) or they can be measured *in situ* by fluorescence densitometry, a technique which is made more sensitive if the esters are converted to Zn-chelates before t.l.c. (Doss 1974). Milligram quantities of porphyrin esters can be purified by t.l.c. (Elder 1972).

None of the solvent systems described above for the t.l.c. of methyl esters separate position isomers. Paper chromatographic methods for the separation of coproporphyrins I and III are given by Fuhrhop and Smith (1975) and a t.l.c. method, similarly using a lutidine–water–NH$_3$ system has been reported by Smith (1975b). Chromatographic methods for the separation of isomers of other porphyrins are less reliable, and the series I and III isomers of uroporphyrin and 7-, 6- and 5-carboxyl porphyrins are customarily identified after acid-catalysed thermal decarboxylation to the corresponding coproporphyrin isomers (With 1975).

(ii) *High-performance liquid chromatography.* The introduction of high-performance liquid chromatography (h.p.l.c.) has been the most important advance in analytical porphyrin chemistry in recent years (Jackson 1977). Methyl ester derivatives of porphyrins from biological samples are readily separated on columns packed with micro-particulate silica using cyclohexane–ethylacetate (Evans *et al* 1976) or heptane–methylacetate (Gray *et al* 1977) mixtures. As with t.l.c., separation in these systems depends largely on the number of methoxycarbonyl groups, methyl esters of dicarboxylic porphyrins having the shortest retention times. Mixtures of porphyrin esters containing from two to eight methoxycarbonyl substituents can be separated within 15 minutes. The eluted porphyrins can be detected and quantified using a spectrophotometric detector set at the Soret band which, in most instances, allows as little as 50 pmol to be detected with ease. Both position isomers and free porphyrins have been separated by h.p.l.c. Although existing methods are slow, they are likely to be improved in the near future.

(c) *Identification techniques*

Comparison of the chromatographic behaviour and absorption spectra of a porphyrin with those of authentic compounds can only provide tentative identification, and then only when such compounds are available. More rigorous identification can be obtained from mass spectra, nuclear magnetic resonance spectra and by chemical modification of substituents (Fuhrhop & Smith 1975; Jackson 1977).

PORPHYRINS AND PORPHYRIN PRECURSORS IN URINE, FAECES AND ERYTHROCYTES

Reference ranges for the concentration of PBG in urine, and of porphyrins in urine, faeces and erythrocytes are given in Table 16.2. Because measurement of the concentrations of these substances is laborious, qualitative screening tests are widely used. Their use is satisfactory provided their limitations are appreciated and provided that each positive test is followed by a quantitative determination made on the same sample.

PBG in urine

The colourless monopyrrole, PBG, is unstable in urine and polymerizes, especially under acid conditions, to form porphobilin and uroporphyrin. This change underlies the characteristic darkening to a reddish-brown colour on standing of urines containing excess PBG. Screening tests for PBG are therefore best carried out on fresh, random specimens of urine. Equal volumes of urine and Ehrlich's reagent (0.28% *p*-dimethylaminobenzaldehyde in 7 M HCl) are mixed. PBG reacts immediately to give a red colour, whereas the identical colour given by urobilinogen takes up to 2 minutes to develop. After neutralization with saturated sodium acetate, the urobilinogen-colour complex can be extracted into organic solvents whereas the PBG-complex remains in the aqueous phase. In order to distinguish PBG from other Ehrlich-reactors, butan-1-ol or an amyl alcohol–benzyl alcohol mixture should be used for the extraction, rather than chloroform with which there are occasional false positives. The lower limit of detection of PBG is about 10 mg/litre, which is considerably higher than the upper limit of normal (Table 16.2).

Quantitative determinations of PBG in urine are best carried out after substances interfering with the Ehrlich reaction have been removed by ion-exchange chromatography as described by Mauzerall and Granick (1956). This technique enables concentrations within the normal range to be measured and can be conveniently combined with the measurement of ALA.

Porphyrins in urine

Urines containing more than 5–10 mg porphyrin/litre are often reddish-brown and show a red fluorescence when examined in ultraviolet light. At lower concentrations excess porphyrin can be detected by shaking 4 ml fresh urine, adjusted to pH 3.5 with glacial acetic acid, with 1 ml amyl alcohol. The phases are separated by centrifugation and examined in ultraviolet light (Wood's filter). Pink or red fluorescence of the upper organic phase indicates the presence of porphyrins. Concentrations above about 500 µg/litre are usually detected by this test but occasional false negatives occur above this limit, due to the presence of compounds which either fluoresce intensely themselves (usually blue-green) or quench porphyrin fluorescence. Marginally increased porphyrin concentrations will not be detected by this test nor does it give any information about the type of porphyrin present, since uroporphyrin and coproporphyrin are both extracted.

Quantitative measurements of urinary porphyrin fractions by solvent extraction and partition techniques of the type described by Rimington (1971) require no special apparatus and, in most instances, are adequate for the investigation of disorders of porphyrin metabolism. However, when available, t.l.c. and h.p.l.c. techniques for the measurement of individual porphyrins allow detailed definition of the porphyrin excretion patterns which characterize the various types of porphyrias (Doss 1974; Gray *et al* 1977). Furthermore, t.l.c. and h.p.l.c. enable abnormal patterns to be detected when total porphyrin concentrations are close to, or within, the normal range.

Porphyrins in faeces

An increase in the concentration of ether-soluble porphyrins in faeces can be detected by a simple screening test. A pea-sized piece of faeces and 0.5 ml glacial acetic acid are ground together with a glass rod. Five ml of peroxide-free ether is added and mixed thoroughly with the faecal suspension. The supernatant is decanted and extracted with 0.5 ml of 5% (w/v) HCl. The presence of porphyrins is indicated by a faint pink to intense red fluorescence in the lower aqueous phase. Red-fluorescing chlorophyll derivatives remain in the upper phase. If this test is negative the porphyrin concentration will be within normal limits. Positive tests are more difficult to interpret. Some normal samples, particularly from constipated patients, may show porphyrin fluorescence. The dicarboxylic porphyrin fraction of faeces comes from biliary protoporphyrin and from the action of bacteria on haem compounds in the gut. The latter may come from the diet or from alimentary tract bleeding, which may increase the faecal porphyrin concentration without being sufficient to give a positive occult blood test.

Quantitative determinations of faecal porphyrins are usually carried out by solvent extraction and partition techniques (Rimington 1971), which divide the ether-soluble porphyrins into coproporphyrin and protoporphyrin fractions. Ether-insoluble porphyrins are best extracted from the faecal residue with urea–Triton X-100 solution, after ether-soluble porphyrins have been removed with ether–acetic acid, and determined as described by Rimington et al (1967). This technique solubilizes all porphyrins remaining in the residue and is not specific for the hydrophilic conjugates found in variegate porphyria and known as X-porphyrin. T.l.c. (Elder 1975) and h.p.l.c. (Gray et al 1977) methods for measuring individual porphyrins in faeces have been described, which are suitable for the determination of isocoproporphyrin. Investigation of the composition of the ether-insoluble fraction is time-consuming and of little diagnostic value.

Porphyrins in erythrocytes

Blood samples for porphyrin analysis should be anticoagulated with heparin or dipotassium-EDTA and protected from the light. Protoporphyrin is stable in EDTA-anticoagulated blood for at least three weeks at 4°C and for several days at room temperature. Screening tests for increased erythrocyte porphyrin utilize either fluorescence microscopy of a saline-diluted unfixed blood smear or solvent extraction. If fluorescence microscopy is used, an iodine tungsten 100-watt quartz lamp is preferable to the more usual mercury vapour lamp, which emits light that rapidly destroys protoporphyrin. Normal blood contains only occasional red-fluorescent erythrocytes and increased numbers, as in protoporphyria, are easily observed. In the solvent extraction test, 0.1 ml of blood is thoroughly mixed with 2.5 ml of peroxide-free ether : acetic acid (5 : 1, v/v). The supernatant is transferred to a thin-walled glass tube and shaken with 0.5 ml of 3 M HCl. The presence of a faint pink to red fluorescence in the lower acid phase indicates excess porphyrin. This test is not as sensitive a screen as fluorescence microscopy and the occasional patient with protoporphyria may be missed.

Techniques for the measurement of erythrocyte porphyrin concentration depend on solvent extraction followed by solvent partition to separate porphyrin from haem, with spectrophotometric (Rimington 1971) or fluorometric determination (Chisholm *et al* 1975). Recently a number of micro-scale fluorometric methods for the measurement of 'free erythrocyte porphyrin' have been described (Chisholm *et al* 1975; Piomelli 1977). Erythrocyte porphyrins may be fractionated by solvent partition (Rimington 1971) or by chromatography.

APPLICATION OF CHEMICAL TESTS TO THE DIAGNOSIS OF THE CUTANEOUS PORPHYRIAS

Demonstration of porphyrin over-production is the first stage in confirming the diagnosis when a patient presents with skin lesions that might be due to porphyria. Screening samples of blood, urine and faeces, using the tests described above, is usually adequate for this purpose. Blood, urine and faeces must be examined in every case. Omission of the faecal tests in an important cause of diagnostic error. The second stage is definition of the pattern of porphyrin over-production (Table 16.3). Here measurement of porphyrin precursors and porphyrin fractions is required, supported by t.l.c. or h.p.l.c. determination of individual porphyrins to resolve diagnostic problems.

Screening tests

(a) *Erythrocytes*

Erythrocyte porphyrin is increased in two types of porphyria: protoporphyria and congenital erythropoietic porphyria. It is also raised in some conditions which are not associated with skin lesions: lead poisoning, iron-deficiency anaemia and sideroblastic anaemias. In these conditions the porphyrin is present mainly as Zn-protoporphyrin, while in protoporphyria it is free protoporphyrin. Chelation of zinc changes the fluorescence emission spectrum of protoporphyrin and spectrofluorometric techniques for the distinction of these compounds have been described.

Erythrocyte porphyrin concentrations are normal in the hepatic porphyrias. Occasional patients have plasma porphyrin levels which are high enough to give positive screening tests and increased porphyrin concentrations when whole blood is used for these tests. This source of error can be eliminated by repeating the test on washed cells.

(b) *Urine*

Urinary porphyrin excretion is increased in the cutaneous hepatic porphyrias and in congenital erythropoietic porphyria. Provided active skin lesions are present, the screening test for increased urinary porphyrins will be positive in all these disorders. In PCT in remission, or in latent PCT, urine porphyrin excretion may not be sufficiently increased to give a positive screening test. In these cases the diagnosis can often be established by showing typical PCT patterns of individual porphyrins in urine and faeces.

The increased porphyrin excretion which may occur in lead poisoning, chronic alcoholism and liver disease is due to coproporphyrin alone. Unlike the coproporphyrinuria of VP and HC, it is not accompanied by increased faecal porphyrin excretion.

(c) *Faeces*

In congenital erythropoietic porphyria, VP and HC, the faeces contain large amounts of porphyrin and positive screening tests are the rule. In VP and HC, cholestatic jaundice from any cause, leads to diversion of porphyrins from their normal biliary route of excretion and is often accompanied by severe photosensitization. A marked decrease in faecal porphyrin excretion has been reported in some of the patients who present with skin lesions and jaundice together. A normal screening test does not exclude the diagnosis of either protoporphyria or PCT, since in both these conditions total faecal porphyrin excretion is normal or only slightly increased in a proportion of patients.

Confirmatory tests

The patterns of porphyrin excretion and accumulation that characterize the cutaneous porphyrias are summarized in Table 16.3. Quantitative measurements of porphyrins are essential for the reliable distinction of the different types. Solvent partition techniques, which measure porphyrin fractions, of which those described by Rimington (1971) are widely used, are usually adequate for this purpose.

(a) *Protoporphyria*

The diagnosis of protoporphyria is confirmed by demonstrating an increased concentration of protoporphyrin in erythrocytes. There is often some increase in erythrocyte coproporphyrin but always to a lesser extent than protoporphyrin. Faecal protoporphyrin concentrations may be increased, but this is not a constant finding. Urinary porphyrin excretion is normal. A small proportion of patients develop severe liver disease and die in liver failure, accompanied by urinary porphyrin abnormalities.

(b) *The cutaneous hepatic porphyrias*

The diagnosis of PCT, VP and HC, which may be clinically indistinguishable, is usually straightforward provided quantitative measurements are made of PBG and ALA in urine and of porphyrin fractions in urine and faeces (Table 16.3). Occasionally in VP the urinary uroporphyrin fraction may be greater than the coproporphyrin fraction so that the urinary findings mimic PCT, due to condensation of PBG to uroporphyrin after the urine has been

Table 16.3 Haem precursor accumulation and excretion in the porphyrias

Condition	Erythrocyte porphyrins	Urine		Faecal porphyrins
		PBG	Porphyrins	
CEP	Increased; copro > proto	Normal	Increased; uro > copro Type I isomers	All fractions increased, especially copro Type I isomers
PP	Increased proto	Normal	Normal	Proto may be increased
AIP	Normal	Increased	PBG polymerises to uro	Usually normal
HC	Normal	Increased during acute attack	Increased copro III; often normal during remission	Increased copro III
VP	Normal	Increased during acute attack	Increased copro III; often normal during remission	All fractions markedly increased proto > copro (about 2:1). Ether-insol. fraction contains X-porphyrin
PCT	Normal	Normal	Increased; 45–80% of total is uro, 15–35% is 7-carboxyl porphyrin I and III isomers	Slight or moderate increase in total porphyrin. Copro fraction often > proto, and contains isocoproporphyrin, 5-carboxyl porphyrin. Ether-insol. fraction contains 7-carboxyl porphyrin

passed or to increased excretion of water-soluble porphyrin conjugates. It is therefore often useful to substantiate a diagnosis of PCT with a test that gives a clear separation between these two conditions. Two are available and convenient: measurement of uroporphyrin and seven-carboxyl porphyrin individually in urine (Doss 1974) or determination of the isocoproporphyrin: coproporphyrin ratio in faeces (Elder 1975).

REFERENCES

CHISHOLM J. J. & BROWN D. H. (1975) Micro-scale photofluorometric determination of 'free erythrocyte protoporphyrin' (protoporphyrin IX). *Clinical Chemistry* **21,** 1669.

DOSS M. (1974) Porphyrins and porphyrin precursors. In *Clinical Biochemistry, Principles and Methods,* Ed. H. C. Curtius, M. Roth, Vol. 2, p. 1326. Walter de Gruyter, Berlin.

ELDER G. H. (1971) Separation of porphyrin methyl esters by two dimensional thin layer chromatography. *Journal of Chromatography* **59,** 234.

ELDER G. H. (1972) Identification of a group of tetracarboxylate porphyrins, containing one acetate and three proprionate β-substituents, in faeces from patients with symptomatic cutaneous hepatic porphyria and from rats with porphyria due to hexachlorobenzene. *Biochemical Journal* **126,** 877.

ELDER G. H. (1975) Differentiation of porphyria cutanea tarda symptomatica from other types of porphyria by measurement of isocoproporphyrin in faeces. *Journal of Clinical Pathology* **28,** 601.

EVANS N., JACKSON A. H., MATLIN S. *et al* (1976) HPLC analysis of porphyrins in clinical materials. *Journal of Chromatography* **125,** 345.

FALK J. (1964) *Porphyrins and Metalloporphyrins.* Elsevier, Amsterdam.

FUHRHOP J-H. & SMITH K. M. (1975) *Laboratory Methods in Porphyrin and Metalloporphyrin Research.* Elsevier, Amsterdam.

GRAY C. H., LIM C. K. & NICHOLSON D. C. (1977) The differentiation of the porphyrias by high pressure liquid chromatography. *Clinica Chimica Acta* **77,** 169.

JACKSON A. H. (1977) Modern spectroscopic and chromatography techniques for the analysis of porphyrin on a microscale. *Seminars in Hematology* **14,** 227.

MAUZERALL D. & GRANICK S. (1975) The occurrence and determination of δ-aminolevulinic acid and porphobilinogen in urine. *Journal of Biological Chemistry* **219,** 435.

MEYER U. A. & SCHMID R. (1978) Diseases of porphyrin and heme metabolism. In *The Metabolic Basis of Inherited Disease.* Ed. J. B. Stanbury, J. B. Wyngaarden, D. S. Frederickson, 4th edn. p. 1166. McGraw-Hill, New York.

PIOMELLI S. (1977) Free erythrocyte porphyrins in the detection of undue absorption of Pb and of Fe deficiency. *Clinical Chemistry* **23,** 264.

RIMINGTON C. (1970) Quantitative determination of porphobilinogen and porphyrins in urine and faeces. *Association of Clinical Pathologists Broadsheet* **70,** London.

RIMINGTON C., LOCKWOOD W. H. & BELCHER R. V. (1968) The excretion of porphyrin-peptide conjugates in porphyria variegata. *Clinical Science* **35,** 211.

SCHWARTZ S., BERG M. H., BOSSENMAIER I. & DINSMORE H. (1960) Determination of porphyrins in biological materials. In *Methods of Biochemical Analysis.* Ed. D. Glick, Vol. 8, p. 221. Interscience, New York.

SMITH K. M. (1975a) *Porphyrins and Metalloporphyrins.* Elsevier, Amsterdam.

SMITH S. G. (1975b Thin layer chromatography of ester and free porphyrins. *British Journal of Dermatology* **93,** 291.

WITH T. K. (1973) On porphyrin esterification and ester hydrolysis. *Scandinavian Journal of Laboratory and Clinical Investigation, Supplement 134.*

WITH T. K. (1975) Decarboxylation of uroporphyrin by heating at atmospheric pressure. *Biochemical Journal* **147,** 249.

17

The measurement of complement and its components in dermatology

R. FIFIELD

INTRODUCTION

The complement system consists of at least thirteen activatable proteins, which are mainly β-globulins, and at least two specific inhibitors. A unique property of complement proteins is their ability to bind to biological membranes when activated. Once membrane bound, a complement protein or series of proteins generates an enzyme function and this activates the next protein in the system. In this way, a whole sequence of components C1, C4, C2, C3, C5, C6, C7, C8 and C9, become successively activated and bound. The attachment of the activated later components (C5–C9) to a cell leads to its lysis. Two distinct phases in complement activation are recognized in this classical numbered complement sequence.

Activation of the complement (C) system (Table 17.1)

In the first phase complement fixation is initiated by antibody/antigen complexes which trigger C1, C4 and C2 reactions which require Ca^{2+} and Mg^{2+} ions. The classical pathway may be activated by antigen-antibody complexes or aggregated immunoglobulins. Human immunoglobulins belonging to the IgG1, IgG2, and IgG3 subclasses and IgM class are capable of initiating the classical pathway, whereas IgG4 subclass and IgA, IgD and IgE classes are inactive in this regard. Among the IgG subclasses, IgG3 is most active followed (in order) by IgG1 and IgG2. Immunologic activation occurs via binding of the first complement component (C1) to a site located in the Fc region of the IgG or IgM molecule.

The classical pathway may also be activated non-immunologically by a number of chemically diverse substances, including DNA, C-reactive protein and certain cellular membranes and trypsin-like enzymes.

The product of these reactions steps is the C42 enzyme which cleaves and activates C3 molecules. Activated C3 molecules (C3b) bind in large numbers to biological membranes and the result is a macromolecular coating of the particle on which complement fixation was initiated. This C3b coating which

Table 17.1

	Classical	Alternative
Immunologic	IgG, IgM	IgA, IgG, IgE
Non-immunologic	Trypsinlike enzymes	Trypsinlike enzymes
	DNA	Lipopolysaccharides
	Staphylococcal	Plant and bacterial
	protein A	polysaccharides
	C-reactive protein	Cobra venom factors

opsonizes complexes for removal by the reticuloendothelial system *in vivo*, is detected in the immune adherence test, when cells with C3b receptors bind to particles or microorganisms coated with C3b.

The second phase of the complement sequence is the lytic or attack phase. A trimolecular complex of $C\overline{567}$ is activated in serum by membrane-bound $C\overline{42}C3b$. The activated complex of $C\overline{567}$ has an evanescent half-life in the 'fluid phase' but can stabilize by binding to any biological membrane within the effective diffusion radius of the complex before it decays. This binding of the activated form of C567 is the principle of reactive lysis exploited in several assays for measuring individual components (e.g. C7, factor B, total alternative pathway). The fixation of C8 and C9 completes the lytic phase. The total haemolytic titre of complement, the CH_{50} is measured as the highest dilution able to lyse 50% of antibody sensitized sheep red cells. The CH_{50} value therefore depends on the correct functional interaction of C1–C9, the whole of the classical complement pathway. Lysis of red cells is a common indicator end-point for several different types of complement tests including the functional measurement of individual complement proteins and the titration of residual complement in complement fixation tests.

There is a second pathway to the C3 conversion and fixation step. This is the alternative pathway containing at least four distinct proteins; properdin, Factor D, Factor B and C3b. It is inappropriate to discuss the interaction of the alternative pathway proteins in detail, but several points are relevant to diagnostic tests. The alternative complement pathway or properdin pathway may be activated immunologically by human IgA and also by some human IgG and IgE molecules. The pathway may also be readily initiated non-immunologically by certain complex polysaccharides, lipopolysaccharides, and trypsinlike enzymes. Unlike the C142 step of the classical pathway it does not require Ca^{2+} ions but does require Mg^{2+} ions in the reaction step where B, D and C3b interact. This property is exploited by selectively chelating Ca^{2+} ions with EDTA in the presence of added Mg^{2+}. Sera treated in this fashion can fix complement via the alternative pathway but not via the classical pathway.

The main consequence of complement activation is the cell lysis caused by antigen–antibody reaction but the activation of the complement system can have other consequences in the biological system i.e. (a) increase in vascular permeability; (b) attraction of polymorphonuclear leucocytes; and (c) enhancement of phagocytes.

The classical pathway

This can be divided into three steps:
1 The initial sequence.
2 The attack sequence.
3 The final sequence.

These steps are illustrated in Figs. 17.1, 17.2 and 17.3 During activation of some of the components, fragments are formed which have biological importance outside the classical or alternate pathway. C3a and C4a when formed cause the release of histamine from mast cells which leads to an increase in permeability and on invasion by white blood cells which can cause an allergic reaction with an increase in IgE and an anaphylactic reaction; while C3b promotes phagocytosis by immune adherence.

The alternate pathway

The alternative pathway was originally described as the properdin system, a group of proteins involved in resistance to infection, which was similar to, but distinct from, complement. The properdin system was found to be involved in

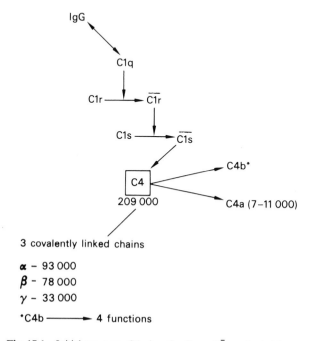

Fig. 17.1 Initial sequence. C1r, inactive form. C̄1s, activated form.

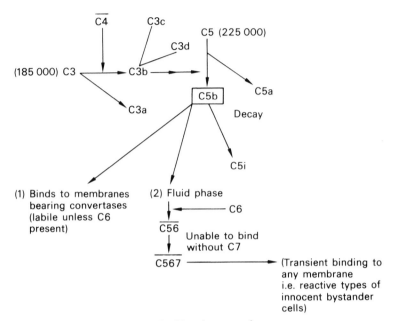

Fig. 17.2   'Attack sequence'.

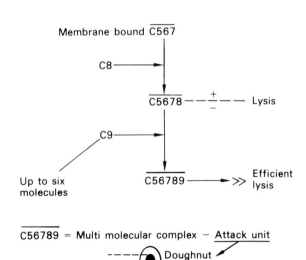

Fig. 17.3   Final sequence.

the destruction of certain bacteria, the neutralization of some viruses, and the lysis of erythrocytes from patients with paroxysmal nocturnal haemoglobinuria. The system did not seem to require specific antibody. It is a single step pathway (Fig. 17.4).

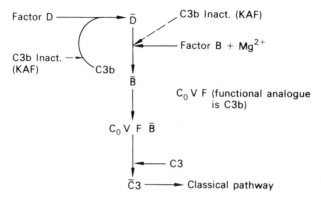

Fig. 17.4   Alternate pathway. C_0VF, Cobran venom factor.

CONTROL MECHANISMS OF THE COMPLEMENT SYSTEM

Uncontrolled activation of the complement system is prevented by the lability of the activated combining sites generated at multiple stages of the complement reaction, including the reaction steps involving C2, C3, C4 and C5, and by time- and temperature-dependent dissociation of some of the active complexes such as the $C\overline{42}$ and $C\overline{423}$ complexes. In addition, several serum proteins have been identified which serve to modulate and limit activation of the complement system. These proteins bind to or enzymatically attack only the specifically activated forms of the components. $C\overline{1}$ inactivator (C1 esterase inhibitor) is a multispecific serum enzyme inhibitor with a molecular weight of 105 000 and the electrophoretic mobility of an α_2-globulin. This enzyme inhibitor inhibitis not only $C\overline{1}$ but also the fibrinolytic enzyme plasmin, the kinin-forming system enzyme kallikrein, and the coagulation system enzymes. $C\overline{1}$ inactivator inhibits the enzymatic activity of $C\overline{1}$ or its $C\overline{1}$s subunit by rapidly forming a firm, essentially irreversible stoichiometric complex with $C\overline{1}$. $C\overline{1}$ inactivator does not bind to proenzyme C1 or C1s. The site of attachment is on the light chain of C1s. Classical pathway activation proceeds past the $C\overline{1}$ inactivator blockade when the stimulus to activation is so intense that $C\overline{1}$ molecules succeed in forming $C\overline{42}$ sites before becoming inactivated by $C\overline{1}$ inactivator molecules or when the available $C\overline{1}$ inactivator has been consumed. However, activation of the kinin-forming coagulation, or fibrinolytic systems would also be expected to facilitate activation of the complement system by consuming $C\overline{1}$ inactivator.

Another key control protein of the complement system is C3b inactivator. This serum enzyme attacks C3b free in solution or on the surface of cells and cleaves the molecule into two or more fragments. The C3b degradation products are unable to function in the $C\overline{42}3$ or $C\overline{3b}$, or B enzymes or to participate in the cyclic C3b-dependent feedback mechanism. Serum also contains an enzyme, possibly the same molecule as the C3b inactivator, which similarly cleaves C4b into fragments and abolishes its biologic activity.

Human serum also contains an enzyme, the anaphylatoxin inactivator, an α-globulin with a molecular weight of 300 000 which destroys the biologic activities of the C3a and C5a fragments of C3 and C5, respectively. Inactivation is accomplished by cleavage of the carboxyl terminal arginine from each of these molecules.

Among the other inhibitors or inactivators of activated complement components which have been described is an inhibitor of C6. This protein is a β_1-globulin.

METHODS OF DETECTION AND QUANTITATION OF COMPLEMENT COMPONENTS

Certain precautions are necessary in the handling of blood specimens for complement studies. The blood should be taken into an EDTA bottle at room temperature (approximately 25°C). Blood should neither be placed in a refrigerator (4°C) nor a water bath (37°C) to achieve separation of plasma and cells. The plasma should be separated as soon as possible and frozen at −20°C if complement studies are not being performed immediately. The plasma should be frozen at −70°C to prevent loss of complement activity in haemolytic tests if the tests are not to be performed within 4 days.

COMPLEMENT PATHWAY ESTIMATIONS

1 Total haemolytic complement (CH_{50}) ——— Haemolysis of sheep red cells

2 C3, C4
$$\begin{cases} \text{SRID} \\ \text{EID} \\ \text{AIP} \end{cases}$$

3 C1q ——— SRID
4 C2, C5, C7, C8, C9 ——— SRID or EID
5 C3/C4 fragments ——— 2 dimensionsal immunoelectrophoresis
6 Alternate pathway fractions e.g. GBG (or C3 proactivator)

——— SRID or EID
——— 2 dimensional immunoelectrophoresis

7   C1 esterase inhibitor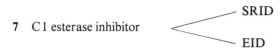

Where SRID = Single radial immunodiffusion.
            = Electro immunodiffusion.
     AIP   = Automated immunoprecipitation.

Total haemolytic complement is a measure of the ability of serum in limiting dilutions to lyse sheep red cells sensitized with rabbit anti-sheep antibody and is defined as the amount of lysis of red cells under optimally controlled conditions. Some drawbacks of this measurement are the problems in controlling the assay i.e. varying batches of sheep cells or the guinea-pig complement used as standards and the loss of complement activity with time; all samples must be assayed quickly or stored at −70°C. The results obtained give no real indication of the method of activation be it by the classical, alternate or both pathways.

COMPONENTS

The most commonly measured components of the classical pathway are C3 and C4 and of the alternate pathway Factor B and C3. These can be measured functionally or immunochemically with the latter method being used more commonly.

Of the available immunochemical methods automated immunoprecipitation (AIP) is only suitable for large batches of samples, but electro-immunodiffusion (EID) or single radial immunodiffusion (SRD) is used for smaller numbers. Electro immunodiffusion or Laurell rockets is the most sensitive and precise method and produces results in 5−6 hours, while SRID may take between 24 and 48 hours to produce complete reaction.

C1 esterase inhibitor (C1EI) and C3b(KAF) are usually measured immunochemically by EID or SRID. Although about 10% of all people genetically deficient in C1EI have normal immunochemical levels but are functionally deficient.

Two dimensional immunoelectrophoresis can be used to show the presence of activated fragments of C3 or C4 or Factor B (see Figs. 17.5 and 17.6).

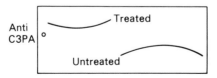

Fig. 17.5   Immunoelectrophoretic analysis of factor B(C3PA) in native form (bottom) and after activation (top). Anti factor B(C3PA) is in the slot and the anode is to the right.

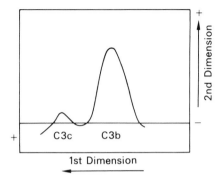

Fig. 17.6 Two-dimensional immunoelectrophoresis of serum whose C3 has undergone activation.

CLINICAL INTERPRETATION

Complement components are acute phase proteins and levels, either of haemolytic complement or the components, are elevated in most inflammatory and infective diseases, and after accidents, operations or myocardial infarction and as such are of no great diagnostic value. However low levels occur most often in renal disease, in the nephritis of SLE, in rheumatoid arthritis and in certain dermatological conditions.

Table 17.2   Approximate sensitivity of some tests for immune complexes

Test	Sensitivity	Reference
C1q precipitation	500 µg/ml	
[125]I-labelled C1q	100 µg/ml	Nydegger et al (1974)
[125]I-labelled Fab (anti-IgG)	100 µg/ml	Ludwig & Cusamano (1974)
C1q deviation	5 µg/ml	Sobel et al (1975)
Polyclonal rheumatoid factor	1.5 µg/ml	Cowdery et al (1975)
Platelet aggregation	1 µg/ml	Penttinen & Myllyla (1968)
C1q binding by ELISA	0.1 µg/ml	Ahlstedt et al (1976)
Anticomplementary activity	0.1 µ;/ml	Johnson et al (1975)

A decrease in serum C3 and C4 and Factor B are indicative of complement activation in both pathways, while low C4, low C3 and normal Factor B indicate classical pathway activation only. Alternate pathway activation on its own is very rare. In dermatology complement component quantitation can be used to show an immune response and an antigen–antibody reaction; the site of this response can sometimes be shown by demonstrating the presence of C3, C4 or Factor B deposited in skin or in blister samples.

The presence of circulating immune complexes or deposition of such complexes at the site of injury has led to many attempts to classify and quantitate such complexes in serum samples, unfortunately due to the varying size and nature of such complexes no single test has yet been devised to do this job accurately.

However, a number of tests have been developed and these generally detect immune complexes by their behaviour as cryoglobulins, their propensity to adhere to cell membranes or their property of interaction with complement components such as C1q (Table 17.2).

REFERENCES

AHLSTEDT S., HANSON L. A. & WADSWORTH C. (1976) A C1q immunosorbent assay compared with thin-layer gel-filtration for measuring IgG aggregates. *Scandinavian Journal of Immunology* **5**, 293.

COWDERY J. S., TREADWELL P. E. & FRITZ R. D. (1975) A radioimmunoassay for human antigen-antibody complexes in clinical material. *Journal of Immunology* **114**, 5.

JOHNSON A. H., MOWBRAY J. F. & PORTER K. A. (1975) Detection of circulating immune complexes in pathological human sera. *Lancet* **i**, 762.

LUDWIG F. J. & CUSUMANO C. L. (1974) Detection of immune complexes using 125 goat anti (human IgG) monovalent (Fab) antibody fragments. *Journal of the National Cancer Institute* **52**, 1529.

NYDEGGER U. E., LAMBERT P. H., GERBER H. & MIESCHER P. A. (1974) Circulating immune complexes in the serum in SLE and in carriers of hepatitis B antigens. Quantitation by binding to radio labelled C1q. *Journal of Clinical Investigation* **54**, 297.

PENTTINEN K. & MYLLYLA G. (1968) Interaction in human blood platelets, viruses and antibodies. I. Platelet aggregation test with micro equipment. *American Medical Experimental Federation* **46**, 188.

SOBEL A. T., BOKISCH V. A. & MULLER-EBERHARD H. J. (1975) C1q deviation test for the detection of immune complexes, aggregates of IgG and bacterial products in human serum. *Journal of Experimental Medicine* **142**, 139.

RECOMMENDED FURTHER READING

LACHMANN P. J. (1974) Complement. In *Clinical Aspects of Immunology*. ed. Gell, Coombs and Lachmann, 3rd Edition. Blackwell Scientific Publications, Oxford.

THOMPSON R. A. (1974) *The Practice of Clinical Immunology*. 1st Edition. Edward Arnold, London.

THOMPSON R. A. (1977) *Techniques in Clinical Immunology*. 1st Edition. Blackwell Scientific Publications, Oxford.

18

Glycosaminoglycans of the skin

F. S. WUSTEMAN

Because of its accessibility mammalian skin has been studied for many years by those interested in all aspects of connective tissue biochemistry. Skin has even been used as a source of glycosaminoglycans (formerly known as mucopolysaccharides; abbreviation GAG) though its content of these polymers is rather low. The quantities are such that, when the available tissue is restricted to the level of biopsy samples, no more than 50 μg of total GAG can be found in whole skin or dermis. Though it contains a similar mixture of GAGs epidermis is an even poorer source and, to obtain approximately the same small yield, 50 mg of dry tissue is needed.

The problems of analysis are further complicated by the fact that the yield of GAG varies considerably depending on the history of the tissue sample [e.g. biopsy material from healthy individuals contains more GAG than post-mortem samples (Van Lis et al 1973)] and on the precise method used for isolation and assay. Variations in the quantities of GAG reported by different laboratories probably result from difficulty reproducible steps in the procedure particularly those (such as dialysis) which separate polymeric from partly degraded GAG. A slight difference in the dialysis tubing pore size, for instance, can lead to inclusion or exclusion of significant quantities of GAG in the final assay.

Though it is widely felt that the anatomical site from which skin is taken has little effect on its GAG content (Van Lis et al 1973, Mier & Wood 1969a) a recent report, while confirming that the composition of the GAG mixture did not vary, describes a significant increase in total GAG of the dermis from weight-bearing sites (Gillard et al 1977).

For these reasons a comprehensive range of control samples must be subjected to any analytical procedure adopted.

In addition to studies on the tissue itself, a considerable amount of work has been done on the GAG produced by cultures of fibroblasts derived from skin. The GAGs secreted into the culture medium of a single dish are in quantities in excess of those found in biopsy samples. Being already in solution they present few difficulties and can be studied by any procedure devised for the parent tissue. There are also GAGs on the surface or inside the cells which are of considerable interest in the study of biosynthetic and degradative processes. They amount to only 10–20 μg GAG per 100 mm dish and therefore also require techniques for assaying GAGs at the lowest levels of detectability.

234

QUANTITATION OF GLYCOSAMINOGLYCANS

The GAGs consist of linear polysaccharide chains in which the repeating unit is a disaccharide residue (see Table 18.1). Hyaluronic acid has the longest chain with several thousands of the disaccharide repeats while the others contain between ten and fifty of these units per chain. Within one sample the molecules occur naturally in a range of sizes so that chain molecular weights, if obtained, would be average values only. For this reason it is more convenient to express GAG concentration in terms of one of its two major monosaccharide constituents. To convert from moles of constituent monosaccharide (hence of disaccharide repeat) to dry weight of GAG it must be remembered that the isolated polymers can contain up to 20% of water. Thus even standard GAG preparations are likely to contain less hexosamine or uronic acid than would be estimated from the sum of the residue weights of acetyl hexosamine, uronic acid, sulphate (if present) and a suitable number of sodium ions. (Theoretically 1 μmole of the sodium salt of hyaluronic acid has a residue weight of 401 μg while the value for dermatan and chondroitin sulphates is 503 μg.)

Since all GAGs contain either glucosamine or galactosamine it would seem most convenient to assay them in terms of this constituent of the disaccharide repeat. The assay of hexosamine residues, however, requires a preliminary acid hydrolysis using milder conditions than those required for peptide bonds (e.g. 4 M HCl/100°C/6 h). Once this is achieved the hexosamines can be separated and measured using a conventional amino acid analyser since they elute as separate peaks between the aromatic and basic amino acids. A modern sensitive automatic analyser would be necessary since quantities of less than 5 nmoles would be available for each assay.

A more convenient alternative is the assay of the uronic acid residue since the one GAG lacking such a component (keratan sulphate) is not a significant constituent of skin. The most reliable assay for uronic acid (which does not require any prior hydrolytic step) is the carbazole procedure as modified by Bitter and Muir (1962). By adopting a microscale version it is possible to assay quantities as low as 5 nmoles in 100 μl aqueous solution with reasonable precision. This has one disadvantage when compared with the hexosamine assay. Each GAG sample (depending not only on its identity by also its source) gives a slightly different colour yield per mole of uronic residue. This depends chiefly on the nature of the uronic acid (glucuronic or iduronic) but also on whether it bears a sulphate group and on the lability of adjacent glycosidic bonds. For this reason it is best to use as reference compounds GAGs which have been isolated themselves from the same tissue in preliminary experiments on a larger scale. Alternatively, results are expressed in terms of glucuronic acid or glucuronolactone with the knowledge that these cannot be converted directly into GAG dry weight figures without the use of a correction factor in addition to the residue weights already mentioned.

Table 18.1 Glycosaminoglycans of the skin

Glycosaminoglycan	Constitutents of the disaccharide repeat		Fractionation as cetylpyridinium complex	Further evidence of GAG identity	Relative quantities found in normal skin
	Hexosamine residue	Uronic acid residue			
Hyaluronic acid	N-Acetyl glucosamine	Glucuronic acid	Complex soluble in 0.4 M NaCl	Depolymerized by testicular hyaluronidase	Approx. 50% of GAG in adult skin
Dermatan sulphate (Chondroitin sulphate B)	N-Acetyl galacto samine 4-sulphate	Iduronic acid	Complex soluble in 1.2 M NaCl	Not depolymerized by testicular hyaluronidase or nitrous acid	Approx. 40% of GAG in adult skin
Chondroitin 4- and 6-sulphate (Chondroitin sulphates A and C)	N-Acetyl galacto-samine 4- and 6-sulphate	Glucuronic acid	Complex soluble in 1.2 M NaCl	Depolymerized by testicular hyaluronidase	Major component before birth but replaced by dermatan sulphate in adults
Heparan sulphate Heparitin sulphate, Heparin mono-sulphate)	N-Acetyl N-Sulphate } Glucosamine	Glucuronic acid or iduronic acid 2-sulphate	Complex soluble in 1.2 M NaCl	Depolymerized by nitrous acid	Minor component in all skin samples
Heparin	N-Sulphate glucosamine 6-sulphate	Glucuronic acid or iduronic acid 2-sulphate	Complex soluble in 2.1 M NaCl	Depolymerized by nitrous acid	Significant in skin (e.g. rat) where mast cells are abundant

GLYCOSAMINOGLYCANS FOUND IN SKIN

In adult human skin only two GAGs are present in sufficient quantities to justify their separation for routine assay at microscale levels (see Table 18.1). Though the absolute levels reported vary considerably, hyaluronic acid and dermatan sulphate are found in approximately equal quantities (a slight decrease has been noted with advancing age in the fraction containing dermatan sulphate (Van Lis *et al* 1973)). They each account for 1–15 μmoles of hexosamine per g dry tissue (Van Lis *et al* 1973; Mier & Wood 1969a; Gillard *et al* 1977). Various laboratories report, in addition to these two major GAG components, minor quantities of heparan sulphate (Van Lis *et al* 1973), chondroitin 4- and 6-sulphates (Gillard *et al* 1977) and particularly in ratskin, heparin. In the fetal skin of man (as with other mammals) hyaluronic acid is more abundant and is accompanied by chondroitins 4- and 6-sulphates which are replaced by dermatan sulphate soon after birth (Breen *et al* 1970).

Mixed total GAG may be assayed directly for hyaluronic acid and dermatan sulphate simply by hexosamine assay provided other hexosamine-containing polymers have been removed. To be sure of this it is necessary to have separated the GAG by virtue of their high density of negatively charged acidic groups. However, once this has been achieved, a simple fractionation into categories based on relative charge density [non-sulphated, monosulphated and 'highly' sulphated GAG (Mier & Wood 1969b)] requires very little extra effort. Unless the quantities of GAG involved are so low that the fractions obtained would be below the level where assay procedures are reliable (approximately 0.05 nmole/μlitre) it is worth proceeding to this fractionation.

ISOLATION OF TOTAL GLYCOSAMINOGLYCANS

The major constituent of skin or epidermis is protein which can be degraded most readily by proteolytic digestion using an enzyme which is active at relatively high temperatures. The tissues must first be obtained in a dry form suitable for weighing. Since lipid interferes with subsequent steps it is convenient to use a defatting solvent at this stage. Immersion in acetone followed by drying in air is sufficient though diethyl ether–acetone (3:1, v/v) or chloroform–methanol (2:1, v/v) have also been used as solvents.

The weighed solid is suspended in an acetate buffer containing cysteine hydrochloride and crystalline papain is added in a further small volume of buffer in which it has been dissolved by warming. The suspension is incubated at 65°C with occasional agitation until the solid is dissolved. If an appreciable residue remains after overnight digestion it should not be discarded until analysis for hexosamine residues confirms that it is virtually freed of any GAG. If this is not so, any GAG remaining in insoluble residues can be rendered soluble by extraction of the solid with 0.2 M alkali at 25°C for 6 h. After this the soluble extract can be adjusted to pH 7 by addition of acetic acid and the solution added to the papain digest for further treatment.

Polymeric protein is precipitated from the papain digest by addition of concentrated aqueous trichloroacetic acid to give a final concentration of 5% (w/v) and, after standing at 4°C for 4 h, it is removed by centrifuging. Though many prefer to remove excess trichloroacetic acid at this stage by dialysis, it is difficult to recover small volumes of solution from dialysis tubing without variable losses. As an alternative, three volumes of ethanol previously saturated with sodium acetate can be added (Celite, an inert solid, can be added when it is feared that a precipitate of this type is in too low a concentration to be collected easily) and, after standing at 4°C overnight, the almost invisible precipitate of crude GAG can be collected by centrifuging.

FRACTIONATION OF GLYCOSAMINOGLYCANS

The separation methods used all exploit the negative charges on the GAG chains by binding them to a positively-charged ion exchange resin (Gillard *et al* 1977) or precipitating them with a positively-charged detergent (Mier & Wood 1969b). Salt solutions of gradually increasing concentrations are used to break the electrostatic bonds and so release the GAGs from the column or the precipitate in sequence determined by their anionic charge density. At pH values around neutrality all the carboxyl and ester sulphate groups are fully ionized so, though it is easy to separate hyaluronic acid (one negative charge per disaccharide unit) from heparin (more than three per disaccharide), intermediate salt concentrations fail to resolve a group of GAGs all bearing approximately two negative charges per disaccharide (dermatan, heparan and chondroitins 4- and 6-sulphates).

The cationic detergent cetylpyridinium chloride has been most widely employed for the fractionation of the mixed GAG (Mier & Wood 1969b). It is added in a concentrated solution to precipitate cetylpyridinium-GAG complexes at 37°C. Celite is added as an inert carrier to help flocculate the precipitate which is then collected by centrifugation. A low salt concentration (0.03 M NaCl) is required for satisfactory precipitation and this must be raised to 0.4 M NaCl (to extract hyaluronic acid), then 1.2 M NaCl (to extract dermatan sulphate but also any heparan and chondroitin sulphates) and finally to 2.1 M NaCl (to extract heparin but also some dermatan sulphate (Van Lis *et al* 1973) probably because it has extra sulphate groups).

To perform each extraction effectively a low concentration of cetylpyridinium chloride must be incorporated in the salt solutions which must each be divided into three portions for successive extractions. After centrifuging the clear supernatants are poured off and pooled for uronic acid or hexosamine assays.

With the quantities available from biopsy samples further fractionation is pointless but semi-quantitative information about minor components can be obtained by cellulose acetate electrophoresis with strip-scanning by densitometer (Van Lis *et al* 1973). A minimum of 5 µg or 10 nmoles of GAG is desirable so it is necessary to concentrate the solutions before they can be applied to the cellulose acetate strip. The simplest way to achieve this is to use the precipitated GAG obtained after adding three volumes of ethanol saturated with sodium acetate to either the mixed GAG or cetylpyridinium-GAG sub-fractions. Electrophoresis for periods of less than one hour (in sodium diethyl barbiturate buffer, pH 8.6) leads to bands which are readily detected by staining with 1% Alcian Blue. By varying the composition and pH of the buffer the resolving power of this technique is sufficient to identify all the major GAG species in a mixture. This requires comparisons with reference compounds which should preferably be those isolation from skin itself and characterized in large-scale experiments. A simpler procedure employs specific pretreatments which depolymerize certain GAG and hence cause their electrophoretic bands to vanish (see Table 18.1). In this way digestion with testicular hyaluronidase can be used to confirm the presence of hyaluronic acid and chondroitin 4- and 6-sulphates but even greater specificity can be obtained using the various bacterial chondroitinases and hyaluronidases which are available commercially. Exposure to nitrous acid (0.2 M $NaNO_2$ in 2 M acetic acid at room temperature for 90 min) degrades both heparin and heparan sulphate and so causes their brands either to disappear or to become severely modified.

Direct assays on samples of abnormal human skin have already indicated changes in the hyaluronic acid content in the lesions of localized (pretibial) myxoedema (Van Lis *et al* 1973), excess chondroitin sulphate in hypertrophic scars (Bazin *et al* 1973) as well as the usual changes in the GAG pattern found in connective tissues undergoing repair processes—elevation of the content of hyaluronic acid, chondroitin sulphate and dermatan sulphate in that sequence (Chvapil 1967).

LABELLING OF GLYCOSAMINOGLYCANS

When faced with the isolation and measurement of such small quantities of GAG it is natural to consider radiolabelling procedures instead of difficult microassays. When applied to tissue samples labelled by incubation *in vitro* they measure the balance between synthesis and degradation during short periods of time following removal from their sites *in vivo*. Incorporation of radioactivity is found to increase with times of incubation up to 4 h (Hervé & Clauser 1969), as would be expected when the GAG have half lives *in vivo* of several days.

The techniques required to achieve this measurement are made easier by the fact that radioactive counting is the final step. Technically difficult procedures such as the precipitation of vanishingly small quantities of GAG are simplified when unlabelled 'carrier' GAGs can be added before addition of ethanol or cetylpyridinium chloride. The alternative approach using ion exchange columns (of 0.5 ml bed volume) (Gillard et al 1977) becomes feasible when it is possible to elute with as much as 2.5 ml of salt solution yet still measure the radioactivity in one scintillation vial. Uniformly-labelled [^{14}C]-glucose and [^{35}S]-sulphate are the most obvious precursors since they give rise to the active intermediates (UDP-uronic acids, UDP-acetylhexosamines and phosphoadenosine phosphosulphate respectively) which donate the basic units required in a GAG chain. Sulphate has the disadvantage of not labelling hyaluronic acid (which is always important in work on skin) while the relatively low specific activities available with ^{14}C-labelled glucose result in GAG derived from them having too few radioactive counts for labelling to lead to work of any greater precision than direct chemical assays. [6-^{3}H]-Glucosamine is available in much higher specific activities (up to 25 Ci/mmole from the Radiochemical Centre, Amersham) and, though this labels the hexosamine residues only, could yield GAGs with specific activities in excess of 10^6 c.p.m./μmole. Using radiolabels such as this accurate measurements could be made on quantities even smaller than 1 nmole of GAG.

This labelling technique has already been used successfully in cell culture experiments with fibroblasts using either the conventional cetylpyridinium chloride fractionation procedure (Bashey et al 1977) or an elegant microversion using a cellulose ester filtration membrane as an alternative method for collecting the precipitate (Saarni & Tammi 1977).

Skin fibroblast culture experiments permit the experimentalist to examine separately the fate of newly synthesized GAG in the cell medium (the bulk), those extracted from the cell surface by trypsin digestion (pericellular GAG) and those remaining inside the cell (presumably a storage pool destined for degradation) whereas these separate pools must be mixed when working up the product from culture of intact tissue. To set against this, the spectrum of GAG produced by fibroblast cultures is more like that of embryonic skin in that hyaluronic acid is the predominant product together with chondroitin sulphates in addition to dermatan sulphate. The exact mixture depends greatly on cell density and on the exact culture conditions such that extensive control experiments must be performed to support any conclusions drawn from fibroblast culture studies.

STUDIES ON INTACT PROTEOGLYCAN

With the possible exception of hyaluronic acid, all the GAGs are synthesized covalently linked to a protein core by bonds which (in the case of dermatan, heparan and the chondroitin sulphates) are of a glycosidic type from the reducing end of the polysaccharide chain to the alcohol group of the side chain of serine residues. This 'proteoglycan' contains a large number of individual GAG chains and forms even larger entities by non-covalent aggregation with hyaluronic acid and specific proteins. These aggregates in turn interact with the fibrous proteins present in the tissue and are thought to influence both the rate of collagen fibre formation and the size of fibre bundles produced. Extraction procedures involving alkali (which breaks the glycosidic bond to serine) or proteolytic digestion (which destroys most of the protein core leaving only a few amino acid residues attached to the serine) though convenient, make it impossible to examine the GAGs in their natural state as part of a larger protein-GAG complex.

To do this it is necessary to use reagents which will break no vital covalent bonds. Recently such a technique has been devised for connective tissues which, like dermis, are relatively low in proteoglycan content (Antonopoulos *et al* 1974). The 'dissociating' solvent (4 M guanidinium chloride) extracts a complex mixture of proteoglycan and other proteins and glycoproteins from which it is separated by ion exchange chromatography on a column of DEAE cellulose. A tissue as difficult as epidermis can be extracted by such dissociating solvent though only with the help of 0.2 M β-mercaptoethanol and ultrasonic disruption (M. Davies, unpublished work).

The further step of examining the intact proteoglycan is desirable since, though the usual sequence of GAG alterations may be seen in many pathological conditions in skin, the initial damage triggering off the repair sequence may result from a defect in the proteoglycan (e.g. as would be caused by degradation by lysosomal enzymes). By measuring only the GAG content or net synthesis and not examining the proteoglycan for evidence of changes it is possible to detect only the consequences and not the initial cause of the disorder. Needless to say the quantities involved are vanishingly small so this approach will become feasible only when radioactive labelling techniques of high specific activity are combined with extraction and purification carried out under the most gentle dissociative conditions.

REFERENCES

ANTONOPOULOS C. A., AXELSSON I., HEINEGÅRD D. & GARDELL S. (1974) Extraction and purification of proteoglycans from various types of connective tissue. *Biochimica Biophysica Acta* **338,** 108.

BASHEY R. I., PERLISH J. S., NOCHUMSON S., STEPHENS R. E. & FLEISCHMAJER R. (1977) Connective tissue synthesis by cultured scleroderma fibroblasts II. Incorporation of ³H-glucosamine and synthesis of glycosaminoglycans. *Arthritis and Rheumatism* **20,** 879.

BAZIN S., NICOLETIS C. & DELAUNAY A. (1973) Intercellular matrix of hypertrophic scars and and keloids. In *Biology of Fibroblast,* Eds. E. Kulonen & J. Pikkarainen, pp. 571–8. Academic Press, London and New York.

BITTER T. & MUIR H. (1962) A modified uronic acid carbazole reaction. *Analytical Biochemistry* **4,** 330.

BREEN M., WEINSTEIN H. G., JOHNSON R. L., VEISS A. & MARSHALL R. T. (1970) *Biochimica Biophysica Acta* **201,** 54.

CHVAPIL M. (1967) *Physiology of Connective Tissue,* pp. 269–72. Butterworths, London.

GILLARD G. C., REILLY H. C., BELL-BOOTH P. G. & FLINT M. H. (1977) A comparison of the glycosaminoglycan of weight-bearing and non-weight-bearing human dermis. *Journal of Investigative Dermatology* **69,** 257.

HERVÉ B. & CLAUSER H. (1975) Biosynthesis of acid mucopolysaccharides by the surviving new-born rat skin. *Biochimie* **57,** 1331.

MIER P. D. & WOOD M. (1969a) The acid mucopolysaccharides of mammalian skin. *British Journal of Dermatology* **81,** 528.

MIER P. D. & WOOD M. (1969b) A simplified technique for the analysis of tissue acid mucopolysaccharides. *Clinica Chimica Acta* **24,** 105.

SAARNI H. & TAMMI M. (1977) A rapid method for separation and assay of radiolabelled mucopolysaccharides from cell culture medium. *Analytical Biochemistry* **81,** 40.

VAN LIS J. M. J., KRUISWIJK T., MAGER W. H. & KALSBEEK G. L. (1973) Glycosaminoglycans in human skin. *British Journal of Dermatology* **88,** 355.

19

Assessment of structure and function of the stratum corneum

R. MARKS

INTRODUCTION

The stratum corneum (SC) is uniquely important to man because of its multi-faceted protective functions. When, because of disease or injury, it fails as a protective membrane the underlying tissue is seriously compromised and indeed if the defect is widespread then death of the organism may ensue. The range of protective functions of the SC is wide and includes protection against fluid and electrolyte loss (or gain from a wet or electrolyte rich environment), protection against microbial attack, mechanical protection and to some extent protection against thermal stress and against incident ultraviolet light. Probably the full range of protection offered by the SC is not yet appreciated and we are even more ignorant concerning the anatomical basis for each protection function. Nonetheless, progress has been made and now at least we have detailed information concerning the anatomy of the SC and have developed methods for examination of this vital part of the skin.

The SC consists of interlocked flattened corneocytes which take on their characteristic shape immediately after leaving the granular cell layer of the epidermis. Fifteen to 20 layers of corneocytes are usually found in the SC but more layers are found on the palms and soles. Between the corneocytes or as an extension of their own cell wall is a poorly characterized substance—the intercellular cement material. This substance seems to contain glycosaminoglycan but detailed knowledge of its chemistry and function are lacking. In lower mammals the corneocytes are stacked one on the other with a 'stacked coin' appearance, each slightly overlapping the other (Christopher 1971). However, this arrangement has not been found in the much more complex epidermis and SC of man and its functional significance in lower mammals is unknown. Corneocytes are continually shed from the surface in the process of desquamation. Normally, solitary or small clumps of two, three or four corneocytes desquamate from the skin surface. As the thickness of the SC remains constant it seems probable that this process of cell loss is not a random or haphazard affair but is carefully regulated.

Individual corneocytes are approximately 30 μm in diameter and 1–2 μm thick although variations occur due to age, sex and site (Plewig 1970). They are irregularly 'shield like' though are often pentagonal or hexagonal in outline. Their surface is broken up into two, three or more major folds. There may, in addition, be other minor folds and some surface irregularity with pits and projections (Barton et al 1978). An outer delicate plasma membrane and an inner tough envelope constitute the corneocyte wall. Within the cell are bundles of proteinaceous keratin filaments set in an amorphous and as yet un-characterized interfibrillary material. There may also be melanin granules and remnants of other cytoplasmic organelles but there are no other coherent and intact structures within the cells.

Sampling techniques

Most structural assessments can be made either on full thickness skin biopsies or skin surface biopsies (Marks & Dauber 1971) (see later). Individual corneocytes may be obtained by a scrub technique (Marks et al 1977) (see later). Surface assessments can also be made from replicas (Nicholls et al 1978b) (see later). For biochemical and certain in vitro functional assessments it may be desirable to use isolated sheets of SC. The simplest method of obtaining such sheets is to pare off areas of callus from the heel but it must be remembered that callus may not be entirely representative of SC from hair bearing skin and anyway represents only partial thickness of the SC. SC may also be obtained from cadaver skin or large specimens removed at operation using the method of metal frame immobilization and trypsinization as has been employed by Ferguson and Agache (1977). But as can be imagined this has very limited application. Stratum corneum may be obtained from subjects or patients by removing a 'split thickness specimen of skin' using a keratotome and then performing a dermo-epidermal split with 0.05% trypsin in Eagles' minimal essential medium and incubation at 37°C for 30–60 minutes. Following separation the epidermal and SC sheet is further prepared by scraping the epidermal cells off the sheet with gauze or a blunt spatula. This technique suffers the profound disadvantage of being an invasive technique and causing pain and discomfort to the subject. In addition, the SC so obtained has been subjected to trypsin and hydration before investigation and these may considerably influence the findings. The cantharidin blister technique (Kligman & Christopher 1963) is another technique for obtaining SC from living donors but causes some discomfort to the donor and the SC may be chemically changed by the application of cantharidin solution.

Assessment of SC structure

The formalin fixed, paraffin embedded and routinely sectioned skin biopsy gives a grossly inaccurate impression of the SC. It is a mere partial skeleton of its in vivo state and no accurate observations can be made of SC thickness and overall arrangement from this type of preparation. To view adequately the SC and to count the constituent corneocytes in its thickness it is necessary to employ a procedure that (a) swells up the corneocytes or makes each corneocyte otherwise readily identifiable and (b) causes little damage to the SC with little loss of the superficial corneocytes. The simplest of these methods is the Christophers and Kligman (1964) technique employing the swelling action of 0.4 N NaOH on the SC in cryostat sections of the skin. The numbers of corneocytes in the SC can be estimated and a rough overall impression of SC architecture can be gained. More information as to structure is given when the techniques of Christophers (1970) or that of McKenzie and Linder (1973) is used. The first employs fluorescein isothiocyanate as a marker for the cornified envelopes of each corneocyte and necessitates an ultraviolet fluorescence microscope. Our group mainly employs the McKenzie and Linder method which is simple and gives adequate and often elegant views of the SC in section (Fig. 19.1). Using this method it was quite easy to demonstrate the desquamative action of salicylic acid (Davies & Marks 1976).

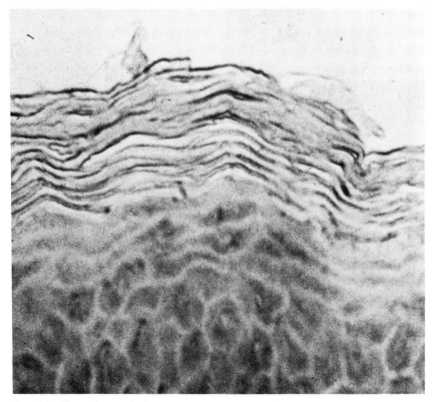

Fig. 19.1 Photomicrograph demonstrating stratum corneum arrangement in vertical section (cryostat section stained by McKenzie and Linder technique, ×45).

Conventional sectioning techniques only give information in the vertical plane and it should be realized that the protective functions of the SC are for the most part dependent on the integrity of its structure in the horizontal dimension. Regardless of this functional consideration, inspection in the horizontal plane enables observations to be made on the surfaces of corneocytes, on the overall surface contour of the skin and on the SC associated with adnexal structures. Two techniques directed to the horizontal plane will be mentioned. The first merely examines the surface of the skin and entails making a replica. In fact, this can be an extremely useful technique where, for example, information concerning pilar or eccrine duct orifices is required. Sarkany (1962) described a simple and useful skin replicating method employing nail varnish. Our group (Nicholls *et al* 1978b) have used a dental silicone rubber impression material to make the 'negative' and then a microscope slide mounting medium consisting of a polysterene (DPX) to make a hard permanent 'positive'. These replicas are capable of a very high degree of resolution (Fig. 19.2) and details on the surface of individual corneocytes can be distinguished in such replicas by scanning electron microscopy (SEM). Skin

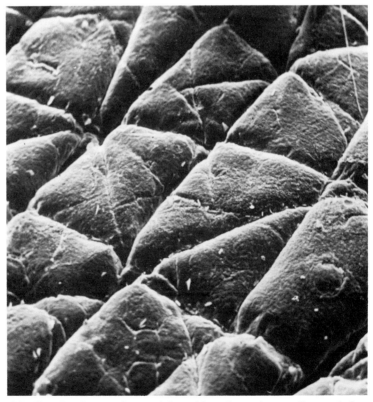

Fig. 19.2   Scanning electron micrograph from skin replica to show excellent resolution possible (×200).

surface biopsy (Marks & Dawber 1971) is also described in Chapter 13. It is a simple method for removing a coherent sheet of SC 3–5 cells thick without disturbing the *in vivo* arrangement. A rapidly bonding cyanoacrylate adhesive is used which has, when polymerized, the same optical properties as glass. A drop is placed on a glass microscope slide which is then pressed onto the area of skin to be examined. After 15–30 seconds the pressure and surface moisture of the skin will have resulted in polymerization and the slide will be stuck to the skin. If the slide is then removed with a 'peeling' motion a layer of SC is easily removed. The act of removal is painless—unless hairs are trapped in the glue when the avulsion of these will, of course, sting. The process of polymerization is exothermic and sometimes a transient sensation of heat is experienced at the site. The method, of course, depends on the bond between glue and glass being stronger than the intracorneal cohesive bond. When attempts are made to sample the palm or sole the manoeuvre may not be successful because of the increased toughness of the SC at these sites actually exceeding the glass-adhesive bond. In most instances this problem can be circumvented by first dampening the surface of the palm or sole thus decreasing the cohesive bond. It should be noted that the adhesive should be stored at 4°C when not in use as it seems to become less efficient after a month of the container being opened. After seven years of continuous use the author has not encountered any adverse reactions from skin surface biopsy (SSB) and has not come across any such reports from others employing the technique. Particular care should be taken when SSB is contemplated on the face to avoid contact with the eyes. If the adhesive spills on the skin or some is left inadvertently after taking an SSB then the dried cyanoacrylate can easily be removed with a little acetone.

The SSB can be used for a wide variety of purposes which include (a) morphological examination of the SC; (b) histochemical investigation of the SC, (c) ultrastructural examination of the SC by scanning electron microscopy (see Chapter 13), (d) microbiological evaluation.

Morphology

Local surface anatomy can be recorded, inspected and quantitated by SSBs employing either transmitted or reflected light microscopy. It must be remembered that the uppermost surface on the slide is derived from a point 3–5 cells down within the SC and that if it is the actual surface required then it is best to obtain replicas (Fig. 19.3).

Histochemical applications

Histochemical applications (Marks 1972) of SSB are wide and by no means completely explored. Staining the SSBs with haematoxylin and eosin demonstrates parakeratotic horn. This will, for example, enable the scattered parakeratotic nuclei of the paralesional, clinically uninvolved areas of psoriatic

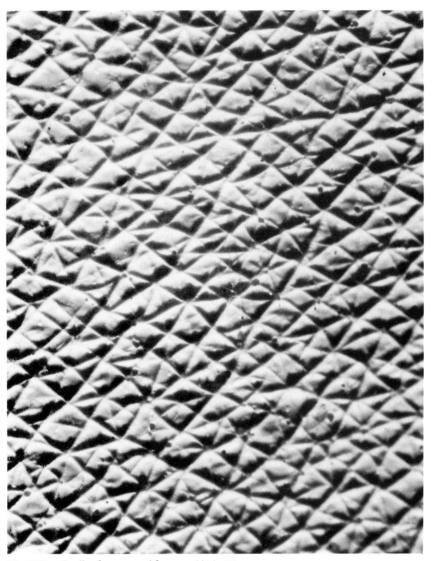

Fig. 19.3a   Replica from normal forearm skin (× 10).

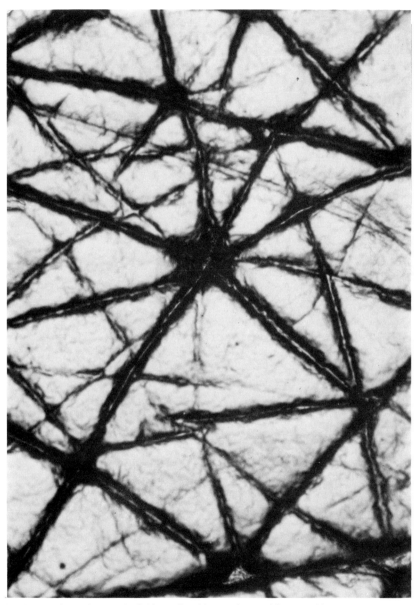

Fig. 19.3b Photomicrograph of skin surface biopsy of normal forearm skin (×40).

lesions to be located (Fig. 19.4) thus demonstrating that the epidermal abnormality is not confined to the lesion. The staining schedule for this and other stains is given in the appendix. Enzymes can be demonstrated within the SC using conventional enzyme histochemical reactions (see Appendix). For this purpose it is more convenient to take the SSBs on microscope cover slips instead of glass slides. In normal SC non-specific esterase can easily be demonstrated around each hair follicle orifice (Fig. 19.5) and sometimes there does appear to be reaction product deposited at the periphery of some of the corneocytes. The enzyme activities associated with Kreb's cycle, the pentose shunt or glycolysis are usually only demonstrable in parakeratotic SC resulting from a rapid turnover and a decreased transit time. In fact, this technique has been used to give a rough and ready estimate of SC transit time (see Chapter 10).

Most of the 'products' of the epidermis can be demonstrated in SSBs using histochemical methods. Melanin pigment granules can be demonstrated using a silver staining technique (Fig. 19.6). The pigment granules often seem to be arranged in a central oval configuration reflecting a previously perinuclear distribution. The density of the pigment granules reflects the degree of melanocyte activity and can be quantitated using the above technique. In addition melanin pigment can be distinguished from blood pigment. Iron in blood pigment can also be identified by employing the Prussian Blue reaction (Perl's stain). On occasions this may be extremely useful clinically—in for example distinguishing a small angiomatous malformation from a melanoma (see Appendix).

The activity of sweat glands can be recorded by first drying off the area to be examined, employing a stimulus to sweating (thermal, emotional, chemical etc.) and then applying to the area of skin a starch iodine mixture, quinizarin or 5% O-phthaldialdehyde in xylene all of which reagents change colour in the presence of sweat. When an SSB is now taken the coloured product is visible at the mouths of each functioning eccrine unit.

Sebum is easily demonstrated in SSBs by first wiping the area to be assessed with ether or acetone and then allowing a period for the glands to secrete before sampling by the SSB technique. The specimens are then stained with either sudan red or black and the extent of the staining can serve as a semi-quantitative estimate of the rate of sebum secretion.

Microbiological assessment

The SSB method allows determination of the *in vivo* colonial arrangement, inspection of the host–parasite relationship as well as quantitation of the numbers of microorganisms present in the SC. It is more suitable for the examination of dermatophytes (Marks & Dawber 1972) than for bacteria although it has proved useful for certain kinds of bacteriological investigation (Marks *et al* 1972). Ringworm fungi, *Malassazia furfur*, *Candida* species and the erythrasma microorganism are all readily demonstrated in SSBs using the

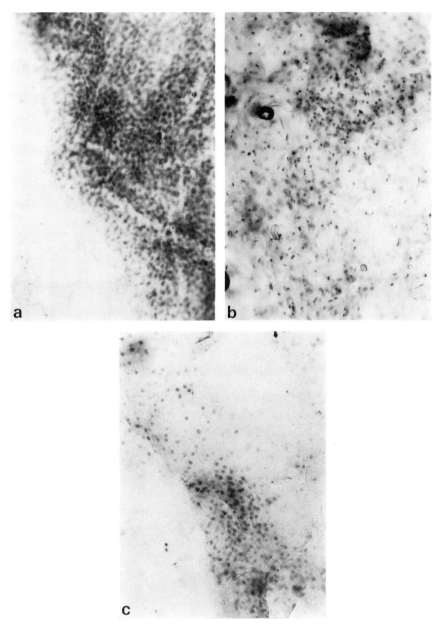

Fig. 19.4 Skin surface biopsies from (a) psoriasis, (b) pityriasis lichenoides chronica; and (c) pityriasis rubra pilaris. H & E, ×16.

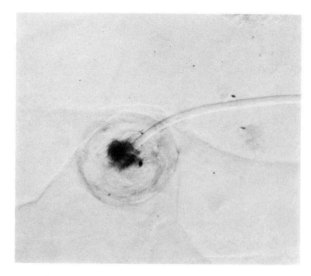

Fig. 19.5   Non specific esterase reaction in skin surface biopsy with reaction product around hair shaft demonstrating hydrolytic enzyme activity of flora of follicle (×25).

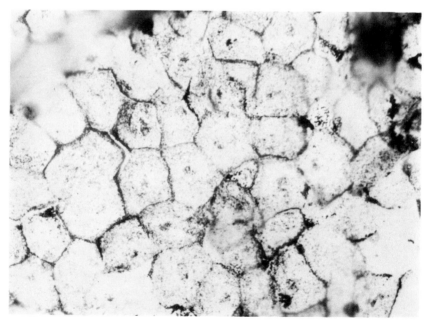

Fig. 19.6   Melanin particles in stratum corneum of negro in skin surface biopsy. Note that many particles are perinuclear (silver stain ×45).

Periodic Acid Schiff reagent (see appendix) (Fig. 19.7). SSBs may also be used for the culture of dermatophytes (Whiting & Bisset 1974) merely by laying the SSB specimen side down on the nutrient medium.

Ultrastructural assessments of structure

Scanning electron microscopy (SEM) has provided much valuable information concerning the overall architecture of the SC as well as the surface structure of individual corneocytes (see Chapter 13). It would be fair to say that the techniques employed in specimen preparation are so easy and the information obtained so useful that all assessments of SC structure should if possible include an SEM report.

Transmission electron microscopy (TEM) of the SC can provide valuable information but the techniques are difficult and require considerable experience before satisfactory results are obtained (see Chapter 12). It is not only a matter of adequate fixation but also extremely careful sectioning in order not to

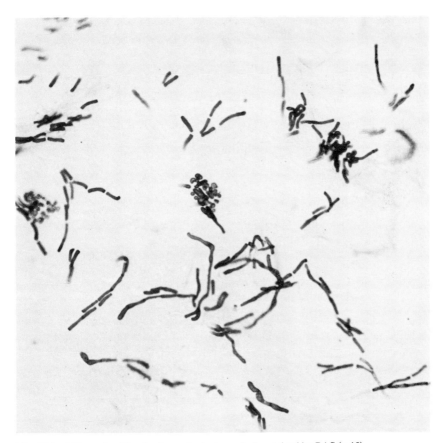

Fig. 19.7 Skin surface biopsies from pityriasis versicolor stained by PAS (×45).

detach the rather tenuously attached superficial corneocytes in the horny layer. The remarkable published electron micrographs of Brody (1970a, b) and Anton-Lamprecht & Schnyder (1974). Anton-Lamprecht (1978) are elegant examples of the high standards that can be reached in TEM of the SC if great attention is paid to detail. Clearly there is no substitute for experience in this field and anyone wishing to be involved in this facet of SC assessment would be well advised to seek the assistance of someone who is continuously and professionally employed in the TEM of SC. In particular, the outer plasma membrane and inner thicker cornified envelope should be separately identifiable in electron micrographs. In addition, the sections should be thin enough and well enough stained to see the fibrillary structure of the keratin bundles (Fig. 19.8).

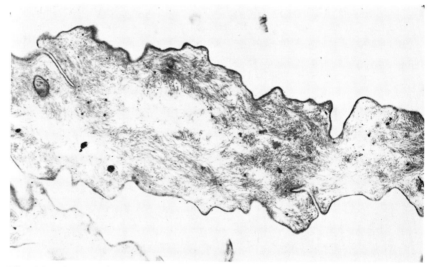

Fig. 19.8   Electron micrograph of corneocyte showing internal fibrillar content. Note a thick outer membrane—this is *not* the plasma membrane (×20 000).

Assessment of structure of individual corneocyte

There is some virtue to isolating and examining the individual corneocyte although it must be admitted this manoeuvre is more pertinent to pharmacological questions than to assessments of the structure of the SC. However, it may be useful for measurements of size and shape of corneocytes and for this reason it is included here. The corneocytes may be obtained using the simple technique of McGinnley *et al* (1969) which has been employed more recently by Plewig (1970), Plewig and Marples (1970). The writers' experience is with a specially constructed 'scrub machine' (Marks *et al* 1977) which has the virtue of delivering a controlled stimulus at the skin surface making quantitation of the numbers of corneocytes removed more accurate and reproducible. The scrub technique employs 0.1% Triton X 100 in 0.06 M phosphate buffer (pH 7.2) in contact with the skin surface. If large numbers of corneocytes are required or it is intended to examine them by SEM or TEM the following procedure is recommended. The liquid product of several 'scrubs' from several different sites are pooled and then packed at the bottom of a tube by centrifugation. The packed corneocytes may then be examined by SEM, TEM or by light microscopy (our group also uses differential phase interference microscopy as this provides an excellent view of the corneocyte wall) (Fig. 19.9). For SEM the cell suspension may be directly smeared on to microscope slides and fixed in 2.5% glutaraldehyde, dehydrated and air dried. Alternatively, the same fixation and dehydration can be followed by critical point drying, the cell suspension being contained within a special chamber (Barton *et al* 1978). The cell preparations are then stuck to stubs and coated with gold in a coating unit before viewing by SEM. For TEM, brief fixation *in situ* using 2.5% glutaraldehyde followed by osmium tetroxide dehydration in graded alcohols is used. The cell pellet is then embedded *in situ* in Araldite. The TEM may be particularly valuable as because of the random distribution of cells in the Araldite mass excellent views of both cell walls and the internal structure may be seen in different sections. One cautionary note must be sounded when it comes to the interpretation of the electron micrographic appearance of the plasma membrane. Unfortunately, the

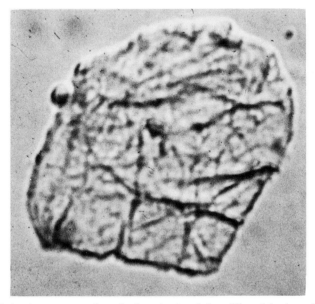

Fig. 19.9 Isolated corneocyte (unstained and viewed by differential phase interference microscope ×400).

detergen 'scrub fluid' seems to remove a considerable proportion of this delicate structure leaving the tougher cornified membrane as the cell wall.

Functional assessment

The investigation of function of the SC is a growth point in modern dermatology but although some progress has been made the techniques are still evolving. In many instances the apparatus required is not as yet commercially available and the 'would be investigator' must arrange for his own to be constructed or develop a link with a group who have an established interest in this field. The 'functions' to be measured are to some extent interrelated and for example any measurement of the mechanical properties of the SC will also give information concerning its ability to prevent fluid loss and its usefulness as a barrier against microbial attack. Another general point should be made concerning *'in vitro'* and *'in vivo'* methods. As with all biological investigations there is no completely satisfactory answer as to which is best. However, the writer prefers *in vivo* techniques for SC evaluation wherever possible because it is immensely difficult to obtain samples (a) which are unaltered by the process of removal; (b) in sufficient amounts for investigation; (c) from all relevant sites. Furthermore, it is difficult to perform serial observations on patients using *in vitro* techniques. In addition, because isolated SC is so deliquescent all investigations must be performed in perfectly controlled environments. Favouring the *in vitro* approach is the 'controllability' of the experiments performed. Clearly it is not easy to ensure 'basal' conditions or to be certain about a pharmacological stimulus when dealing with living subjects.

Assessments of function should include a measurement of water permeability and an estimate of SC mechanical strength. If possible, an attempt should also be made to obtain an index of the rate of desquamation.

Measurement of permeability to water

This measurement *in vivo* is intended to provide information about the rate of loss of fluid from insensible perspiration. Clearly, it is a most important index of competence of the SC as a barrier and could serve as a valuable indicator as to the progress of skin disease and the results of treatment. The techniques for making the measurement are not easy and the interested reader is referred to an excellent review of the topic by Idson (1975). There are both 'open' and 'closed' methods. The 'closed' methods were the earliest techniques available and usually depended on measuring the amount of water coming from a cup of known area of contact with the skin in a known period of time. Using this approach it is of course necessary to ensure lack of sweating in the area examined and one of the anti-cholinergic drugs such as poldine methanesulphonate (5% poldine methanesulphonate in 95% ethanol) is satisfactory for this purpose. The most accurate of these techniques drew dry air or nitrogen over the test site and carried the water vapour to a trap where it was estimated either gravimetrically or electronically (Baker & Kligman 1967; Grice & Bettley 1967). The disadvantages of this method include not knowing the effect that 'zero humidity' itself has on the rate of transepidermal water loss, the cumbersome nature of the apparatus, and the comparatively long time each determination takes. 'Open' methods are quicker and interfere less with the local physiology. They depend on the flux of water vapour from the test site and the apparatus used is termed an 'evaporimeter' (Nilson & Oberg 1975). The electronic sensors are quite sensitive and in our experience great care must be taken in handling and storing them between experiments. Using this technique it is necessary to ensure that the ambient temperature and humidity are, within reasonable limits, controlled. In our hands this has proved a most satisfactory method for testing the water barrier function of the SC *in vivo*.

Measurement of mechanical strength

Mostly the assessment of mechanical strength has been restricted to determinations of 'breaking strain' and elasticity of SC *in vitro* and in the horizontal plane. Either an 'Instron' (Middleton 1969) or 'textile dynamometer' (Agache *et al* 1973) has been used for this purpose. Because of the ease with which SC takes up water from the atmosphere this type of investigation must be performed in a completely controlled atmospheric environment after a period of equilibration. Our group has concentrated on the measurement of intracorneal cohesion *in vitro* and in the vertical dimension (Marks *et al* 1977). We routinely use a direct method employing an apparatus termed a cohesograph (Fig. 19.10). The piston of this machine is stuck to the skin surface with the same cyanoacrylate adhesive (Permabond—Staines, Middx) as is used to produce skin surface biopsies (see previously). The force required to distract the piston with attached SC from the skin surface is the 'intracorneal cohesion'. It is recorded in grams automatically by a force transducer and direct writing recorder. In our experience this technique is simple, accurately reproducible and moderately sensitive. Using this apparatus we can detect sex and site differences and changes after hydration of the SC. We have also used an 'indirect technique' in which the surface contour of the rupture plane of skin surface biopsies is measured using an instrument that is commercially available called the surfometer (GV Planer Ltd). The area under the curves of the contour is regarded as a function of the intracorneal cohesion. The technique is neither as accurate nor as sensitive as the direct method—and it is more time-consuming and difficult to perform.

There is a wide range of other tests of SC strength which in the author's opinion are more likely to be of use in asking very specific questions. Because space does not permit and because of their highly specialized nature only brief reference will be made to them. Our group have developed a technique for determining the force required to produce a point deformation in the SC *in vivo* (Nicholls *et al* 1978a). This may be of considerable use in the future to answer pharmacological questions. Thermo-mechanical analysis (Humphries &

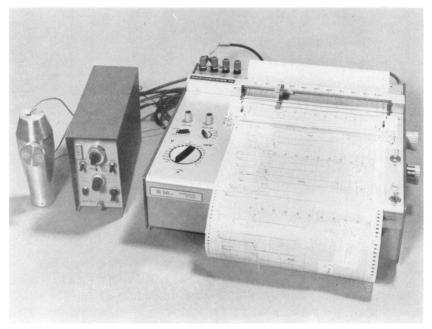

Fig. 19.10 Cohesograph apparatus.

Wildnauer 1971) is performed on samples of SC *in vitro* and can give considerable information as to the physical state of the material examined.

Measurement of desquamation

There are two types of approach that have been adopted for this assessment. The first relies on the rate of disappearance of dyestuffs on (and sometimes in) the SC. This approach is utilized in determinations of the turnover time of the SC. It is more fully described in the chapter on epidermal cell kinetics (Chapter 10). The other approach attempts to quantitate the actual number of squames leaving to SC surface per unit area per unit time. The scrub technique (Marks *et al* 1977) previously described in this chapter describes *forced* desquamation and although the values obtained by counting the numbers of squames in the fluid may bear a relationship to the normal rates of corneocyte cell loss we are ignorant of it. Our group have recently devised a chamber (Fig. 19.11) which we believe may give a more accurate estimate of the rate of desquamation. The chambers are attached to the skin surface with a non irritant adhesive material used for colostomy appliances and known as Stomahesive (Squibb Surgicare Ltd). The chambers remain in place for 48 hours after which time they are filled with phosphate buffer. The buffer is withdrawn and the corneocytes within it are counted in a haemocytometer chamber. This technique is still being developed but promises to be of great value.

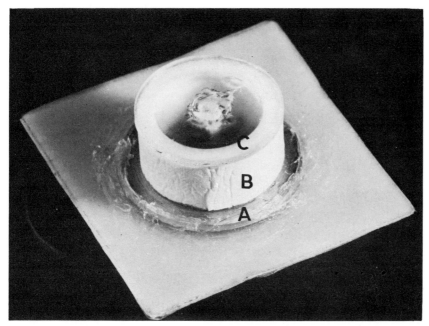

Fig. 19.11 Chamber used for collecting corneocytes from skin surface. Aluminium ring (A) with cylinder of porous nylon mesh (B) sealed by Perspex disc (C) set in the disc is an area of silicone rubber. The chamber is stuck to a rectangle of the stoma dressing material 'Stomahesive' which has a hole cut from its centre portion.

APPENDIX

Haematoxylin and eosin stain for skin surface biopsies

1. Place skin surface biopsy (SSB) in Harris's haematoxylin for 10 minutes.

2. Rinse in distilled water and 'blue' in tap water for 5–10 minutes.

3. Differentiate in 1% acid alcohol for no more than 5 seconds. (The SSB may become detached from the slide—if this happens carry on with the staining procedure but take care not to lose or mix the specimen with any others.)

4. 'Blue' again in tap water for as long as necessary.

5. Place in 1% aqueous eosin for 2–5 minutes.

6. Rinse in several changes of distilled water.

7. Take rapidly to absolute alcohol and leave in absolute alcohol for 5 minutes.

8. Clean in xylene, mount in DPX (mounting medium). An excessive amount of DPX will be necessary due to the thickness of the specimen.

PAS technique for skin surface biopsies

1. Cover SSB with 1% periodic acid for 10 minutes.

2. Wash in several changes of distilled water.

3. Cover with Schiffs reagent* for 15 minutes.
4. Wash in tap water for 5 minutes.
5. Dehydrate, clear and mount in DPX giving specimen 5 minutes in absolute alcohol to ensure complete removal of water.

Perls' Prussian blue reaction

1. Place SSBs in fresh solution of equal parts of 2% aqueous potassium ferrocyanide and 2% hydrochloric acid, for 60 minutes. With a doubtful result, the reaction may be carried out at 60°C, but this is not usually necessary.
2. Wash thoroughly in several changes of distilled water.
3. Conterstain lightly with 1% neutral red or safranine for 10–15 seconds.
4. Wash in water, dehydrate for at least 10 minutes, clear and mount in DPX.

Silver impregnation method for melanin granules (Fontana's technique)

Silver solution: To 25 cm^3 of 10% aqueous silver nitrate add strong (0.880) ammonia drop by drop until the precipitate which first forms has almost disappeared; then add 25 cm^3 of distilled water. This solution should be left for 24 hours, stored in a dark bottle and filtered before use. It is better to renew this solution after 14 days but it may be used for 1 month.

1. Cover SSBs in Gram's iodine for 10 minutes.
2. Transfer to 3% sodium thiosulphate for 5 minutes.
3. Wash in several changes of distilled water.
4. Transfer to the silver solution in a covered container and leave in the dark for 24 hours at room temperature.
5. Rinse in several changes of distilled water.
6. Tone in 0.2% gold chloride (or Cajal's toner) for 15 minutes.
7. Rinse in distilled water.
8. Fix in 3% sodium thiosulphate for 4 minutes.
9. Wash in running tap water for 4 minutes.
10. Counterstain with 1% safranine for 1 minute.
11. Wash in tap water for $\frac{1}{2}$ minute.
12. Dehydrate for at least 10 minutes, clear and mount in DPX.

Enzyme histochemical tests on SSBs

SSBs taken for enzyme histochemical investigation ought to be kept at a temperature of −20°C until the reactions have been completed.

---

* Schiffs reagent is available commercially, but it is recommended to be made up as follows: 1 g basic fuchsin; 2 g potassium metabisulphite; 2 cm^3 concentrated hydrochloric acid. Add fuchsin to 200 cm^3 boiling distilled water (remove from heat first)—cool solution to 50°C and add potassium metabisulphite while mixing—cool to room temperature—add hydrochloric acid—stand overnight in dark and add activated charcoal while shaking (0.2 g) filter through Whatman no. 1 paper. Store at 4–8°C.

Non-specific esterase

Method

1. Incubate SSB in reaction media for 2 hours at 37°C.

2. Rinse in distilled water, fix in 10% formal saline for 10 minutes. Rinse in water.

3. Counterstain lightly with neutral red if desired.

4. Rinse in distilled water.

5. Dehydrate for at least 10 minutes, clear and mount in DPX.

Reaction medium

5-Bromo-4-chloro-indoxyl acetate: 2 mg
Ethyl alcohol: 0.2 cm^3
Tris buffer pH 7.2, 0.2 M: 10 cm^3
Water distilled: 9.8 cm^3
Potassium ferrocyanide (0.5 M): 0.42 cm^3
Potassium ferricyanide (0.05 M): 0.32 cm^3
Calcium chloride (0.1 M): 0.42 cm^3
CONTROL—incubate without substrate.

Succinate dehydrogenase

Method

1. Cover SSBs with reaction mixture and incubate in hydrated oven at 37°C for 2 hours.

2. Rinse with several changes of distilled water for 10 minutes.

3. Mount in glycerine jelly.

Reaction mixture

Glycyl-glycine PVA buffer pH 8.0[1]: 10 cm^3
Sodium succinate: 0.136 g
Nitro blue tetrazolium (2 mg/ml): 20 mg
Dissolves with stirring
Just before use add PMS solution[2]: 1 cm^3
(1) Glycl-glycine PVA buffer
50 cm^3/0.1 M glycyl-glycine.
× cm^3 0.1 M NaOH.
Make up to 100 cm^3. Check pH 8.0.
Add 25 g PVA to this—dissolve with stirring and gentle heating.
(2) Phenazine methosulphate (PMS) solution
10 mg PMS in 10 cm^3 distilled water.
Use very fresh.

Lactate dehydrogenase

Method

As for succinate dehydrogenase but incubate for 30 minutes.

Reaction mixture
Glycyl-glycine buffer pH 8.0: 10 cm^3
Sodium lactate: 0.080 g
Nitro blue tetrazolium (2 mg/cm^3): 20 mg
β-nicotinamide adenine dinucleotide (NAD)
(3 mg/cm^3): 30 mg
PMS solution: 1.0 cm^3

Glucose-6-phosphate dehydrogenase

Method
As for succinate dehydrogenase—incubate for 40–60 minutes.

Reaction mixture
Glycyl-glycine buffer: 10 cm^3
Glucose-6-phosphate (substrate, 1.5 mg/cm^3): 15 mg
Nitro blue tetrazolium (3 mg/cm^3): 30 mg
Nicotinamide adenine dinucleotide phosphate (NADP 2.5 mg/cm^3): 25 mg
PMS solution: 1.0 cm^3

REFERENCES

AGACHE P., BOYER J. P. & LAURENT R. (1973) Biomechanical properties and microscopic morphology of human stratum corneum incubated on a wet pad in vitro. *Archives Dermatologische Forschung* **246,** 271.

ANTON-LAMPRECHT I. (1978) Ultrastructural criteria for the distinction of different types of inherited ichthyoses. In *The Ichthyoses,* Eds. R. Marks & P. Dykes, pp. 71–87. MTP Press.

ANTON-LAMPRECHT I. & SCHNYDER U. W. (1974) Ultrastructure of inborn errors of keratinization VI. Inherited ichthyoses—a model system for heterogeneities in keratinization disturbances. *Archives Dermatologische Forschung* **250,** 207.

BAKER H. & KLIGMAN A. (1967) Measurement of transepidermal water loss by electrical hygrometry. Instrumentation and responses to physical and chemical insults. *Archives of Dermatology* **44,** 961.

BARTON S. P., KING C. S., MARKS R. & NICHOLLS S. (1978) Ultrastructural studies on isolated normal human corneocytes (in preparation).

BRODY I. (1970a) An electron microscope study of the fibrillar density in the normal human stratum corneum. *Journal of Ultrastructure Research* **30,** 209.

BRODY I. (1970b) Variations in the differentiation of the fibrils in normal human stratum corneum as revealed by electron microscopy. *Journal of Ultrastructure Research* **30,** 601.

CHRISTOPHERS E. (1970) Eine neue Methode zur Darstellung des Stratum corneum. *Archiv für klinische und experimentelle Dermatologie* **237,** 717.

CHRISTOPHERS E. (1971) Cellular architecture of the stratum corneum of mammalian skin. *Journal of Investigative Dermatology* **56,** 165.

CHRISTOPHERS E. & KLIGMAN A. M. (1964) Visualization of the cell layers of the stratum corneum. *Journal of Investigative Dermatology* **42,** 407.

DAVIES M. & MARKS R. (1976) Studies on the effect of salicylic acid on normal skin. *British Journal of Dermatology* **95,** 187.

FERGUSON J. & AGACHE P. (1977) Influence of site, storage and trypsin treatment on the mechanical properties of the stratum corneum. *Journal of Investigative Dermatology* **68,** 256.

GRICE K. A. & BETTLEY R. (1967) The effect of skin temperature and vascular change on the rate of transepidermal water loss. *British Journal of Dermatology* **78,** 582.

HUMPHRIES W. T. & WILDNAUER R. H. (1971) Thermomechanical analysis of stratum corneum I. Technique. *Journal of Investigative Dermatology* **57,** 32.

IDSON B. (1975) Percutaneous absorption. *Journal of Pharmaceutical Sciences* **64,** 901.

KLIGMAN A. M. & CHRISTOPHERS E. (1963) Preparation of isolated sheets of human stratum corneum. *Archives of Dermatology* **88,** 702.

MCGINLEY K. J., MARPLES R. R. & PLEWIG G. (1969) A method for visualizing and quantitating desquamating portion of the human stratum corneum. *Journal of Investigative Dermatology* **53,** 107.

MACKENZIE I. C. & LINDER J. E. (1973) An examination of cellular organization within the stratum corneum by a silver staining method. *Journal of Investigative Dermatology* **61,** 245.

MARKS R. (1972) Histochemical applications of skin surface biopsy. *British Journal of Dermatology* **86,** 20.

MARKS R. & DAWBER R. P. R. (1971) Skin surface biopsy: an improved technique for the examination of the horny layer. *British Journal of Dermatology* **84,** 117.

MARKS R. & DAWBER R. P. R. (1972) In situ microbiology of the stratum corneum. *Archives of Dermatology* **105,** 216.

MARKS R., NICHOLLS S. & FITZGEORGE D. (1977) Measurement of intracorneal cohesion in man using in vivo techniques. *Journal of Investigative Dermatology* **69,** 299.

MARKS R., RAMMARAIN N., BHOGAL B., MOORE N. (1972) The erythrasma micro-organism in situ: Studies using the skin surface biopsy technique. *British Journal of Clinical Pathology* **25,** 799.

MIDDLETON J. S. (1969) The effect of temperature on extensibility of isolated stratum corneum and its relation to skin chapping. *British Journal of Dermatology* **81,** 717.

NICHOLLS S., KING C. S., GUIBARRA E. & MARKS R. (1978a) Measurement of point deformation of human skin in vivo—contribution of stratum corneum. *Journal of Investigative Dermatology* **70,** 227 (Abstract).

NICHOLLS S., KING C. S. & MARKS R. (1978b) Morphological and quantitative assessment of physical changes in the horny layer in ichthyosis. In *The Ichthyoses,* Eds. Marks, R. & Dykes, P. p. 95. MTP Press.

NILSON G. & ÖOBERG (1975) A new method for measurement of transepidermal water loss. Transactions III. Nordic meeting on medical and biological engineering. Tampere, Finland, January 1975.

PLEWIG G. (1970) Regional differences of cell sizes in the human stratum corneum II. Effects of sex and age. *Journal of Investigative Dermatology* **54,** 19.

PLEWIG G. & MARPLES R. R. (1970) Regional differences of cell sizes in the human stratum corneum. *Journal of Investigative Dermatology* **54,** 13.

SARKARY I. (1962) A method for studying the microtopography of the skin. *British Journal of Dermatology* **74,** 254.

WHITING D. A. & BISSET E. A. (1974) The investigation of superficial fungus infections by skin surface biopsy. *British Journal of Dermatology* **91,** 57.

Index